Americans in
Occupied Belgium,
1914–1918

ALSO BY ED AND LIBBY KLEKOWSKI

Eyewitnesses to the Great War: American Writers, Reporters, Volunteers and Soldiers in France, 1914–1918 (McFarland, 2012)

Americans in Occupied Belgium, 1914–1918

Accounts of the War from Journalists, Tourists, Troops and Medical Staff

ED KLEKOWSKI *and*
LIBBY KLEKOWSKI

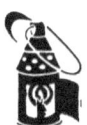

McFarland & Company, Inc., Publishers
Jefferson, North Carolina

LIBRARY OF CONGRESS CATALOGUING-IN-PUBLICATION DATA

Klekowski, Edward J.
　Americans in occupied Belgium, 1914–1918 : accounts of the war from journalists, tourists, troops and medical staff / Ed Klekowski and Libby Klekowski.
　　p.　cm
　Includes bibliographical references and index.

　ISBN 978-0-7864-7255-0 (softcover : acid free paper) ∞
　ISBN 978-1-4766-1487-8 (ebook)

　1. Belgium—History—German occupation, 1914–1918. 2. World War, 1914–1918—Belgium. 3. World War, 1914–1918—Personal narratives, American. 4. Americans—Belgium—History—20th century. I. Klekowski, Libby, 1941– II. Title.
　D623.B4K45 2014
　940.3'493092313—dc23　　　　　　　　　2014004102

BRITISH LIBRARY CATALOGUING DATA ARE AVAILABLE

© 2014 Ed Klekowski and Libby Klekowski. All rights reserved

No part of this book may be reproduced or transmitted in any form or by any means, electronic or mechanical, including photocopying or recording, or by any information storage and retrieval system, without permission in writing from the publisher.

On the cover: Mrs. Winterbottom, née Gladys H. Appleton, in her Minerva driving to one of the outer Antwerp forts to retrieve wounded (*Le Miroir*, 1914); background map of Belgium (© Hemera Technologies/Getty Images/Thinkstock)

Manufactured in the United States of America

McFarland & Company, Inc., Publishers
　Box 611, Jefferson, North Carolina 28640
　　www.mcfarlandpub.com

To Amanda, Ulrich, Philip and Alexandra,
our companions in exploring Belgium

Table of Contents

Preface 1
Introduction 5

1. The Attack 9
2. Book Burning 30
3. Murder and Mayhem on the Meuse 50
4. Besieged Antwerp 67
5. The Last Ditch in Belgium 91
6. Prussian Belgium 113
7. Is Food a Weapon? 131
8. Feeding the Etappen Zone and Social Darwinism 151
9. Battles Around Ypres 169
10. Medieval U-Boat Nest 190
11. Americans Going and Coming 208
12. Final Acts 227
13. After the War 244

Chapter Notes 259
Bibliography 275
Index 279

Preface

Belgium in the First World War — the first country invaded, the longest occupied, and when the war finally ended, the first forgotten. More than four years of carnage on the Western Front displaced from memory what happened behind the lines in Belgium. This is unfortunate because Belgium was, in many respects, a dress rehearsal for the civilian terrors of the Second World War. Nevertheless, for most Americans the history of Belgium during the Great War is only the history of the bloody battles around the Ypres Salient between the British and German armies. The authors were like most Americans regarding Belgium and the war, that is, until we got an opportunity to live there.

Our home for six months was the university town of Leuven (Louvain). Soon after arriving, as we explored our new home, we noted that most of the buildings in the town center had stone plaques affixed to their fronts with two dates inscribed: 1914 and a date in the early 1920s. We learned that the Imperial German Army had sacked the town in August 1914, and that the buildings with the dates were those destroyed during the sack and rebuilt in the 1920s. You could follow the extent of the destruction by following the plaques up and down the streets. Then there was our first visit to the university library. The building seemed old, but it was not. As we waited to enter, a university student asked us if we were Americans and if we knew the story of the library. We said yes to the first question and no to the second. She then gave us a brief guided tour. Covering the building's façade were hundreds of stone memorial plaques with the names of American schools, colleges, associations, clubs, municipal departments, scientific and engineering societies. She explained these donors rebuilt the university library after the German Army burned the original library during the sack of 1914. One could say her tour was the inspiration that ultimately led to this book.

Before the war, Belgium had a large American colony, which included representatives of American companies, artists, writers and diplomats with the American Legation. When the war began, American journalists flocked to Belgium. There was more freedom of movement for the foreign press in Belgium than in either France or England. Perhaps the strangest American visitors in the early days of the war were war tourists, their passion being to witness battles and gore — they were, admittedly, a bit insane, but they left interesting memoirs. During the German occupation of Belgium, many Americans lived in Belgium and northern France supervising the activities of the Commission for the Relief of Belgium (C.R.B.). Other Americans volunteered as soldiers in the Canadian Army, became pilots in the Royal Flying Corps, or served as medical staff in the British Army; all saw action in the Ypres Salient battles. Remarkably, even after America entered the war on the side of the Allies and most of the non-military Americans left Belgium, a small group remained, tolerated by the German occupiers. Fortunately, many Americans left written accounts of what transpired in Belgium during the German invasion, occupation and final retreat. Their first-hand accounts are the basis of this book.

Since memoirs, magazine articles and newspaper reports from the war years were so important in understanding American experiences in Belgium, our first acknowledgment must be to the W.E.B. Du Bois Library at the University of Massachusetts Amherst. We especially thank Melinda McIntosh, reference librarian extraordinaire, for her enthusiasm and skills in researching our often obscure queries; Diane McKinney, interlibrary loan coordinator; Barbara Morgan, law reference librarian; Laura Quilter, copyright policy librarian; Robert Cox, head of special collections and archives; and the university librarians of the post-war years for assembling an incredible collection of First World War memoirs. Special thanks to the University of Massachusetts Biology Department for providing Ed a post-retirement office, his former department head James Walker for help with funding and Charlene Coleman for keeping track of the funds, and Thomas Carpenter for computer assistance.

We thank Nicole Milano of the Archives of the American Field Service, New York, for copies of letters by A. Piatt Andrew written during the Second Battle of Ypres, and Jean Paul De Vries and Brigitte De Vries of the Romagne '14–'18 Museum in Romagne, France, for making available to us all the wartime issues of *Le Miroir*. Rainer Hiltermann of Brussels deserves very special thanks for his tireless help. Rainer is the authority on all things pertaining to the German occupation of Belgium. He was generous with period pictures from his collection and gave us a bound set of *Illustré 1914*, a rare pictorial magazine published in occupied Brussels. We acknowledge the skill of Meg Clark, our graphic artist, who brought the photographs in *Le Miroir* and *Illustré 1914* back to life. Maps are original and drawn using Inkscape software.

Of course, our special thanks to Amanda Klekowski von Koppenfels and Ulrich von Koppenfels for their generous hospitality in Brussels and their suggestion we spend time in Leuven, and to Ulrich for reading the entire manuscript and for help in exploring Antwerp and Charleville (the latter always in the rain).

Regarding Belgian place names, memoirs and histories of the First World War use the French names for cities, towns and villages in Flanders. We have retained that convention but include the contemporary Flemish name in parentheses, e.g., Louvain (Leuven), Ypres (Ieper), Bruges (Brugge).

Introduction

> If one examines the European War from the standpoint of pure reason, both its origin and development seem a chaos of improbabilities which could not have been foreseen by the most sagacious mind.— Gustave Le Bon, war psychologist, 1916[1]

The First World War caused the premature deaths of 9.5 million combatants and wounded 15 million.[2] It was one of the deadliest wars in human history. So why was it fought? Moreover, why was Belgium so important?

The crisis began with the assassinations of Archduke Franz Ferdinand and his wife Sophia in Sarajevo, Bosnia, on June 28, 1914. Since the archduke was next in line to the Austro-Hungarian throne, his death had consequences; unfortunately, the consequences far exceeded his importance. In the United States, newspapers noted the royal murders but went on to more interesting news.

> On the last Sunday morning of June, 1914, early in California, and a bit later in Kansas and Ohio, when the sun was sending up the thermometer and flies droned lazily in and out opened windows, a rumor clicked over telegraph wires that a Duke had been murdered, with his Duchess, at an unimportant town in Central Europe. Compared with battery announcements for the day's baseball games, it was of slight interest.[3]

Austro-Hungarian Emperor Franz Josef held Serbia responsible for the deaths. He vowed retaliation; military and clerical parties in Vienna agitated for a punitive war on Serbia. Through the summer, the diplomatic stew simmered until finally brought to a raging boil by the arrogant, bungling and sometimes malicious behavior of Europe's leaders and their underlings. By the end of July, war became inevitable. Citizens who would soon become cannon fodder rallied to their leaders in nationalistic hysteria, egging them onward toward the cataclysm, viewing war as a nation's spiritual regeneration.

> The present contest has more than one analogy with the religious wars of olden times. It is begotten of the same illusions and shows traces of the incoherence,

frenzy, and brutality. It is ruled exclusively by irrationality, for if reason had been able to dominate the aspirations of kings and nations, there would have been no war to-day.[4]

In revenge for the murder of Archduke Franz Ferdinand in Sarajevo, Austria attacked Serbia; Russia came to Serbia's defense as a fellow Slavic nation, but, unfortunately, the Czar made the fatal mistake of mobilizing the entire Russian Army for what should have been a trivial military confrontation. The Kaiser, in fear of being caught off guard by the war footing of his large neighbor to the east, ordered German mobilization and the Imperial German Army went into action. Its plan was to quickly defeat the French, who were allied with the Russians, and then turn the army east on the Russians. By launching an unprovoked attack in the west, followed by a speedy victory, the plan would prevent a two-front war — but the plan failed. The Germans also hoped that the British would be neutral in the conflict and not aid the French — another hope that fell by the wayside.

In August of 1914, Kaiser Wilhelm II "let slip the dogs of war" in Aachen (Aix-la-Chapelle),[5] a German city near Belgium. It was to be a quick incursion, an easy military lark through topographically unchallenging real estate situated between Germany and France. However, that particular real estate belonged to the small neutral country of Belgium. Crossing it would turn out to be a bit more challenging than initially imagined. First, the Belgian Army resisted the German juggernaut with more vigor than anticipated and second, the violation of Belgian neutrality brought in the British as allies of the Belgians and French.

> By the Treaty of the 18th of April, 1839, Prussia, France, Great Britain, Austria, and Russia declared themselves guarantors of the treaty concluded the same day between His Majesty the King of the Belgians and His Majesty the King of the Netherlands. This treaty states: "Belgium will form an independent and perpetually neutral State."[6]
>
> To say that a State is protected by Permanent Neutrality is to say that it is excluded from any war whatsoever.
>   Permanent Neutrality tends essentially, as has been said, to safeguard small States against the encroachment of powerful neighbours in such a way as to maintain equilibrium between the great countries.[7]

In 1914, in direct violation of a treaty endorsed by his great grandfather in 1839, Kaiser Wilhelm II ordered the invasion of Belgium. On August 3, 1914, the German Chancellor, Theobald von Bethmann-Hollweg, addressed an enthusiastic Reichstag:

> Gentlemen, we are in a position of necessity [energetic assent]; and necessity knows no law (*Not kennt kein Gebot*). [Energetic applause]. Our troops have occupied Luxemburg [energetic "Bravo!"]; perhaps they have already entered

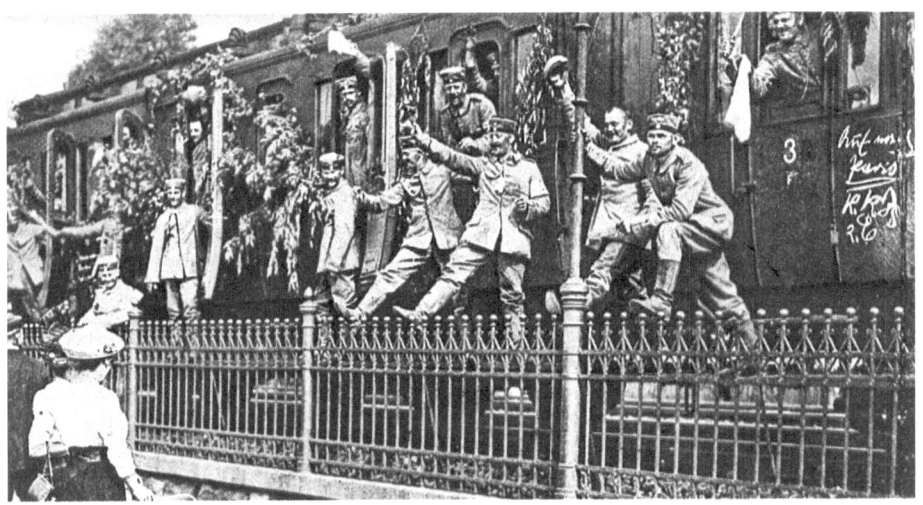

German recruits leaving for the front. War hysteria swept through Europe in August 1914. The most expendable, those who would later refer to themselves as cannon fodder or as sheep being led to slaughter, were often the most enthusiastic when the war began (*Hamburger Fremdenblatt*, 1914).

> Belgian territory [energetic applause]. Gentlemen, this is in contradiction to the rules of international law.[8]

On August 4, Germany invaded Belgium; in response, Great Britain declared war against Germany. In Berlin, learning of the British response to the invasion, the German Chancellor accused the British Ambassador of going to war over a mere technicality.

> He said the step taken by His Majesty's Government (the British Government) was terrible to a degree: just for a word — "neutrality" — a word which in wartime had so often been disregarded — just for a "scrap of paper," Great Britain was going to make war on a kindred nation.[9]

In addition to being the cause of Britain's entry into the war, the invasion of Belgium had another consequence. It biased many Americans against Germany. "It was to be expected that public opinion in America would range itself overwhelmingly on the side of the Entente [Great Britain, France, Russia]. As a result of the violation of Belgian neutrality, this happened far in excess of expectation."[10]

"Perpetually Neutral" Belgium became the unwilling crucible of the war in the west, where the Imperial German Army went from success to success in 1914 until finally stopped by the Belgian, British and French armies along a narrow sliver of Belgium bordering France. Nearly all of Belgium was under German occupation for most of the war. Its liberation occurred in the fall of 1918.

Chapter 1

The Attack

> Liège seems to be holding out still. The Belgians have astonished everybody, themselves included. It was generally believed even here that the most they could do was to make a futile resistance and get slaughtered in a foolhardy attempt to defend their territory against invasion. They have, however, held off a powerful German attack for three or four days. It is altogether marvelous.[1]— Hugh Gibson, secretary of the American Legation in Brussels, August 7, 1914

> The whole world seems to be changing place like sand on a moving disc and my mind is losing its grip on what is real.[2]— Glenna L. Bigelow, an American in Liége[3] on August 4, 1914

On August 4, 1914, the Imperial German Army crossed the German frontier and invaded Belgium, a country about the size of Vermont. The army jumped off from Aachen, a small German city near the Belgian border. Its first objective was the Belgian city of Liège (Luik), 35 miles (56.3 km) to the west. A major railway hub with more than 400 trains passing through each day, Liège was the key to the Belgian rail system. Because railroads would play such an important role in moving men and munitions during the war, the speed and success of the German drive toward France depended on taking Liège. "Liège, therefore — a great industrial center and junction of railways, roads and rivers, guarded by a ring of twelve forts extending across a diameter of eight miles — must first be reduced: it would then be possible to break westward."[4]

An American woman, Miss Glenna Lindsley Bigelow[5] from New Haven, Connecticut, was a guest of Monsieur X and Madame X in the Château d'Angleur in the village of Angleur, a commune near Liège and within the ring of forts. When Miss Bigelow published her war memoir in 1918, the German Army still occupied Belgium so she preserved the anonymity of her Belgian hosts for fear of reprisals. However, before publication, an anonymous writer

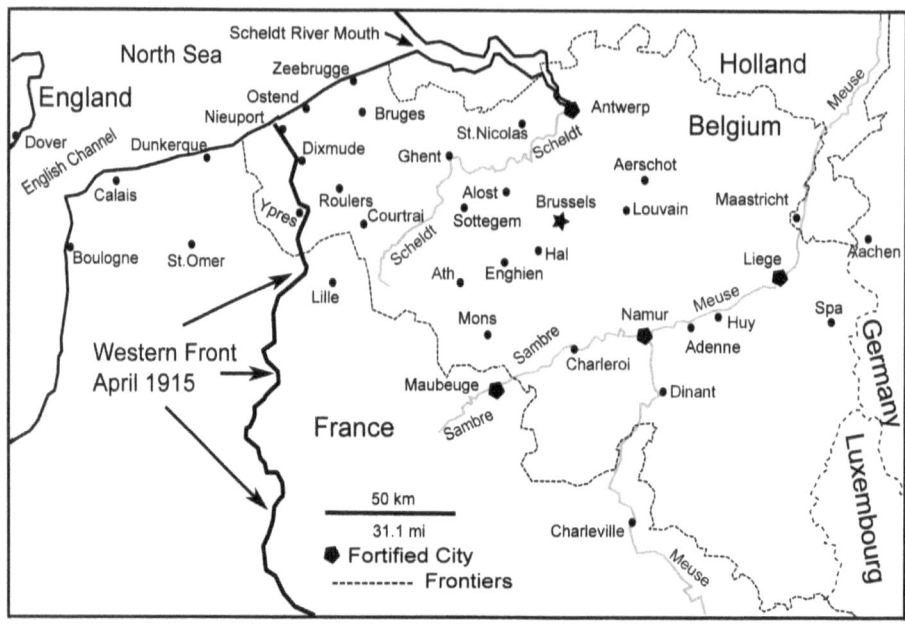

added a forward that included clues to the identity of Monsieur X. He was purportedly president of the International Sleeping Car Company of Europe, which his brother had founded. The Liège-born banker, Georges Nagelmackers, founded the *Compagnie internationale des Wagons-lits*, a company that included the famous Orient-Express. In 1914, his brother was head of the company and probably Bigelow's Monsieur X, Château d'Angleur being Château Nagelmackers. Monsieur Nagelmackers was very well connected; his cousin was the wife of a member of the Kaiser's Imperial Court. Consequently, General von Moltke, the Chief of the General Staff, issued written orders protecting the château and its owners during the invasion and occupation.

The Germans attacked Liège on August 4 but were repulsed, at considerable cost, by the city's defenses. Liège's twelve forts—a concrete and steel necklace designed to defend it from invaders—took twelve days to break (August 4–16, 1914). Completed in the 1890s and armed with Krupp fortress guns, the forts exacted heavy German losses early in the attack. Interestingly, Kaiser Wilhelm was a major Krupp investor; in fact, according to the *Wall Street Journal* (August 20, 1915), he owned $5,000,000 worth of stock. One might say guns made with his investments were responsible for much of what his soldiers suffered taking Liège. While laying siege to the forts, the German Army broke through the connecting defenses and managed to take the city proper on August 7. "Some of the Prussians have succeeded in penetrating into the city, tho' the forts have not surrendered, and are already establishing martial rule. Aeroplanes, with the wings turned back, Taubes, have been flying about all the morning."[6]

A Dutch journalist, entering Liège on August 8, described the first day of "martial rule": "Crowds of soldiers moved through the main streets, reveling, shouting, screaming in their mad frenzy of victors. They sat, or stood, or danced in the cafés, and the electrical pianos and organs had been started again 'by order.' Doors and windows were opened wide, and through the streets sounded forth the song 'Deutschland über Alles' (Germany before all others)."[7]

With the center of the city in hand, the German command now turned to the problem of the forts. The forts were mostly underground structures with concrete carapaces through which rose steel cupolas containing artillery guns, the cupolas moving up and down before and after firing. Machine gun positions behind solid masonry emplacements accessed from underground galleries protected the forts from infantry attacks. Under the forts, tunnels led to cellars for ammunition and stores. A deep dry moat and fields of barbed wire surrounded each fort. Originally designed and constructed in the eighteen-eighties, the forts were still deadly but obsolete in 1914. Although these forts were generally impervious to conventional artillery bombardment, the Germans possessed new weapons that would crack them open. Two types of giant siege mortars were brought into play: the Škoda 30.5 cm (12 in) mortar and the Krupp 42 cm (16.5 in) mortar, famously known as *Dicke Bertha* (fat or big Bertha) for Krupp heiress Bertha von Krupp und Bohlen-Halbach.

The Czech Škoda Works developed the Škoda 30.5 cm siege mortar for the Austro-Hungarian Army. Although designed as a mobile weapon, moving a twenty-ton mortar into position for an attack was no easy task. The monster mortar moved by train from Aachen to the vicinity of Liège. From there, a specially designed Škoda-Daimler tractor, which itself weighed fifteen tons, towed three trailers with mortar components to the firing site. Glenna Bigelow probably witnessed a Škoda road convoy on the move. "Austrian artillery was passing today with their great cannon drawn by automobiles. The wheels of the gun carriages are enormous and the cannon are the biggest things we have yet seen."[8]

Each shell the mortar fired weighed nearly 1,000 pounds (with propellant); since the mortar could fire 10 rounds per hour, an hour's shooting weighed 5 tons. Thus for a single mortar to destroy a fort, the Germans had to move at least 40 tons of materiel (tractor 15 tons, mortar 22 tons, plus munitions) along unpaved roads from a railroad siding—a major engineering effort in itself! Although the occupation of the city began on August 7, it took another nine days to subdue the forts, most of that time probably spent positioning the mortars.

On the evening of August 12, more firepower became available. Two big Berthas arrived by railroad from the Krupp factory in Essen. Tractors, augmented

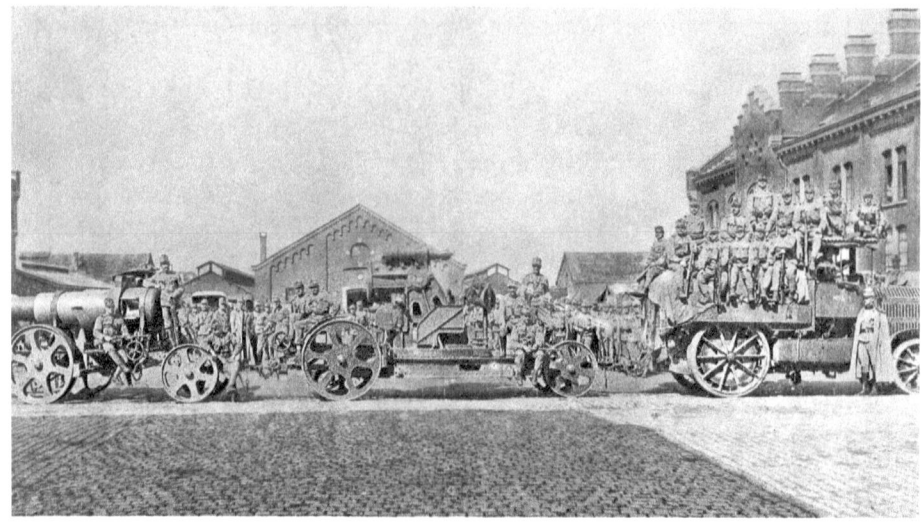

A Škoda 30.5 cm mortar on the move. Three wagons carried the mortar's components: one carried the barrel, another the carriage and another the platform. Typically, a battery (two mortars) traveled together in three road trains of two wagons per train, each towed by a 120 horsepower Austro-Daimler tractor. The photograph shows a barrel wagon, a carriage wagon, the tractor and the battery crew. When Glenna Bigelow wrote, "Austrian artillery was passing today with their great cannon drawn by automobiles," she was probably describing a Škoda road train (*Illustré*, 1914).

by teams of horses from a circus, pulled the two super heavy mortars (totaling 42 tons) into firing positions.[9]

The Škoda fired a special armor piercing shell that weighed 850 pounds, the Krupp fired an armor piercing shell that weighed 1,700 pounds; either could penetrate between 6 and 7 feet of reinforced concrete, but the Krupp made a bigger bang! A delayed action fuse ignited the shell after it had penetrated, resulting in a massive underground explosion that roared through a fort. The defenders were roasted, asphyxiated, or knocked unconscious from the shock waves. Miss Bigelow's journal entry for August 10 probably describes the beginning of the end of the forts:

> A heavy cannonading began at 4.30 a.m.—it literally tore us from sleep, for it seemed as if the very house were tumbling down about our ears and the singing and whizzing of those big shells was *bizarre*, to put it mildly. One did not know whether to get up or efface one's self in the blankets. I remember having the utmost confidence in the headboard of my bed, which was toward the window. But that did not obliterate the siren whistle of those big shells and the moment of suspense between the lightning and the thunder. After each deafening burst I kept reiterating to myself, "Saved again."[10]

1. The Attack

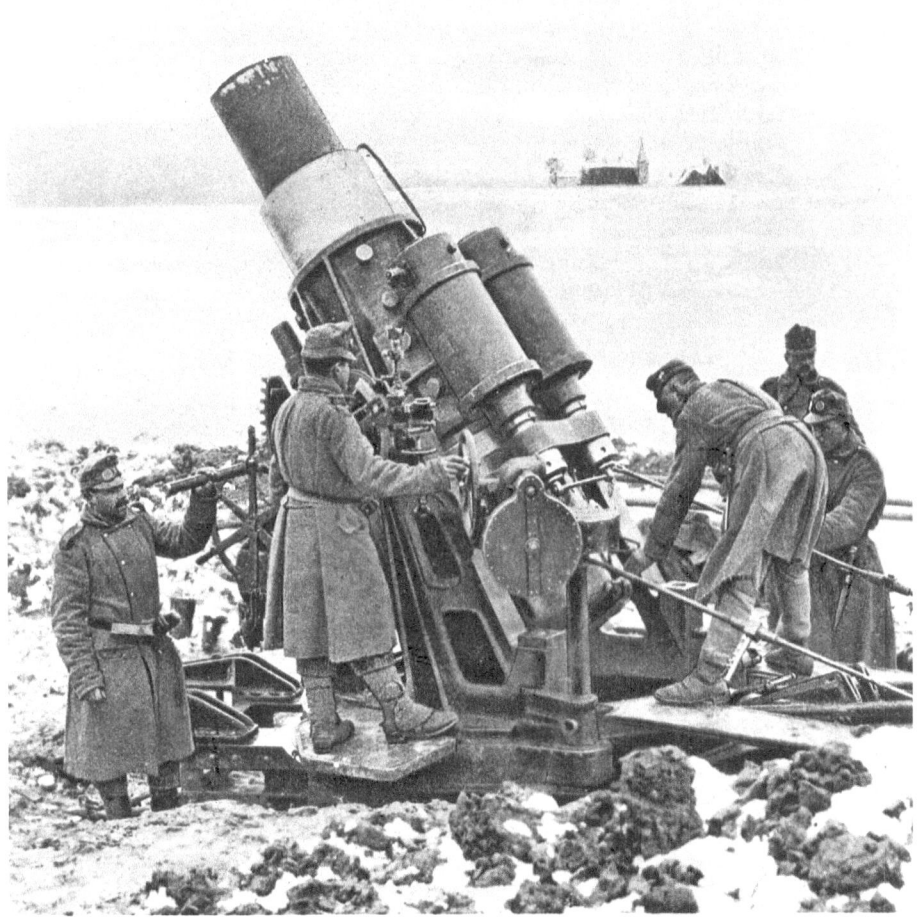

A Škoda 30.5 cm mortar assembled and ready to fire. With a well-trained crew, a mortar battery could be in action six hours after the road trains reached the firing site. The German Army's high praise for the mortar in the early months of the war resulted in honors for Karel Škoda, the president and CEO of Škoda Works. In December 1914, Emperor Franz Josef made him a baron. In the spring of 1915, the German High Command gave Baron Škoda a special tour of the captured Belgian and French forts so he could personally see the destruction wrought by his mortars (*Hamburger Fremdenblatt*, 1914).

Most of the forts withstood bombardment for less than a day before throwing in the towel. After a couple of Škoda 30.5 cm hits, the structures were burning inside and full of asphyxiating smoke. The forts were death traps. A Belgian officer in one of the forts described the consequences of a 42 cm shell:

> A tremendous explosion shook the fort to the foundations; the powder-magazine had caught fire. It is impossible to describe the appalling results of that explosion; the entire middle-part of the fort collapsed in a stupendous cloud of flames, smoke and dust; it was an awful destruction, an immense avalanche of masses of concrete, fragments of armour, which in their fall crushed to death nearly the whole of the garrison. From this fantastical, confused mass, overwhelming clouds of suffocating smoke escaped through some crevices and holes.
>
> After this infernal rumble, deadly silence followed, interrupted only by the groans of the wounded. The German artillery ceased to fire, and from all sides their infantry came rushing on, their faces expressing the terror caused by such great calamities. They were no longer soldiers longing to destroy, but human beings hurrying to go to the assistance of other human beings.[11]

Wounded from a nearby fort were moved to a convent in Angleur where Glenna Bigelow and others went to help. The sights she witnessed staggered her.

> August 13 ... charred bodies with no suggestion of faces — just a flat, swollen, black surface, with no eyes, nose nor mouth. Some of the wounded lay on beds, others in the middle of the floor or wherever there was space, and each was holding up hands burned to the bone.[12]
>
> August 14 ... we nursed the soldiers all day — if last night was horrible I could not find the words to describe what the daylight revealed, or the awful odor of burned flesh when the wounds were redressed.[13]

That evening Glenna met the invaders. After nursing the wounded, she was now required to dine and make small talk with the officers responsible for the horrors. Château Nagelmackers, where Voltaire had once stayed, where Liszt had composed, now hosted the masters of the new "German *Kultur*."

> At eight o'clock dinner was served. Madame X.'s daughter and I, after such a scrubbing and disinfecting, came down the last ones and stepped into a veritable playworld of the Middle Ages with the most beautiful setting — a large salon, opening out onto the terrace, with old Flemish-wood fire-place and raftered ceiling, Japanese bronzes, rugs from the Orient, soft lamps and portraits of dear grandmothers, in the beauty of their youth, smiling out from their golden frames on the walls. As we came into the room from the brightly lighted hall, a semi-circle of gray-green coats rose right up out of the dimness and we were blinded by a vision of shining buttons, polished boots, gleaming swords and a military salute accompanied by clinking spurs. At the end of the room stood Madame X. and her sons waiting for us. Naturally there were no presentations and the moment was unique in the extreme — nobody moved for a second which seemed like a decade and nobody spoke, so all there remained to do was to acknowledge the salute with a semi-circular bow.[14]

Dinner conversation was tense, everyone skirting around the fact that the officers were not really guests but invaders. Among the tidbits Miss Bigelow learned from her Prussian guests was that Germany printed three newspapers — one for officers, one for soldiers, and one for imbeciles. Since all the officers fervently believed they would be celebrating in Paris within two weeks, Bigelow believed they must have been reading the one for imbeciles! It had taken nearly two weeks just to subdue Liège. One time, seated next to an elderly officer whose language skills were limited to a few French phrases and a straggle of English words, her attempt to fill a conversational void led to a startling admission:

> I wanted to get him started on "War" without precipitating an international difficulty and I asked him as stupidly as possible (perhaps I did not need to simulate that) if he liked "War." He hesitated just a second and I was prepared for the usual self-respecting denial when he horrified me by answering a simple "Yes."
> Viola, le sentiment prusse![15]

After dinner, all adjourned to the salon for a bit more inane chit-chat until finally the officers kicked their spurs together, kissed the ladies' hands, and bid all good night. The Imperial German Army, under their leadership, was soon to be off to Brussels, with a few stops in between.

While the German Army marched toward Brussels and points west, Glenna Bigelow sought to escape Belgium. She encountered only one problem — the German authorities held her passport. She approached the American Consul in Liège to act on her behalf and get her passport. However, she soon concluded he was hopeless, either an incompetent or a fool, or both. She went directly to the German authorities and managed to brow-beat her way through the Teutonic red tape. On November 7, 1914, she crossed the frontier into neutral Holland. From there she took a boat to England. Landing in Folkstone, she immediately re-crossed the English Channel to France where she served as a nurse for the war's duration.

In Brussels, another American, Brand Whitlock, awaited the invaders at his post as head of the American Legation. The forty-five-year-old American Minister and his wife Nell Brainerd Whitlock arrived in Brussels in February 1914 and would remain until April 2, 1917.

Whitlock came to Belgium from the Mid-West; he served as mayor of Toledo, Ohio, for four terms, 1905 to 1912.[16] As a progressive, he fought corruption, big business, political bosses and other special interests. He was against prohibition (working men should have their beer as long as there was no rowdiness in saloons), advocated decriminalizing prostitution (believing the oldest profession could be eliminated by alleviating the conditions that forced women into the life), and was against capital punishment (considering it indefensible on ethical and religious grounds). For these "radical" views, he often incurred attacks from Toledo's pulpits.[17] Mayor Whitlock, defender of the underdog and elected to office four times, decided on a career change in 1912. He had had enough of politics; his passion was to be a literary man and he longed for the public to remember him as such. Today, only scholars interested in him and folks hoping to cure insomnia read his novels. Photographs of Whitlock in Brussels reveal a thin, almost effete looking, middle-aged man with hair parted in the middle, wearing wire-rimmed glasses. His suits were elegant, even a bit foppish — he looked like a literary man. In 1902, Whitlock saw his first novel published.[18] Although he continued publishing during his terms in office, he felt he needed a sabbatical, preferably in Europe, so his literary creativity could really bloom. The dream of a sabbatical became reality, at least so he thought, when at the end of 1913 President Wilson appointed him United States Minister to Belgium.[19]

Soon after his arrival in Brussels, Whitlock received an invitation to the Royal Palace for an audience with Albert, King of the Belgians; this would be the beginning of an enduring friendship between the two men. The February 14, 1914, meeting was to be a formal presentation of papers of the new American Minister to the King. The problem was "What to wear?" The previous American Minister had cooked up an ambassadorial uniform with lots of gold braid, knee breeches and silk stockings. To Whitlock, this was symbolic of flunkeyism, and for an ex-mayor of Toledo, accustomed to fighting for the common man, dressing like a flunkey was out of the question. He opted for the simple garb of an American citizen, or as Hugh Gibson, his pithy Secretary of Legation, put it, "the simple garbage of an American citizen."[20] The King was relieved; evidently, the previous minister's theatrical costume had been the joke of the court.

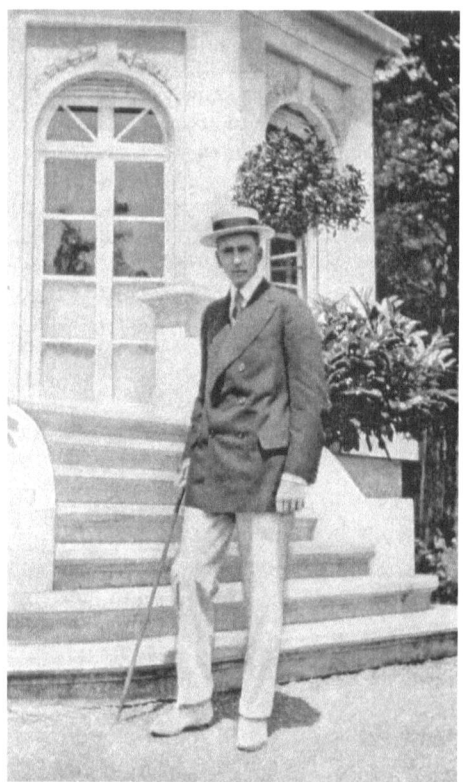

Brand Whitlock photographed in Brussels in 1914. The former Toledo, Ohio, mayor saw his Brussels assignment as a relaxed European sabbatical. He anticipated that his ministerial duties would take a couple of hours a day at most, thus leaving lots of time to write his great American novel and play golf for inspiration. Whitlock's Belgian sojourn turned out to be slightly different from what he had envisioned (Hugh Gibson, *A Journal from Our Legation in Belgium*, 1917).

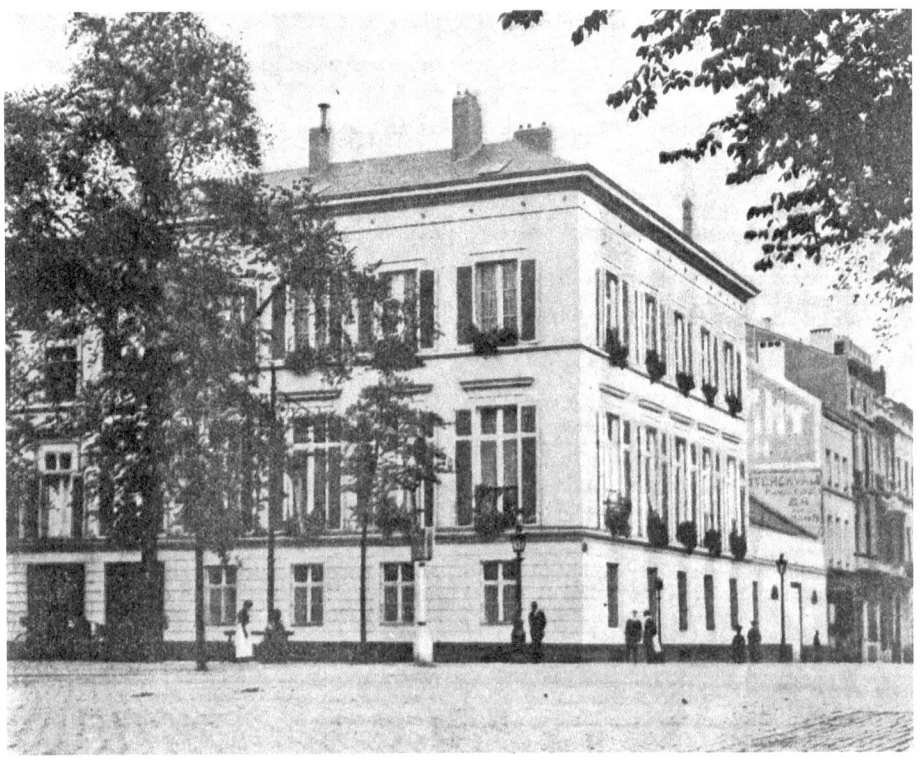

The American Legation in Brussels during the war years. Demolished in the latter part of the twentieth century, the Legation gave way to a modern office building. Considering the importance of the Legation during the First World War, it is remarkable that no plaque marks its former location (*Everybody's Magazine*, 1918).

The formalities over, Whitlock settled into his sabbatical, but first he and Nell had to rent an inexpensive residence. The Whitlocks were not poor, but nor were they diplomats from the moneyed set. In those days, a Minister covered much of the cost of representing his country. The Whitlocks were not in that league. After much and often frustrating searching, they were finally able to rent a fully furnished four-story house from an army colonel who was transferring from Brussels. Located on the corner of rue de Treves and rue Belliard, the house evidently was charming and had the added attribute of being in the Quartier Léopold, the diplomatic quarter of Brussels. As they say, location is everything, and sure enough, 74 rue de Treves was everything, that is everything American in Brussels from 1914 to 1917. The annual rent was $2,400, of which the U.S. government paid $1,600 for use of the bottom floor as a chancellery. For six months, from February until August 1914, Whitlock's day consisted of perhaps an hour or two on Ministry business, the rest of the morning working on his novel, then lunch, a drive into the country, and, weather permitting, a round of golf. In the evening there were diplomatic dinners and balls to attend. It sure beat Toledo!

Hugh Gibson, Whitlock's Secretary of Legation, assisted in ministerial duties, what few there were. A thirty-one-year-old bachelor, Gibson also looked forward to an easy time in Brussels. He recorded in his journal his hopes about the new diplomatic posting.

> Brussels, July 4, 1914. — After years of hard work and revolutions and wars and rumours of war, the change to this quiet post has been most welcome and I have wallowed in the luxury of having time to play.[21]
>
> For the last year or two I have looked forward to just such a post as this, where nothing ever happens, where there is no earthly chance of being called out of bed in the middle of the night to see the human race brawling over its differences.... I have thought that I should like to have a long assignment to just such a post and become a diplomatic Lotus Eater.[22]

Gibson's favorite haunt in Brussels was the restaurant of the Palace Hotel.[23] Here he often dined, exchanging news and gossip with diplomats from other legations. During the war German officers, members of the German aristocracy

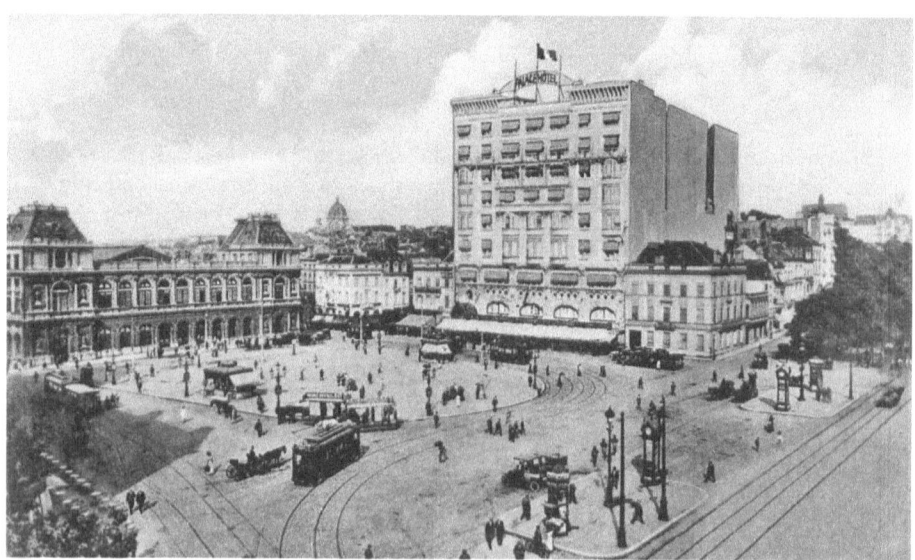

Place Rogier, Brussels, in 1913. The building on the left, spanning the entire side of the square, is the Gare du Nord, then the main Brussels railroad station. This station was the entry point for nearly all wartime visitors. The very large multistory building on the right with the Belgian flag is the famous Palace Hotel. Convenient to the station and very luxurious, Palace guests included almost everyone of importance who visited Brussels during the war (Rainer Hiltermann collection).

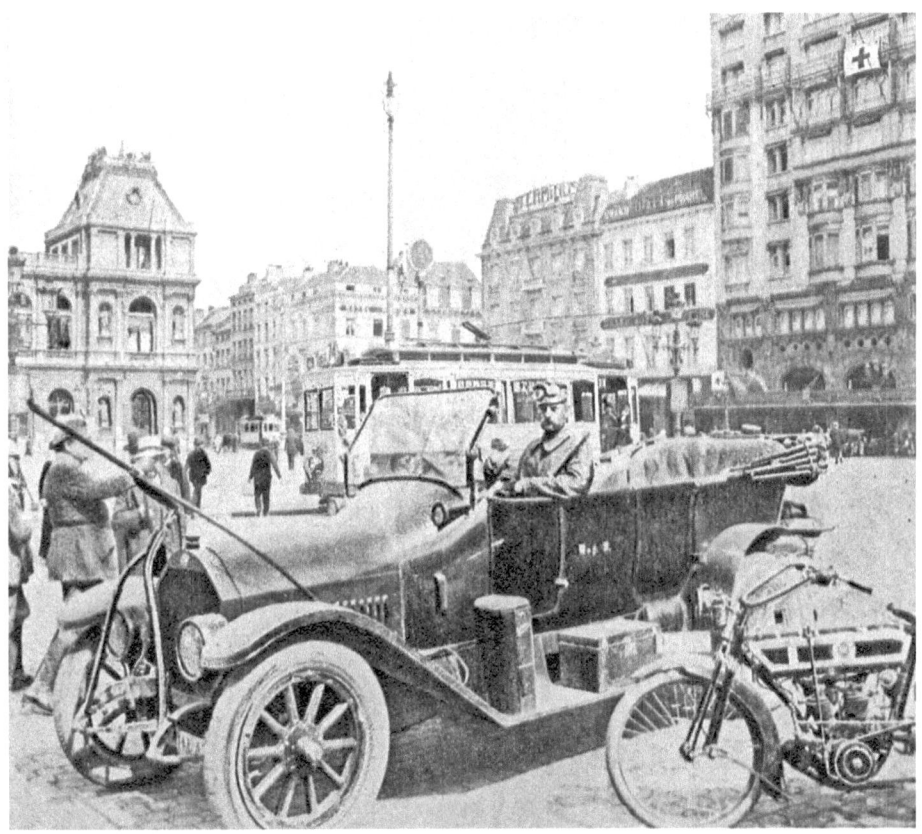

Place Rogier, Brussels, during the German occupation. A German military auto has a device affixed to its front to cut chin-high wires stretched across roads. On the extreme left in the background is the Gare du Nord. On the far right, the building with the Red Cross flag is the famous Palace Hotel, which at the time was probably housing war wounded (*Illustré,* 1914).

visiting Brussels and American reporters stayed at the hotel. Gibson remarked that his primary source of news about how the war was going came from table talk in the Palace dining room. Nearly all Brussels wartime memoirs mention Le Palace. Completed in 1908, the Art Nouveau-style hotel was the most modern and luxurious accommodation in Brussels, boasting among its luxuries the innovation of *en suite* bathrooms. It fronted the Place Rogier near the North Station (Gare du Nord), then the main rail terminus for visitors coming to Brussels.

Gibson and Whitlock often visited the Spanish Legation at 69 rue Belliard, only two short blocks from the American Legation. Whitlock's closest friend in Brussels, the Marquis de Villalobar, served as the Spanish Minister. Since

Villalobar was not married, Nell Whitlock often acted as hostess at his legation.

The German Legation was nearby at 58 rue Belliard. Whitlock and the German Minister, Herr von Bellow-Saleski,[24] had both arrived in Brussels in early 1914, and being new men on the scene, often socialized together. At a dinner party at the German Legation in May of 1914, von Bellow-Saleski told Whitlock, "I have never had a post where there has not been trouble; in Turkey it was the Revolution, in China it was the Boxers. I am a bird of ill omen. But now ... I have the most tranquil post in Europe; nothing can happen in Brussels."[25]

He was so very wrong.

Von Bellow-Saleski was keenly interested in spreading German *Kultur* in Belgium and, to this end, he intended to set out a new German-style formal garden behind the Legation. He never got the chance, Belgium got German military *Kultur* rather than botanic! Today the old German Legation building still stands and still represents German interests in Brussels. It houses the Goethe Institute, an organization promoting German language and culture — the mission Herr von Bellow-Saleski had for the building in 1914.

Herr von Bellow-Saleski gave an interview to the *New York Times* on August 2, 1914, in which he categorically stated that Germany would never violate Belgium's neutrality — German troops would not cross into Belgium.[26] They did, of course, on August 4.

The invasion ended Whitlock's sabbatical. As news of the invasion spread, Americans soon over-ran the American Legation. "All day the Legation was crowded with frightened Americans, who continued to pour into Brussels and remained there hesitant, undecided, bewildered, loath to brave the Channel-Crossing to England, hoping for some miracle that would arrest the war or spare them its discomforts."[27]

Only gold coins had any value; banks refused American banknotes, letters of credit and checks. The Legation found itself deluged with American tourists and expatriates. "There was another type, more worldly-wise, with manner and sophistication; they had lived in Europe long years, and had not been reminded of their nationality until the income-tax summoned them; now they came in eager haste for passports to establish an identity that they had not always, perhaps, cared to own."[28]

An American reporter in Brussels at the time left a more cynical account of his fellow Americans:

> When the war broke loose those persons in Europe it concerned the least were the most upset about it. They were our fellow countrymen. Even to-day, above the roar of shells, the crash of falling walls, forts, forests, cathedrals, above the scream of shrapnel, the sobs of widows and orphans, the cries of the wounded

and dying, all over Europe, you can still hear the shrieks of the Americans calling for their lost suit-cases.[29]

Immediately after the German Army entered Belgium, Berlin recalled von Bellow-Saleski. Before leaving his post, he convinced Whitlock to look after German interests, as there were numerous German nationals living in Belgium. Whitlock helped assure they were not abused and repatriated hundreds of businessmen and their families. This aid won him points when he later negotiated with the German occupation authorities to ease the plight of the Belgians.

On the evening of August 17, the Belgian government, King Albert and Queen Elizabeth and the Belgian Army abandoned the capital for the fortified city of Antwerp. Nearly all foreign legations followed in their wake. Whitlock cabled Washington asking whether he should remain or leave Brussels for Antwerp; his instructions were to do what he thought best. He opted to remain, as did the Spanish Legation. When the German Army finally arrived and occupied Brussels, only Brand Whitlock and Hugh Gibson, as representatives of the most powerful neutral, remained to negotiate with the German high command on behalf of the Belgian citizens.

However, not everyone was leaving. American reporters, sensing a big story, immediately booked passage for Europe on the Cunard luxury liner *Lusitania*, scheduled to depart New York bound for Liverpool on August 4, the day Britain declared war against Germany. On board she carried the first contingent of American newspaper correspondents to cover the European war, their ultimate destination, Belgium. Authorities believed three German cruisers, *Dresden*, *Karlsruhe*, and *Straßburg*, lay outside New York harbor, intending to attack the British liner once she cleared U.S. waters. The threat delayed *Lusitania's* departure until 1:00 a.m. on August 5. She slipped out of her berth with "all lights out" except for running lights on masthead and sides. The black silhouette glided out of the harbor where three British cruisers waited to serve as escorts for the voyage across the Atlantic.[30] Americans followed *Lusitania's* voyage almost as a sporting event, i.e., German hounds chasing a British fox.[31] She arrived safely in Liverpool on the evening of August 11.[32] *Lusitania* continued to cross the Atlantic monthly during the war until sunk by a German submarine on May 7, 1915.

Among the passengers who disembarked August 11 was the American reporter and celebrity Richard Harding Davis.[33] By 1914, he had already published 24 books, one of which, *Soldiers of Fortune*, became a motion picture in 1913. He had written countless newspaper and magazine articles and was America's most well-known and well-paid war correspondent, having covered 6 international conflicts.[34] He crossed the English Channel and took a train for Belgium to report on his final war; Davis arrived in Brussels on August 17, the same day the Belgian national government abandoned the capital for Antwerp. Gibson describes Davis's stylish entrance:

> I went to the Palace [Hotel] to dine with Palmer and Blount. We had hardly got seated when in walked Richard Harding Davis and Gerald Morgan, and joined us. I had not expected Davis here so soon, but here he is. He was immaculate in dinner jacket and white linen, for war does not interfere with his dressing.[35]

Frederick Palmer and Gerald Morgan were American journalists; both had traveled with Davis on *Lusitania*. D.I. Blount was an American businessman living in Brussels. Blount owned an automobile and often he and Gibson motored around Brussels, especially to *Le Palace* to dine. Richard Harding Davis was much impressed with his Palace accommodation and said so in a letter to his wife, "Gerald Morgan and I got in last night; this is a splendid new hotel; for $2.50 I get a room and bath like yours on the 'royal suite,' only bigger."[36]

The occupational imperative of a war correspondent is to find the fighting and describe what he sees in newspaper dispatches. A war correspondent must see battles, or, at best, recent carnage caused by battles. Editors expect descriptions of gore and heroism. Dallying over drinks at the terrace café of the Palace Hotel was pleasant but would not bring in a paycheck. Thus the Americans set about renting cars with drivers to take them to the front, which was somewhere between Liège and Brussels. Unfortunately for the journalists, large battles never materialized, the Belgian Army simply melted away when engaged. As Frederick Palmer put it, "the Belgian army, in a professional sense, was hardly to be considered as an army."[37]

> One of the puzzling things about the early mid–August stages of the war was the almost instantaneous rapidity with which the Belgian army, as an army, disintegrated and vanished. To-day it was here, giving a good account of itself against tremendous odds, spending itself in driblets to give the Allies a chance to get up. To-morrow it was utterly gone.[38]

With so little to write about, the Americans retreated to the comforts of the Palace and waited for the Germans to come to them. And come they did.

A string of atrocities marked the German Army's progress through Belgium; at the slightest provocation, or sometimes without any provocation at all, they burned towns and villages and shot innocent civilians, including women and children. For all its vaunted discipline, the German Army often disintegrated into a hoard of barbarians. What Attila and the Huns did in Europe in the fifth century, the Germans were doing in Belgium in the early twentieth. When German cavalry patrols appeared in Brussels' outskirts, everyone believed the Imperial German Army, with all its unstoppable might, would shortly take the city. Would the city defend itself? Would city officials order a suicidal and pointless defense? After all, the Belgian Army had already departed for Antwerp, leaving only the Garde Civique, supplemented by citizen volunteers, including Boy Scouts, to mount a defense, a defense hardly adequate to stop or even slow the most powerful army in Europe. Brand Whitlock and the Spanish Minister Marquis de Villalobar realized if the Germans encountered any resistance, Brussels would be the setting for numerous atrocities. They managed to convince King Albert, currently in Antwerp with his army, that a defense of Brussels would only result in the destruction of the city and the deaths of countless of its citizens. Resistance would be futile and spark grave consequences. The King agreed and ordered Burgomaster Adolphe Max to declare Brussels an open city to the invaders. On August 19, just a day before the Germans arrived, Burgomaster Max issued a proclamation to the citizens of Brussels; the following was the most important part of the text: "As long as I live and am free to do so, I will protect to my utmost the rights and honour of my fellow-citizens. I beg you to help me in this work by refraining from any hostile acts, carrying of arms, and joining in disturbances."[39]

The American journalists now had something to report. They would finally see the Imperial German Army. Everyone attended the triumphal entry. It turned out some of the German troops were a bit confused geographically, thinking they were actually marching into Paris rather than Brussels — well, the Kaiser had promised a speedy victory and both cities did speak French.

The Germans arrived on August 20, 1914. Hugh Gibson and Richard Harding Davis watched the entering columns march (swagger) into the city. What the Americans saw was the first modern army of the twentieth century.

> We watched the passing of great quantities of artillery, cavalry and infantry, hussars, lancers, cyclists, ambulance attendants, forage men, and goodness only knows what else. I have never seen so much system and such equipment. The machine is certainly wonderful; and, no matter what is the final issue of the war, nobody can deny that so far as that part of the preparation went, the Germans were hard to beat.... The men's kits were wonderfully complete and contained all sorts of things that I had never seen or heard of, so I turned for explanation to Davis, who had come along and was lost in admiration of the equipment and discipline. He said he had been through pretty much every campaign for the last twenty years, and thought he knew the last word in all sorts of equipment, but that this had him staggered.[40]

The triumphal entry lasted three days; day and night, it went on and on. Finally, overwhelmed and bored after hours of watching the endless parade of field-grey uniforms, Davis returned to his suite at the Palace to attempt to describe the scene for his American readers. Many considered the resulting article the finest piece of writing of World War One.

After an hour, from beneath my window, I still could hear them; another hour and another went by. They were still passing. Boredom gave way to wonder. The thing fascinated you, against your will, dragged you back to the sidewalk and held you there open-eyed. No longer was it regiments of men marching, but something uncanny, inhuman, a force of nature like a landslide, a tidal wave, or lava sweeping down a mountain. It was not of this earth, but mysterious, ghostlike. It carried all the mystery and menace of a fog rolling toward you across the sea. The uniform aided this impression. In it each man moved under a cloak of invisibility.[41]

Davis was most impressed by the new German uniform, for in contrast to the gaudy and impractical outfits the Belgian and French soldiers were forced to wear into battle, the German soldier's uniform helped him to survive.

After you have seen this service uniform under conditions entirely opposite you are convinced that for the German soldier it is one of his strongest weapons. Even the most expert marksman cannot hit a target he cannot see. It is not the blue-gray of our Confederates, but a green-gray. It is the gray of the hour just before daybreak, the gray of unpolished steel, of mist among green trees.[42]

Later, he described a scene in the Jardin Botanique, just across the road from the Palace Hotel, "Later, as the army passed under the trees of the Botanical Park, it merged and was lost against the green leaves. It is no exaggeration to say that at a few hundred yards you can see the horses on which the Uhlans ride but cannot see the men who ride them."[43]

A German officer speaking to an American journalist disparaged the Napoleonic uniforms of his enemies, especially the French uniform that made men living targets. "*Ach*, but it was shameful that they should have been sent against us wearing those long blue coats, those red trousers, those shiny black belts and bright brass buttons! At a mile, or even half a mile, the Germans in their dark-gray uniforms, with dull facings, fade into the background; but a Frenchman in his foolish monkey clothes is a target for as far as you can see him."[44]

Not every American visitor in Brussels stayed at the fashionable Palace Hotel that fateful August; four young American women, members of a dance quartet performing at the Gaiety Theater in the city, probably had less opulent digs. The dancers, caught by the invasion, remained in Brussels for a month before making their escape. "The day after we appeared at the Gaiety[45] in Brussels the theatre was transformed into a hospital. Two of our party served as nurses for several weeks. The suffering they saw was frightful. French, English and German wounded were treated alike."[46]

The German authorities in Brussels, anxious to help the stranded dancers, provided a horse and cart and the necessary permit allowing them to travel through the battle line to Ostend and cross to England. They loaded the cart with their baggage and the foursome trudged alongside, walking all the way to the coast. As they traveled, other Americans attempting to get out of Belgium joined the procession. There was comfort in numbers. "We went very slowly, for on all sides of us there was battle or had been fighting. There were lines of baggage wagons, soldiers hurrying to the front, and ambulances and carts of every description carrying the wounded back from the firing line. Twice we were under fire."[47]

The Americans reached a small village near Ghent (Gand) just as their money ran out, stranding them in the middle of nowhere. An unlikely happenstance saved them. An automobile driven by E. Alexander Powell, a correspondent for the *New York World*, with his photographer Donald Thompson and Julius Van Hee, the American Vice-Consul for Ghent, as passengers, entered the village. Powell picks up the story.

> As we came thundering into the little town of Sotteghem, which is the Sleepy Hollow of Belgium, we saw, rising from the middle of the town square, a pyramid, at least ten feet high, of wardrobe trunks, steamer trunks, bags, and suitcases. From the summit of this extraordinary monument floated a huge American flag. As our car came to a halt there rose a chorus of exclamations in all the dialects between Maine and California, and from the door of a near-by café came pouring a flood of Americans. They proved to be a lost detachment of that great army of tourists which, at the beginning of hostilities, started on its mad retreat for the coast, leaving Europe strewn with their belongings. This particular detachment had been cut off in Brussels by the tide of German invasion, and, as food supplies were running short, they determined to make a dash — perhaps crawl would be a better word — for Ostend, making the journey in two lumbering farm wagons.... When we arrived they had been there for a day and a night and had begun to think that it was to be their future home. It was what might be termed a mixed assemblage, including several women of wealth and fashion who had been motoring on the Continent and had had their cars taken from them, two prim schoolteachers from Brooklyn, a mine owner from West Virginia, a Pennsylvania Quaker, and a quartet of professional tango dancers — artists, they called themselves — who had been doing a "turn" at a Brussels music-hall when the war suddenly ended their engagement.[48]

Powell and Van Hee gave the group four hundred francs. They last saw their compatriots leaving the village with two creaking wagons and the huge American flag flying above. They were singing in loud voices, *We'll Never Go There Any More*. All made it to Ostend and eventually home.[49]

Back in Brussels, military jurisdiction replaced civil law; Field Marshal General Colmar von der Goltz, governor-general of Belgium, became the country's virtual dictator, with General von Jarotzky serving as his military governor of Brussels. Gibson found that even his favorite restaurant had changed.

> I went down to the Palace Hotel on the chance of picking up a little news, but did not have much luck. The restaurant was half filled with German officers,

who were dining with great gusto. The Belgians in the café were gathered just as far away as possible, and it was noticeable that instead of the usual row of conversation, there was a heavy silence brooding over the whole place.[50]

General von Jarotzky controlled the issuance of travel permits for diplomats and correspondents as well as almost anything else regarding officialdom in the city. Hugh Gibson got to know him well.

> The General himself is a little, tubby man, who looks as though he might be about fifty-five; his face is red as fire when it is not purple, and the way he rages about is enough to make Olympus tremble,.... He switched languages with wonderful facility, and his cuss words were equally effective in any language that he tried. Just as with us, everyone wanted something quite out of the question and then insisted on arguing about the answer that they got.... As he talked, the General would be getting redder and redder, and when about to explode, he would spring to his feet and advance upon his tormentor, waving his arms and roaring at him to get the ____ out of there. Not satisfied with that, he invariably availed of the opportunity of being on his feet to chase all the assembled crowd down the stairs and to scream at all the officers in attendance for having allowed all this crowd to gather.[51]

Calm would preside for about four minutes as the General's office refilled with petitioners, and the comedy act would begin anew. The planning and discipline that characterized the German entry into Brussels seemingly was lost in administering the place. Gibson thought visits to von Jarotzky's office would have been "screamingly funny" had it not been that some of the General's decisions affected human lives. Although treated with dignity as a representative of America and a fellow government official, Gibson sometimes waited hours for a meeting with the busy general and thus observed the administrative turmoil surrounding the man. Gibson noted, "Our little German General, von Jarotzky, has kept clicking his heels together and promising us anything we chose to ask."[52] However, as Gibson learned, promises made were not necessarily kept, and if kept, could be delayed. The General's acquiescence often was just a way to get Gibson to stop pestering him and get him out of the office.

American journalists implored Gibson for German travel permits allowing visits to the active front, but the answer was always negative. At best, Gibson obtained permits for them to travel to the outskirts of Brussels—but what defined the outskirts? Armed with Brussels environs travel permits, four journalists rented a taxi in front of the Palace Hotel, determined to find out how far they could go. The quartet headed out of town looking for a war story— and vanished. Their disappearance caused a bit of angst at the American Legation.

> About four o'clock, McCutcheon, Irwin and Cobb[53] breezed in, looking like a lot of tramps. Several days ago they had sailed blissfully away to Louvain [Leu-

1. The Attack 27

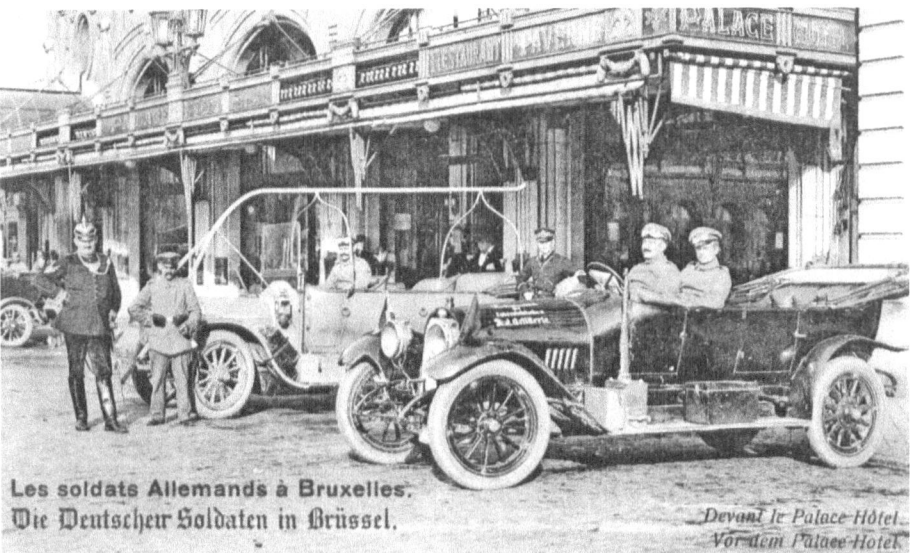

Les soldats Allemands à Bruxelles.
Die Deutschen Soldaten in Brüssel.
Devant le Palace-Hôtel.
Vor dem Palace-Hotel.

German military autos parked in front of the terrace restaurant of the Palace Hotel. The auto on the left has a frame affixed to deflect potentially decapitating wires stretched across roads, evidently a not uncommon road hazard in Belgium. The restaurant at the Palace Hotel must have been extraordinary as many war memoirs mention it. The autos probably await officers dining there (Rainer Hiltermann collection).

ven, a small city 15 miles east of Brussels] in a taxi, which they had picked up in front of the hotel. When they got there, they got out and started to walk about to see what was going on, when, before they could realize what was happening, they found themselves in the midst of a Belgian retreat, hard-pressed by a German advance.[54]

Caught between the two armies, the Americans barely escaped with their lives and were later arrested by the Germans for being in the wrong place and for lacking the appropriate documents to be there. They were sent back to Brussels and ordered to remain in the city — or else.

The most brazen correspondent without documents was, as one would expect, Richard Harding Davis. His antics nearly got him shot as a spy. He inadvertently wandered into the path of the Imperial German Army as it marched to engage the British Expeditionary Force at Mons. The fighting began August 22 and lasted until August 24 when the British retreated. On August 23, Davis set off for the front in a Brussels taxicab with fellow journalist Gerald Morgan. Their German passes were, of course, only valid for the environs of Brussels. They reached the town of Hal (Halle), about 10 miles (16.1 km) southwest of Brussels. Hal is on the main railway line between Brussels and Mons, about 22 miles (35.4 km) from Mons. At Hal the cab turned back, Davis and Morgan continued on foot in the midst of the German Army. "The column stretched for fifty miles. Where it was going we did not know, but, we argued, if it kept on going and we kept on with it, eventually we must stumble upon a battle."[55]

Almost immediately, a German officer arrested the Americans, but they managed to lose their captor in the gray mass of men marching by. At this point, Morgan thought it was insane to continue and turned back for Brussels. Davis foolishly continued and faced arrest once again. This time his captor pushed an automatic deep into his stomach to make the point and escorted him to a German colonel who signed a pass for Davis to go to the village of Enghien, spend the night there and return to Brussels the next day. Enghien is about 17 miles (27.4 km) from Mons. The next day, August 24, as the battle of Mons was in full swing, Davis continued his trek following the German Army. "The gray tidal wave was still roaring past. It was pressing forward with greater speed, but in nothing else did it differ from the tidal wave that had swept through Brussels."[56]

Davis could not speak a word of German and only the most rudimentary French. He reached the vicinity of the small town of Ath, about 15 miles (24.2 km) from Mons, where his luck finally ran out. The arresting officer, who fortunately spoke English, questioned why Davis was wearing a British uniform in the photograph in his American passport. Davis tried to explain that he was photographed in his war correspondent's uniform, a uniform he had copied from the British when he covered the Boer War. "Sure, sure," thought the German and promptly arrested Davis as a British spy. Taken to Ath and then to Ligne, a small town about a half dozen miles north of Mons, he was locked up under guard while the Germans considered whether or not to shoot him as a British spy.

The Germans reached a decision; they would not shoot Davis but would give him a chance. He had 48 hours to report to the German commander of Brussels; his pass indicated that if he was still on the road after 2 days whoever captured him could shoot him summarily. His pass stated (in German, of course):

> The American reporter Davis must at once return to Brussels via Ath, Enghien, Hal, and report to the government at the latest on August 26th. If he is met on any other road, or after the 26th of August, he will be handled as a spy. Automobiles returning to Brussels, if they can unite it with their duty, can carry him.[57]
>
> Chief of General Staff,
Von Gregor, Lieutenant-Colonel

Davis had two days to cover about 50 miles (80 km) on foot, a challenge even for someone fit, but Davis was nearly 50 years old and had decades of fine dining behind him. Besides that, his foot was bleeding from blisters caused by a split shoe. He began his trek, hobbling along the road, stopped every few miles by soldiers checking his pass. In desperation, Davis flagged down a car traveling in the right direction; it carried a German general. Fortunately, the general took pity on the straggler along the road and, after reading the pass, offered a ride. He was going to a meeting in Hal; he would take Davis that far. As the car pulled into Hal, the general changed his mind. "I go on to Brussels," he said in fractured French. "Desire you to accompany me?" The Palace Hotel restaurant saved Davis from walking the last 10 miles (16.1 km) to Brussels; the general had decided to lunch there rather than in Hal. He dropped Davis off as they entered the city and Davis made for the American Legation.[58] Brand Whitlock picks up the story:

> I was standing in my window that Tuesday morning, ... when I heard cries as of glad welcome in the next room. I went in, and there sat Richard Harding Davis. He was extended in one of the Government's big leather chairs, with an air of having collapsed in it. He was sunburned and unshaven, powdered grey from head to foot with dust, and beside him on the floor lay his bundle, a khaki bag, part of his correspondent's kit. Despite his good looks, his indubitable distinction in any emergency, he looked like a weary tramp, and he lifted his tired eyes drolly, humourously, to me.[59]

Chapter 2

Book Burning

"The people build cities," wrote Erasmus, and added, only too truly, "while the madness of princes destroys them."[1] — Foster Watson

Over a period of five days, from August 25 to August 29, 1914, the Imperial German Army systematically destroyed the center of Louvain,[2] a university city of 42,000 located about 16 miles (25.8 km) east of Brussels. When the burning and shooting finally ended, the city was a smoking ruin of gutted buildings and collapsed masonry walls. Of the medieval cathedral, only standing walls remained; the wooden interior was just a pile of burned timber. The Catholic University, where Erasmus lectured from 1517 to 1521,[3] also disappeared in the inferno, as did the university library with its famous collection of books and manuscripts dating from the Middle Ages. "In the streets of the ruined and deserted city, where the soldiers were completing their work of pillage, and further on even into the country, leaves of manuscripts and books fluttered about, half burned, at the mercy of the wind."[4]

To understand what happened in Louvain and its significance, it is necessary to consider events occurring prior to its sack. The story begins with a foray from Brussels to Louvain by four American reporters. On August 19, a day before the Germans entered Brussels, the quartet hired a taxi outside the Palace Hotel and instructed the driver to take them to Louvain (see Chapter 1). They had heard there might be some fighting going on between the Belgians and Germans near the town; maybe they would find a battle in Louvain. Their editors were clamoring for an exciting war story.

> So we started — Cobb, Dosch, McCutcheon, and I[5] — in a Brussels city taxicab whose driver was willing to take a chance for an extra tip. We had just arrived; we knew nothing of Belgian geography; only one of us had any knowledge whatever of French. We did not even know where we were going.[6]

When the Americans left Brussels, plans were still afoot to defend the city with makeshift defenses hastily erected on the principal roads leading into the city and streetcars flipped on their sides to block thoroughfares, forcing taxis to weave slowly through the obstacles to get past. Presumably, the barricades might just slow a German cavalry charge, a tactic not much used in the First World War. Here and there new trenches defaced parks, but the reporters noted "the turf carefully cut away in blocks and stacked for future use."[7] Napoleonic-vintage cannons poked their "stupid noses" from embrasures in the new earthworks. A few barbed wire entanglements hanging from recently planted posts complemented the fortifications. A Belgian forlorn hope of half-trained, listless citizen soldiers, the *Garde Civique*, anxiously manned their city's imaginary defenses. A dispirited sentry stopped the taxi, refusing to let it pass. His fellow citizen soldiers argued successfully that he allow the driver to complete the journey and get his fare. Finally, the Americans continued their journey, a lack of passes less important than payment of the driver's fare. Then, for the next mile or two, they passed many people reading or strolling in the parkway, along the roads, even nurses pushing baby carriages. Brussels was obviously ready for war. Fortunately, it would capitulate without an angry shot fired.

Leaving the environs of the city, the Americans soon encountered the other side of the German invasion — refugees fleeing before the invaders. In the lead were young men and women, the fast walkers, each carrying a suitcase or a bag of necessities. All walked briskly with some chatting and laughing as if on an outing. Then came everyone else — the slow walkers. Old women, children, whole families trudged past, each carrying what they could and some more than they should.

> A young boy struggled with a child's wagon, full to overflowing. A whole family passed. The children grouped around an overburdened mother, each carrying a bundle. The father trundled a wheelbarrow, shaded by an umbrella, and containing among much bedding, a pair of baby twins, sound asleep.
>
> No one spoke, but no one wept either. The world was struck silent, dumb. The only sound was the shuffling of their feet along the dry pathway.[8]

The Americans' taxi nudged past hundreds of refugees fleeing Louvain and neighboring villages, all seeking safety in Brussels. Unfortunately, Brussels would come under German control the next day, and many would join the throngs evacuating that city. No place was really safe. After a few more miles, the taxi blundered into the Belgian Army, which, of course, was retreating or just plain vanishing. At this point, the taxi driver refused to go any farther, correctly fearing the German Army would commandeer his cab. The four reporters now continued on foot toward the university city of Louvain, a place they envisioned to be similar to Ann Arbor (University of Michigan) or Ithaca (Cornell) or Cambridge (Harvard) but with a Catholic twist! The four were in many ways "babes in Belgium." They entered Louvain from the west just as the German Army entered from the east — two very different entries. The four foot-sore Americans wandered in asking anyone who would listen, and in very rudimentary high school French, "Is this Louvain?" It certainly did not look like Ann Arbor, or Ithaca, or even Cambridge. They eventually settled into an open-air café, *Le Lion Rouge*, on the southern edge of Louvain, for some cheese sandwiches and coffee served by a 300-pound proprietress. From there they watched the entry of the German Army into Louvain. The advance guard came on bicycles, followed by a troop of Uhlan lancers on coal-black horses, riding as if on parade. The cavalry's mission, almost their only mission, in the First World War was to look intimidating on parade. The reporters established a camaraderie with some of the advance guard, buying the hungry soldiers beer and sandwiches. A surprising number of the Germans had spent time in America and were eager to speak to the Americans.[9]

Then they heard a strange sound:

> But as we listened there came a sound heavier than the ring of hoofs on the macadam roads; and then — singing. Round the corner swung the head of an infantry brigade giving full voice to "*Die Wacht am Rhein*." They were singing in absolute time; they were singing in parts, like a trained chorus! Never have I heard anything quite like the beat and ring of their marching. They wore heavy, knee-high cowhide boots; and those boots, propelled by heavy, stalwart German bodies, struck the roads with a concerted shuffling thump which shook the earth.... Intent on their singing and their marching, looking neither to right nor left, they shuffled and stamped on to conquest and death. It had become a horde by now — cavalry, infantry, artillery, cavalry, infantry, artillery, rolling, pouring toward Brussels and toward France.[10]

> And every other man, regardless of his breed, held a cheap cigar between his front teeth; but the wagon drivers and many of the cavalrymen smoked pipes — the long stemmed, china-bowled pipe, which the German loves. The column moved beneath a smoke-wreath of its own making.[11]

As the town filled with troops, the Americans became very uncomfortable, feeling that they should make themselves known to a senior officer. They approached three who had just stepped out of a staff car and seemed to be in good spirits. Fortunately, one of the officers spoke English. Upon learning that the four American reporters had successfully passed through the battle lines in a Belgian taxi, he burst into laughter. He translated the tale to his brother officers who also thought the story a great joke. A captain who had spent time in New York and spoke English joined the party; he also cracked up in laughter. For reasons not completely clear to themselves, the Americans were the funniest thing in Louvain. The officers bought them a round of beer; the reporters seemed to be the toast of the town! The captain guided the Americans to the General Staff headquarters at the Palais de Justice. They were to meet Major Renner, the Adjutant, there the following day. In the meantime, they took rooms in a small fourth-rate hotel near the railroad station — German officers occupied all the better hotels. The Americans' hotel had a pretentious name, but that was all.

> It called itself by a gorgeous title — it was the House of the Thousand Columns, which was as true a saying as though it had been named the House of the One Column; for it had neither one column nor a thousand, but only a small, dingy beer bar below and some ten dismal living rooms above.[12]

The execution ground was nearby, behind the station. The seriousness of their situation came home whenever they heard shots and saw a corpse carried off.[13]

The following day, the Americans picked Irvin Cobb, the most cordial and wittiest of the group, to interview the Adjutant and report back.

> "Well, boys," he said, "we're still the wheeze of the German army!" The Adjutant, too, had roared when he heard of the taxicab. He, too, had translated, and the Palais de Justice had rung with Germanic laughter.
>
> "I should say, gentlemen," Cobb quoted the Adjutant, "that you owe your present delicate situation to an inordinate desire for travel or to an excessive appetite. You know we have no correspondents with the German army."
>
> "Well, you've got four now!" said Cobb.
>
> "I know — and it's not your fault, since we came to you, not you to us," said the Adjutant. "At the same time it would be dangerous for you, and certainly indiscrete for us, to send you through our lines to Brussels now. There have been reprisals along the road. Some of our men become brutes when their comrades are attacked, and some fool lieutenant might exceed his authority." The Adjutant spoke perfect English — even a little American slang.[14]

Later the Adjutant got more serious; the Americans should remain quietly in their hotel on the Rue de la Station, although they could venture out for meals. They were to show no curiosity about army movements, not speak to officers or men, and definitely take no notes. The German Secret Service was aware of the foursome and watching. The Americans were essentially under house arrest. In the meantime, the situation in Louvain grew dangerous with the occupiers becoming more and more paranoid, issuing proclamation after proclamation concerning the behavior of the inhabitants. Offenses that appeared threatening to the army carried a dire penalty; the execution ground near the hotel was busy. Everyone was to be in bed by eight, their windows closed, doors unlocked, and there was to be a light in every window. The Adjutant explicitly warned the Americans to be watchful.

> But this shooting from ambush by civilians; this murdering of our people in the night — that we cannot endure. We have made a rule that if shots are fired by a civilian from a house then we shall burn that house; and we shall kill that man and all the other men in that house whom we suspect of harboring him or aiding him.
>
> We make no attempt to disguise our methods of reprisal.[15]

Soldiers entered houses near the hotel searching for arms; a detail searched the Americans' rooms. "Taking no chances on firing from our hotel, we made the proprietor, regardless of expense, give us all the front rooms."[16] After three days, the weary and nervous foursome returned to Brussels; it was August 22, 1914 — three days later Louvain burned.

Probably the first journalist to see the burning town was the Dutch reporter Lambertus Mokveld. The athletic twenty-four-year-old pedaled his bicycle 45 miles (72.5 km) from the Dutch/Belgian border when he learned Louvain was burning, probably arriving in Louvain in the afternoon of August 26. He cycled past the spoor of the invading army: burned villages, terrorized villagers and roads strewn with glass from broken wine and beer bottles. The German Army seemed to be drinking its way across Belgium. Several miles from Louvain, Mokveld began to smell smoke.

> The town was on fire, and ruddy smoke hovered over it. Deserted like a wilderness, not a soul moved in the streets. The first street I entered was the Rue de la Station. Large, imposing mansions used to stand here, but the devouring fire consumed even the last traces of greatness.
>
> All houses were on fire, and every now and then walls fell down with a roar of thunder, shrouding the greater part of the street in a thick cloud of suffocating smoke and dust. Sometimes I had to run to escape from the filthy mass.[17]

Mokveld entered the ruins of what had been Louvain, engulfed in the scorching heat from the flames. Debris, glass and hot cinders made bicycling impossible; shouldering his bike he worked his way farther into the smoldering wreckage of the town. Streets were barely recognizable. At a corner three soldiers emerged from a burning building. Startled by the young man carrying a bicycle, they brought up their rifles and ordered him to halt.

> I explained who I was, and was then allowed to come nearer. They were drunk, and with glassy eyes talked about francs-tireurs [guerrilla snipers], the friendship Germans felt for Netherlanders, and so on. One of them entered the still burning corner house and returned with three bottles of wine, one a bottle of Champagne; corks were drawn and one of the bottles handed to me.[18]

Nearby rifle fire interrupted the strained bliss of alcohol-fueled fellowship; the Germans brought their rifles at the ready to defend their new friend from Holland — Holland was after all neutral and traded with Germany. Just then, a troop of German soldiers, wildly drunk, swung around the corner, taking random potshots at the burning houses. They joined the drinking party. Mokveld was able to slip away and was soon at the Grand Place, the town center from which the major streets radiated. There he saw the fifteenth century Gothic cathedral of St. Pierre — or what was left of the noble pile. It was now a smoking ruin with collapsed roof, burned altar and pulpit, and jagged walls with stained glass windows blown out. Across from the cathedral was one of

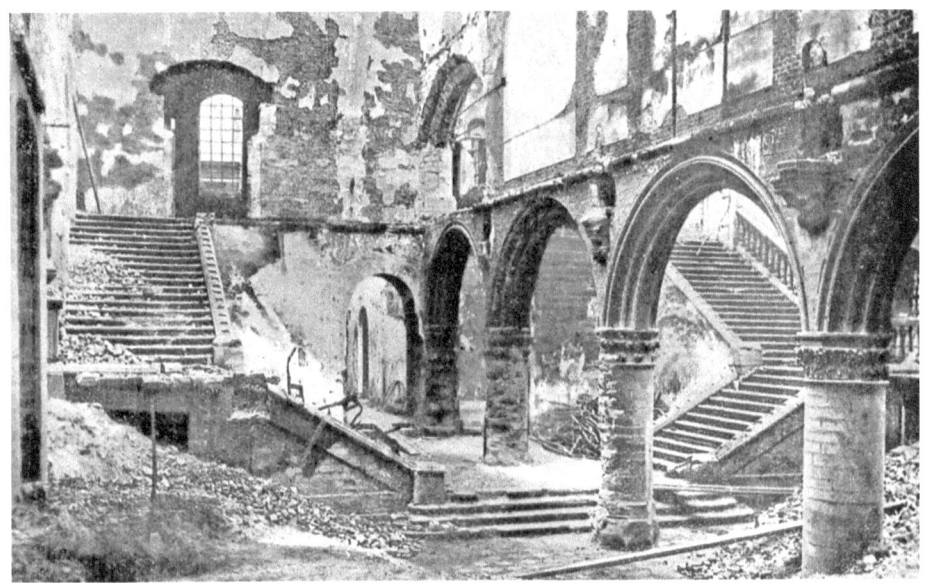

The fire-gutted interior of the Louvain University Library (Halles de l'Université). The photograph shows a "cleaned-up" interior, Belgian laborers having cleared the building of burned timbers and piles of charred books and manuscripts. The library was part of the itinerary for tourists visiting Louvain during the war (*Album de la Guerre*, 1922).

the most magnificent civic buildings in Europe, the fifteenth century Hotel de Ville. It survived untouched, serving as the headquarters for the Imperial German Army in Louvain. The three-story building appeared as an anomalous architectural jewel standing in a sea of devastation. The next stop on Mokveld's tour was the university quarter and its famed library.

Founded in 1425, the University of Louvain was similar to the universities at Cambridge and Oxford with its profusion of colleges, which by the eighteenth century numbered forty-two. The seat of the university until 1914 was the Halle aux draps or Cloth Hall, a building begun in 1317 and completed in 1345. Known as the Halles Universitaires, the structure grew with the addition of a large building in 1723. This complex housed the university library with its 230,000 books, 800 incunabula (books printed before 1501) and 950 manuscripts as well as lecture halls and a large reading room. On the night of August 25, 1914, the Halles Universitaires went up in flames. The following week Father Paul Delannoy, Librarian of the University of Louvain, returned to his beloved library to see what remained.

> I saw the ruins of the Library again eight days after the fire, and even then I was only able to look at them from a distance and at considerable risk. Broken

pillars, an impassable heap of bricks, stones, and beams smouldered in the fire which slowly consumed thousands of volumes between huge portions of dangerous and threatening walls: that was all that remained of the majestic building known as the *Halles Universitaires*, and of the rich treasure it contained.[19]

As soon as they could, the university's faculty scattered, finding positions lecturing in France, England, Holland and America. For some, the escape from provincial Louvain into the broader secular world was life-changing. Father Delannoy, University Librarian, went to Paris where he gave lectures at the Collège de France. In Paris, he met a woman, abandoned his celibacy and left the priesthood.[20]

However, for many citizens of Louvain escape was impossible. The forcible evacuation of the city's 42,000 inhabitants began on August 27. The invaders separated men from women and children, parents from their children and husbands from their wives, treating the conquered like cattle. The Germans seemed unable to make up their minds what to do with their captives. Some served as human shields for the German Army as it marched into battle. Some marched aimlessly around the countryside for days, driven by rifle butts and threats, before being released and told to return to Louvain. Those without families headed for neutral Holland, but those separated from their families returned to the ruins and hoped and waited. The Germans executed over two hundred for trivial offenses. More than a thousand Louvainers began a strange odyssey into Germany: initially crammed into filthy boxcars that had previously transported horses, they then suffered a fifty-hour journey to Cologne without food or drink and they finally marched through jeering crowds in Cologne while hysterical mobs of men, women and children hurled vile epithets and shouted "Zum Tod! Zum Tod!" (Kill them! Kill them!). After a night in the open under guard, with a small portion of black bread to curb their hunger, the bewildered and terrorized captives were off again. German authorities changed their minds and packed the Louvainers into a slow train back to Belgium. The trip lasted two days and three nights without food and only a mouthful of water. Finally released somewhere in Belgium and told they were free, the half-dead captives trekked to anywhere not yet under German control.[21]

An American teenager from Illinois, Marguerette Uyttebroeck,[22] was in Louvain visiting Flemish relatives when the terror began. Her father and fifteen-year-old brother disappeared, taken captive and transported to Germany. The sixteen-year-old Ms. Uyttebroeck somehow made her way to Cologne aboard a German prison train, loaded with British and Belgian prisoners of war, to search for her family. There she learned her brother and father were in a concentration camp.[23] Eventually the entire family managed to return to Illinois. However, the Midwest had links to Louvain that were much deeper than Flemish immigrants. In 1857, the bishops of Detroit and Louisville had founded the

American College of the Immaculate Conception[24] in Louvain. The college's purpose was to train seminarians to become pastors in the newly settled territories of America's heartland. The American College was almost the only refuge when the university precinct burned, and although the Germans killed some of its priests and drove the others away, the college buildings survived to become one of the city's primary relief centers during the German occupation. It was the only college to open for students (six seminarians) for the 1914-1915 academic year.[25]

In Brussels, the German authorities imposed tight restrictions on telegraphic communications as a way of keeping reports of events in Belgium from reaching the outside world. Even the American Legation found it impossible to send diplomatic cables. The Germans were very agreeable in allowing use of their military wire, but nothing got out of Brussels to the outside. It was all ja, ja, ja but really nein, nein, nein. To circumvent delays and restrictions, Minister Whitlock obtained permission from the Germans to send diplomatic telegrams via an automobile link to Antwerp, then under Belgian control and still connected to the international cable. On August 25, the date of the burning of the Louvain library, Hugh Gibson and his American friend, Daniel Lynds Blount, set out in Blount's little racing car for Antwerp with the diplomatic post. The trip was not without danger, as the travelers would cross both German and Belgian battle lines.

> While we were waiting for the final formalities for our trip to be accomplished, I invested in a wrist watch and goggles. We also bought a fuzzy animal like a Teddy bear, about three inches high, and tied him on the radiator as a mascot. He made a hit with all hands and got a valuable grin from several forbidding-looking Germans. We had signs on the car fore and aft, marking it as the car of the American Legation, the signs being in both French and German. As we were the first to try to make the trip, we thought it up to us to neglect nothing that would help to get us through without any unpleasant shooting or bayoneting.[26]

The 35 miles (56.4 km) journey was relatively uneventful, given where and when Gibson and Blount traveled. A couple of times German officers stopped the duo. However, after close inspection of their diplomatic documents, the Germans saluted and, in response, Gibson and Blount took off their hats and bowed as gracefully as one could within the confines of the racing car. Their instructions were to drive slowly and cautiously, stopping every several hundred yards in order to present a calm and unthreatening demeanor to soldiers at the checkpoints. After leaving the German lines, the car went into high gear until reaching the Belgian lines, when progress slowed again. They arrived in Antwerp in early evening. They booked into a hotel housing many of the Brussels' diplomats who had evacuated the city as the German Army approached. Everyone wanted to learn the news of Brussels. Gibson sent off his cables. With official duties discharged, he enjoyed dinner, drinks and endless war gossip with old diplomatic friends before going to bed. Gibson's sleep was so sound he slept through a nighttime bombing raid by a German Zeppelin, only learning of the event the next morning. He had been wondering why his bed shook in the middle of the night.

> The first bomb was in a little street around the corner from the hotel, and had fallen into a narrow four-story house, which had been blown to bits. When the bomb burst, it not only tore a fine hole in the immediate vicinity, but hurled its pieces several hundred yards. All the windows for at least two hundred or three hundred feet were smashed into little bits. The fronts of all the surrounding houses were pierced with hundreds of holes, large and small.[27]

The following morning, Gibson and Blount, along with many others, took the Antwerp Zeppelin tour. When the Zeppelin entered Antwerp airspace, it cut its engines and drifted silently over the city, dropping bombs as it went; blown out buildings and craters in parks and streets marked the path of the drift. Following the consequences of drift on the ground was the Zeppelin tour. Although killing ten people outright, the bombing attack achieved little else. Nevertheless, it was the talk of the town. That night Antwerp was on alert for another Zeppelin attack, but the Zeppelin stayed home. The following day Gibson and Blount packed their little car with diplomatic messages, letters and newspapers and drove back to Brussels without incident. The American Legation was again in contact with the rest of the world.

That was not the case for the American reporters in Brussels; they had stories but no way to get them out of occupied Belgium. From the very first days of the occupation, outside communication nearly ceased. For example, the Richard Harding Davis article describing the German entry into Brussels, probably the most famous descriptive writing of the war, had to be smuggled out of Brussels.

> T.A. Dalton, a young Englishman, dressed in riding breeches, puttees and dark coat was the courier who brought the Davis message. He left Brussels Friday evening (Aug. 21) at dusk, marching out of the city on the road to Ghent beside long lines of German infantry. Dalton continued on the main road to Ghent, walking most of the way and sometimes getting a short lift on wagons or automobiles.
>
> When he came to the point where the German main body turned off from the road to Ghent, Dalton hid in the brush beside the road and crept along on his hands and knees before he took the road again. He finally reached Ostend and crossed today to Folkstone on the government refugee boat, arriving at London at 2:30 p.m. and at the Tribune office a quarter of an hour later.[28]

However, what worked once would not again. As the Germans established themselves in Brussels and the countryside, communication with the outside

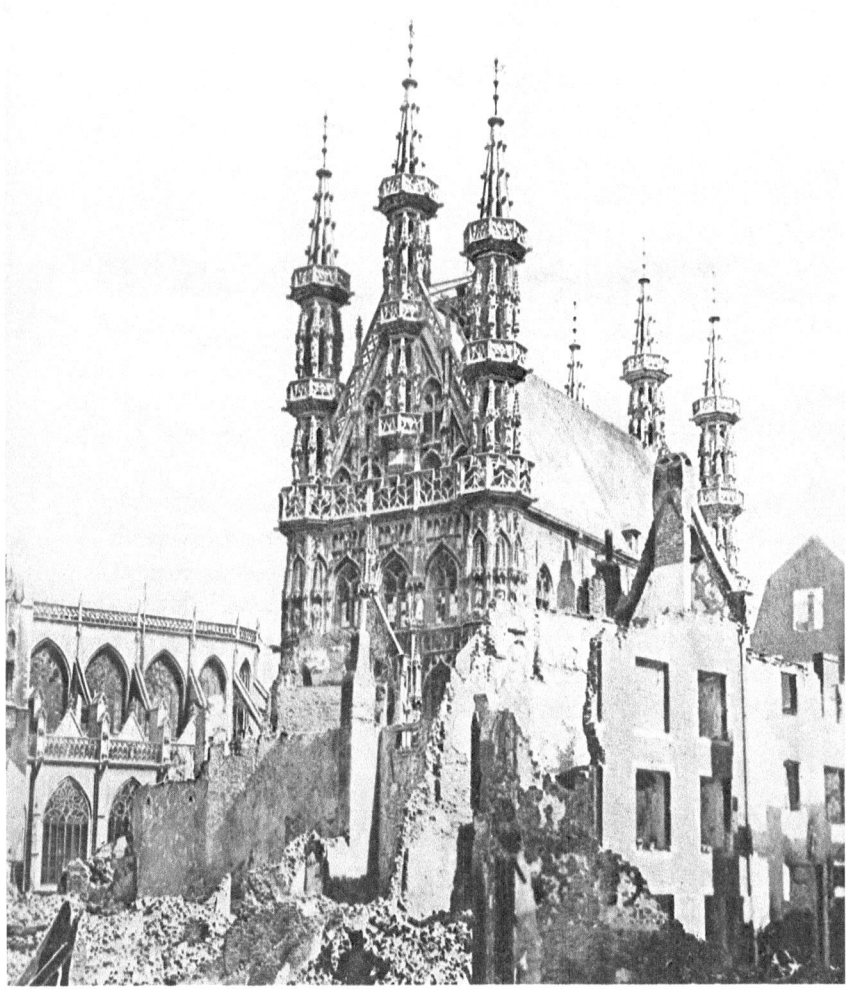

The Louvain town hall or Hôtel de Ville seems to rise from the ruins of the city. The building is probably the most magnificent example of secular medieval architecture in Belgium. It housed the German command during August 1914 and thus escaped destruction. The arched walls on the left are the remains of the fire-gutted cathedral (*Illustré*, 1914).

became more and more difficult for the journalists, and then nearly impossible. Two things became clear: the Germans did not want the journalists there and the Americans did not want to stay.

> The mail-trains and the telegraph office were in the hands of the invaders. They accepted our cables, censored them, and three days later told us, if we still wished, we could forward them. But only from Holland. By this they

accomplished three things: they learned what we were writing about them, for three days prevented any news from leaving the city, and offered us an inducement to visit Holland, so getting rid of us.[29]

Richard Harding Davis (Wheeler Syndicate), Gerald Morgan (*London Daily Telegraph*), Will Irwin (*Collier's Magazine*) and Arno Dosch (*World's Work*) were among the first to leave. They boarded a train carrying German wounded and British prisoners of war, scheduled to leave at 8:00 a.m. from the Gare du Nord on August 27. The train's destination was Aachen, Germany. From there, it was an easy connection to neutral Holland. The Gare du Nord[30] was on Place Rogier, as was the Palace Hotel. After breakfasting at the hotel, the Americans walked to the station. German soldiers filled the place: infantry regiments rested on straw along the platforms, a battery of artillery took over the entire central platform, and a field kitchen occupied one corner where a cook in his undershirt shoveled breakfast into waiting mess cans.[31] Upon learning that the Americans were traveling to Germany, soldiers crowded around, all wanting to talk. Very soon, the linguistic deficiencies of the Americans greatly curtailed discourse, but this did not discourage the soldiers, who only spoke louder — as if deafness, not an insufficient German vocabulary, were the problem. Fortunately, English speakers surfaced: a soldier who had been a waiter in New York, another who had relatives in San Francisco and even an officer with an Oxford degree. It was all very cordial. At four that afternoon, the train left the station. "When the train started at last, fifty soldiers scrambled for the honor of carrying our bags. They refused tips. An excited little private came along, waving a bottle of port. He threw it into the window of our compartment, and stood bowing with his hat off. When we finally gathered speed, the whole station rose up and cheered madly."[32]

After about 15 miles (24.2 km), the train slowed and pulled into, of all places, the Louvain station, an unscheduled two-hour stop. The heavy odor of smoke filled the air. By the strangest luck, the reporters landed in Louvain at the height of its incineration — it was the story of the year. The area near the station had burned the day before; its smoking ruins still smoldered. Beyond the immediate vicinity, the streets were still burning, the houses in flames with smoke pouring from broken windows. The reporters heard explosions out of sight and deeper in the city. Soldiers surrounded the train; everyone must remain onboard; the city was off limits. The story of the year lay in front of them, limited to the view from their carriage windows; the reporters were beside themselves.

> A private thrust his head into our window; we talked no German, but he yelled and babbled on and on. From the distance came regular explosions. He waved his hand in the direction of the sound; he made pantomime of shooting, cutting, thrusting, with a bayonet. There was no liquor on his breath; but he

2. Book Burning

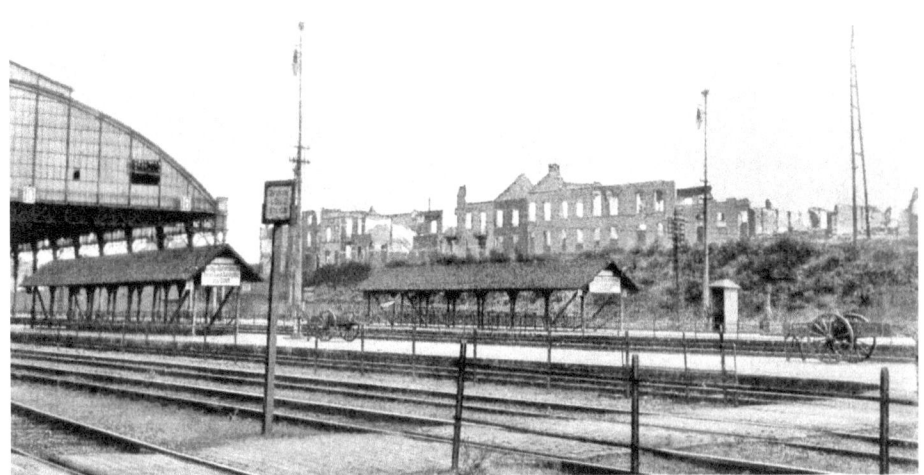

A view of the ruins of Louvain. The German soldier who took this photograph likely shot it from a coach window after his train stopped at the Louvain railroad station. This was probably the same scene witnessed by the American journalists when their train made an unscheduled stop at Louvain on August 27, 1914; however, at that time, the city was in flames (*Kriegs-Album des Marinekorps Flandern 1914–1917, 1918*).

> reeled and weaved in all his movements. A detail strung along the station railing took up the conversation. And all gave play to those same exaggerated gestures, as of drunken men.[33]

A Dutchman at the station translated for the Americans.[34] Was this the intrepid bicyclist Lambertus Mokveld? He was certainly there at the time.

Richard Harding Davis began writing immediately, with the flaming city as a backdrop. His story made the front page in many American newspapers and was instrumental in bringing the Louvain tragedy to the American public's attention. The barbarism of making war upon defenseless civilians shocked the seasoned war correspondent. This was something new. He called it the "War on the Defenseless."

> At Louvain it was the war upon the defenseless, war upon churches, colleges, shops of milliners and lacemakers. War was brought to the bedside and the fireside, against women harvesting in the fields and against children in wooden shoes at play in the streets.
>
> At Louvain that night the Germans were like men after an orgy.
>
> You felt it was only a nightmare, cruel and uncivilized. And then you remembered that the German Emperor has told us what it is. It is his holy war.[35]

Another American also on board that train was Mary Boyle O'Reilly of Boston. An activist in Catholic charitable organizations, intensely keen on helping the poor and downtrodden, a lecturer in sociology and a writer of note, she arrived in Brussels to do charitable work in early August 1914, just as the invasion began. She immediately linked up with Brand and Nell Whitlock, who knew her father. Brand Whitlock even arranged for her to have an audience with Elizabeth, Queen of the Belgians, at the royal palace in Brussels.

The train left Louvain on the evening of August 27 for Aachen, Germany, where the five Americans changed trains for Holland. Once in Holland, Ms. O'Reilly determined to return to Belgium and see Louvain up close. She convinced an adventurous Dutchman with an automobile to attempt the journey, even though they lacked the proper permits. She crossed into Belgium disguised as a peasant[36] and, facilitated by distributing German newspapers and cigarettes at German checkpoints, the pair reached Louvain, probably on August 28. The city burned from August 25 to August 29. O'Reilly wrote of her adventures in Louvain in a letter to an Irish missionary order, which published it in the *Missionary Record of the Oblates of Mary Immaculate* for January 1915, printed in Dublin. Unfortunately, the issue with the letter is not extant. A Boston newspaper republished excerpts of the O'Reilly letter in 1915; she was the only American journalist to witness Louvain's destruction from within the city.

> Through the sunlit, still undemolished streets (it was two days since the fire started), shooting parties of three men walked abreast on patrol, or paused to confer and to fire into cellar windows. Behind them came the raiders, picked men from the 9th German Army Corps.
>
> Each scout carried a small note book, which he consulted before inscribing [with chalk on the door] certain houses with the German of "Good people," "spare the house." I offered these fellows newspapers and they let me watch them at their work. Then they passed on.
>
> Files of 20 soldiers followed, lined up and were told off to as many doorways. At an order 20 axes broke into 20 homes and the sappers brought out blankets and food. Again the soldiers lined up and German officers inspected the loot.
>
> At an order, each sapper took a bomb and a box of petrol, ran to a doomed house, placed his bomb, sprinkled the petroleum, and dashed out to observe the result. During the time I sat watching, bands of sappers devastated nine streets: they worked with military precision.[37]

After seeing what she could in Louvain, without being arrested, O'Reilly rushed to Brussels to report to Brand Whitlock. Whitlock thought it very dangerous for her to continue her personal investigation of the Louvain tragedy; she had after all entered Belgium illegally. The best she could hope for was to get out of Belgium before the German authorities realized she was there. She crossed back into Holland that night. Why she did not publicize her observations is a mystery. After all, she was a writer and journalist, and she had one of the biggest stories of 1914. All she ever wrote of what she saw was that letter to an obscure Irish religious house.

In Brussels, reports reached the American Legation that there was serious trouble in Louvain. On August 28, the same day Ms. O'Reilly was prowling around Louvain, Hugh Gibson and his friend Blount decided to drive to Louvain to check on the validity of the horror stories reaching the Legation. The group grew as the Chargés d'Affairs of Sweden and Mexico joined them. They entered Louvain along one of its outer boulevards.

> About half way around the ring of boulevards we came to the burning houses. The outer side of the boulevard was a hundred feet or so from the houses, so the motor was safe, but it was pretty hot and the cinders were so thick that we had to put on our goggles. A lot of the houses were still burning, but most of them were nothing but blackened walls with smouldering timbers inside. Many of the front doors had been battered open in order to start the fires or to rout out the people who were in hiding.[38]

Confirming Miss O'Reilly's observations, Gibson reported that the houses were first broken into, then systematically looted for valuables, food and wine, and finally the furniture and hangings piled in the central room and torched. "It was all most businesslike."[39] Because the houses were substantial stone structures, the fires did not spread from one house to another; each had to be set alight separately. Destroying Louvain turned out to be more difficult than the Germans first thought. However, with organization and enough men anything was possible. Before they finally gave up on the task, they managed to destroy about 1,100 houses, approximately 20 percent of the city. On August 28, 1914, the Germans optimistically believed they could erase the entire place. Responding to international pressure, the Kaiser would cancel orders for the city's destruction on August 30. Before that order came down, a German officer told Gibson what Louvain would be like in the future.

> We shall make this place a desert. We shall wipe it out so that it will be hard to find where Louvain used to stand. For generations people will come here to see what we have done, and it will teach them to respect Germany and to think twice before they resist her. Not one stone on another, I tell you — *kein Stein auf einander*!
>
> I agreed with him when he remarked that people would come here for generations to see what Germany had done — but he did not seem to follow my line of thought.
>
> While we were talking about these things and the business of burning and looting was pursuing its orderly course, a rifle shot rang out near by.[40]

The group retreated to the railway station, believing it would be safer. At the station, soldiers were herding several hundred people, mostly women and children, into trains. Then more shots rang out and all was chaos. Civilians and soldiers scrambled for cover.

> Apparently a number of civilians, goaded to desperation by what they had seen, had banded together, knowing that they were as good as dead, and had determined to sell their lives as dearly as they could. They had gathered in the ruins of the houses fronting on the station and had opened up on us. There was a brisk interchange of shots, with an occasional tinkle of broken glass and a good deal of indiscriminate cursing by the soldiers who had taken refuge with us.[41]

After the firing died down, Gibson and his friends retrieved Blount's car, which had sat in the open during the firefight but not been hit, and started back to Brussels. Passing through the outskirts of Louvain, where the fires had not yet reached, they witnessed another aspect of the German terror. As the motor car passed civilians, mostly women and children, the Louvainers stopped whatever they were doing, turned toward the auto and raised their hands over their heads, showing they were unarmed and defenseless. It was a silent plea or supplication, "Please don't harm me."

> Our worst experience of this was when in coming around a corner we came upon a little girl of about seven, carrying a canary in a cage. As soon as she saw us, she threw up her hands and cried out something we did not understand. Thinking that she wanted to stop us with a warning of some sort, we put on the brakes and drew up beside her. Then she burst out crying with fear, and we saw that she was in terror of her life. We called out to reassure her, but she turned and ran like a hunted animal.[42]

Once Gibson asked a German officer about the provision of The Hague Conventions that stated there be no collective penalty on innocents for the lawless acts of individuals.[43] The officer's response was to dehumanize Belgians. "All Belgians are dogs," he said. They were beasts and thus outside the Conventions. That evidently included little girls.

Incredibly, several weeks later German authorities promoted the ruins of Louvain as a tourist destination![44] Gangs of laborers began clearing the streets of debris and stabilizing the ruins of the cathedral and university library. Restored train links between Brussels and Aachen encouraged visitors to come for a day or two. A special Sunday schedule allowed for daytrips from Brussels. Visitors could explore the miles of ruins and perhaps find a souvenir to take home — maybe even a charred book! Enterprising photographers set up cameras in front of the more "picturesque" ruins. Printed as postcards and mailed to Germany, photographs of grinning soldiers posed in front of gutted buildings showed the folks at home the fun of being in Belgium.

Sometimes the Belgian photographers got a bit too creative. An American tourist with strong German sympathies visited the city in 1915 and expressed great displeasure at a postcard he purchased. "One of the favorite postal card pictures of Louvain, which has been widely circulated, shows the Town Hall with its east façade in ruins. This was evidently obtained by pointing the camera at the Town Hall across the débris of a house that had been blown up by dynamite."⁴⁵

Another postcard that raised the ire of the same American was a sketch that showed a party of German soldiers "drinking champagne in a motor car which stands in the Grand Place, while the Town Hall burns and German soldiers slaughter innocent women and children."[46] One just could not trust Belgian photographers! This postcard is still available in Leuven (Louvain) antique stores.

The American reporter Irvin Cobb also visited as a tourist. Cobb had been one of the four reporters who stayed in the city for three days prior to its sack. He searched for the fourth-rate hotel where he and his colleagues had remained under house arrest for three days, the fabled House of the Thousand Columns.

> Its site was a leveled gray mass, sodden, wrecked past all redemption ... I looked for the little inn at which we had dined. Its front wall littered the street and its interior was a jumble of worthlessness. I wondered again as I had wondered many times before what had become of its proprietor — the dainty, gentle little woman whose misshapen figure told us she was near the time for her baby.[47]

Near the railway station, a recent widow who had lost her husband during the sack of the city begged Cobb to buy her postcards with views of the desolation. She pointed to some nearby soldiers. "They did," she said; "they killed him! Will you buy some postal cards, m'sieur? All the best pictures of the ruins!"[48]

Now come the hard questions: why did the Imperial German Army attempt to destroy the university city of Louvain, and especially why did it torch the university library? Strategically, these actions turned out to be calamitous in terms of international public opinion. Louvain became the poster child of German aggression and barbarism in Belgium. The burning of the library with its collection of rare books illustrated German *Kultur* at its worst, the land of Goethe and Beethoven now burned books. Prussian militarism trumped European heritage. The British especially seized upon the Kaiser's blunder in Louvain. British newspapers portrayed the Kaiser and his army as savages from the east (Huns) slaughtering innocents, desecrating churches and erasing European cultural landmarks — not to mention burning books! England used events in Louvain and Belgium to rally the British people in support of the war, using the subliminal message, What happened in Louvain could happen here. The real, but of course unintended, consequence of the German Army's actions in Louvain was to facilitate recruitment for the British Army. The sack of Louvain

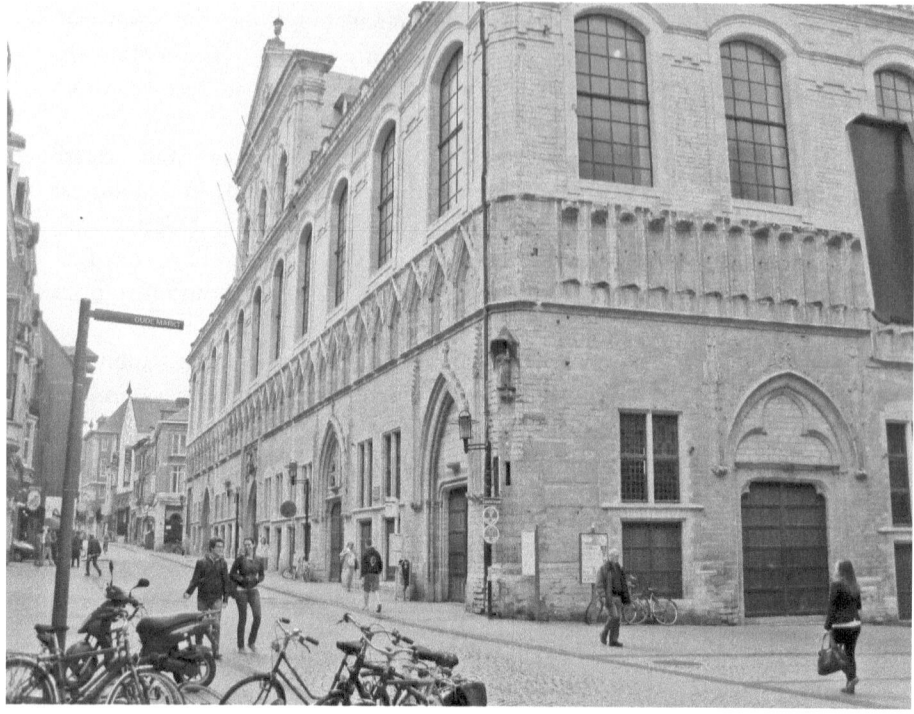

The Louvain University Library (Halles de l'Université) today. The walls survived the conflagration of 1914, and the restored building, although no longer a library, still serves the university (photograph by Libby Klekowski).

was a publicity bonanza for the British and became part of the propaganda campaign that helped turn America to the side of the Allies.

Trying to understand the cause (or causes) of the Prussian blunder at Louvain became a cottage industry for post-war historians. Most concluded that the primal cause traced back to the Franco-Prussian War of 1870-1871. In that war, the Prussian Army encountered an unplanned-for aspect of French resistance, the *francs-tireurs*, civilians who took up arms against the invaders, ambushing patrols and sniping from villages. Today governments call these groups *guerrillas*, or sometimes even terrorists. To the Prussians, the actions of *francs-tireurs* seemed somehow unfair, outside the rules of war; civilians should not fight, that was the army's job, and only the army's. Although *francs-tireurs* caused less than 1,000 casualties in the Franco-Prussian War, time magnified that number. Many of the senior officers of 1914 had been junior officers in 1870, and they inculcated the fear of *francs-tireurs* into the Imperial German Army invading Belgium.[49] American reporters all commented on the anxiety both officers and men had to the unseen menace, the *francs-tireurs*. The Germans were always on their guard; even the pop of a wine cork could unleash a fusillade of return fire.

The tactic devised to deal with *francs-tireurs* was simple, direct and brutal; kill or severely maltreat all, or at least a lot, of the civilians in the vicinity of the imagined or real event. Thus began the reprisals against innocent men, women and children; and if only women and children were available — they would have to do. The German authorities never seemed to understand that their tactic of reprisals against innocent civilians was "beyond the pale" in the eyes of the Allies. After the war, Brand Whitlock recounted the experiences of some women from Louvain.

> German soldiers beat on the door of her home in Louvain, and her father and brother ran to open it, [she] heard shots and had not seen her father or brother since. She took her eight-weeks-old baby in her arms and climbing the garden wall, found refuge in the home of a friend for a night and a day, while on all sides the houses were in flames, and finally, carrying her child, she dodged from street to street, holding up one arm and waving a white handkerchief.[50]

The woman and her child, seeking safety in village after village, finally reached Brussels where they came to Whitlock's attention. He also learned that even pregnant women were not safe from German abuse.

> It was so with the widow of sixty; German soldiers at five o'clock on Wednesday morning turned her and her niece, a young woman about to become a mother, out of her house, and they were driven half-clad from place to place — [guard houses and barracks]. They were forced every now and then to kneel on the ground and to raise their arms above their heads, while the Germans pressed the muzzles of guns against their breasts, or kicked them or struck them; then, holding them as prisoners in the barracks until Thursday, allowed them to return home to find their house burned to the ground.[51]

Reprisals, of course, included the destruction of all nearby buildings. One shouted phrase, "*Man hat geschossen!*" (They are shooting!), and all hell broke loose: murder, pillage, fire, rape and massacre. Whitlock noted that priests were special targets. Here he describes the experience of a young Louvain priest he knew.

> He had been seized with others, made to march in front of the troops [a human shield], kicked, and cuffed, and spat upon, struck with the butts of guns; his hands were tied behind him with barbed wire and there at the Place de la Station he was forced to remain standing, not even allowed to lean against the wall; and this for hours, with repeated insults and personal outrage, while his townsmen one by one were led out and shot, there at the side of the Square.[52]

The Allies simply could not understand the senseless cruelty.

The question has always been whether an act by misguided Belgian *francs-*

tireurs sparked the Louvain outrage. The answer depends on whom one asks — a Belgian or a German. Both agree the trouble began on August 25, when the Belgian Army attacked from Antwerp in the direction of Louvain, supposedly to help relieve pressure on the English retreating from Mons. The Belgians pushed the Germans out of Malines (Mechelen) 30 km (18.6 mi) northwest of Louvain and advanced to within 10 km (6.2 mi) of the city. Whitlock gives the Belgian explanation for what caused the sack of the city.

> That afternoon the Belgian army made a sortie from the defenses of Antwerp; there had been a sharp fight at Malines, and the Belgians had had the better of it, driving the Germans out of Malines and back along the road toward Louvain.... The Germans retiring on Louvain, had reached the Porte de Malines; night was falling and German reinforcements, just then leaving Louvain, met them ... and the two parties, each mistaking the other for Belgians, opened fire. There was instant panic, the usual cry, "They're shooting!" Riderless horses and terror-stricken soldiers streamed into the town and then, and in that manner, the awful tragedy began.[53]

Thus, the Belgians claim that confusion in the German Army rather than *francs-tireurs* caused the tumult on August 25 and the continued sack of the city was a cover-up to pass the blame to the Belgians.

George B. McClellan, the son of an American Civil War general, presented the German explanation in a notorious article published in the *New York Times*.[54] McClellan and his wife had toured Belgium under the auspices of the German government. The resulting article was a Pollyanna-puff-piece arguing that things were in many ways actually better in Belgium than before the invasion! This article included the German view of what happened on August 25 and probably held the distinction in 1915 for generating the most rebuttal letters.

> It is believed that the Belgian authorities expected the sortie from Antwerp on Aug. 25 to be successful, and through agents in Louvain organized a revolt among the citizens for the same night.
> When the townspeople saw the Landsturm company marching through the city from the direction of Antwerp, they thought the sortie had been successful and the troops were the head of the German retreat. They struck at an appointed signal under the impression that they would be able to destroy a demoralized and retreating enemy.[55]

From almost every house around the railway station and the great square near the cathedral came "a fusillade from rifles, shotguns and mitrailleuses [machine guns], most of the firing coming from the upper floors. The firing killed or wounded a number of soldiers, and stampeded the horses hitched to the supply and ammunition wagons."[56]

Thus, the Germans claimed that their actions in Louvain were a consequence of the concerted attack by Belgian *francs-tireurs* on the evening of August 25. The reason the library burned that night, according to the German explanation, is that German soldiers could not find the keys to the building. "It is said that at the university the librarian and his assistants all deserted their posts, locking the library behind them and carrying off the keys. It was not possible to save either building or books, for when the doors were at last battered down the interior had been gutted."[57]

So what actually happened on August 25, 1914, in Louvain? Even after a century, the answer is still nearly impossible to disentangle from the conflicting German and Belgian accounts.[58] The only point of agreement seems to be that the German Army did sack the city.

Chapter 3

Murder and Mayhem on the Meuse

> The Germans enter a town, take hostages — the burgomaster, some councilmen, one or two notables; they demand money, food, wine and forage. All goes well for a few days. The army moves on. There is a reverse, and soldiers swarm back into the town crying "*Man hat geschossen!*" (They're shooting!) Then murder, pillage, fire, rape, massacre. This happened again and again.[1]
> — Brand Whitlock, 1918

> It struck me always that as soon as something took place anywhere which might lead to disorder, the method adopted was as follows: first a fusillade in order to scare the inhabitants, secondly looting of numberless bottles of wine, and finally cruel, inhuman murders, the ransacking and the wrecking.[2] — L. Mokveld, 1917

Unbelievable as it may seem, Louvain was not the only, or the worst, atrocity in Belgium. In the late summer and early fall of 1914, the German Army went crazy in a number of towns. It was as if a blood lust would infect both officers and men, sending the army on a rampage. Often what incited the rampage was a set back or reverse on a nearby battlefield. If the Belgians or French gave the Germans a drubbing, Belgian civilians would pay in blood. Unable to punish the enemy forces, the Germans took vengeance on innocents. The American Legation learned of mass killings all through the early months of the invasion. "The tale is unending; horror piles on horror. We heard them every day all that autumn, all that winter; every refugee who came to Brussels, every one who came."[3]

The worst of the atrocities occurred in and around Dinant, a small town of 7,500 inhabitants on the Meuse River in southeastern Belgium. Picturesquely situated on the right bank[4] of the Meuse at the base of barren limestone cliffs, Dinant was a tourist destination for walkers and anglers, the nearby waters noted for pike and chub fishing. Astride the cliffs, a ruined fortress overlooked the town. Interestingly, Dinant was no stranger to sack and pillage. In 1466, Philippe le Bon, Duke of Burgundy, may have been the first to put it to fire and sword.

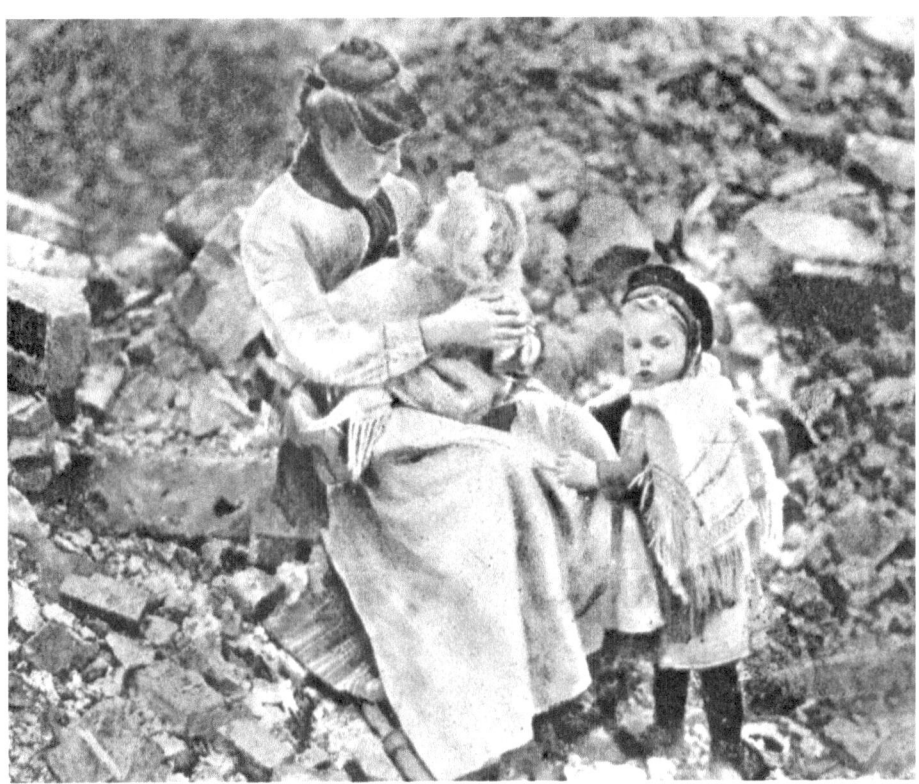

With most men either conscripted into the army and fighting or simply executed as hostages, the women held families together when the Germans arrived. The invaders reduced homes and often whole villages to piles of rubble whose only living inhabitants were women and children numb with shock. Here a Belgian woman attempts to comfort her two small children, pretending, for their sake, that all will be fine (*Illustré*, 1914).

> Duke Philip the Good, irritated by some act of aggression, besieged Dinant with 30,000 men. The inhabitants, when summoned to surrender, replied by hanging the messengers sent with the proposals. The Duke, enraged at this outrage, was preparing to take the town by assault, when it surrendered. He gave it up to pillage for 3 days, and then set fire to it; and while the flames were still raging, ordered 800 of the inhabitants, bound two and two, to be thrown into the Meuse.[5]

In 1914, the German Army nearly surpassed Philip the Good (a.k.a. Philippe le Bon). Although the destruction took place from August 21 to August 25, the scene was set on August 15. On that day, a fierce fight took place between French troops on the left bank and German troops on the right bank, the Germans attempting to cross the river.

Granville Fortescue, an American reporter for the London *Daily Telegraph*, got to Dinant a couple of days before the Germans appeared. He had arrived in Brussels as the war began and stayed, of course, at the Palace Hotel with the gang of other American correspondents. In contrast to his colleagues, who usually went out in the field in groups, Fortescue was a "lone wolf" correspondent, traveling in Belgium by himself and getting stories that the Palace Hotel pack missed. His background is not without interest. He dropped out of the University of Pennsylvania in 1897 to join the Cuban insurrection. In May 1898, he enlisted in the First U.S. Volunteer Cavalry (the Rough Riders), led by his first cousin Colonel Theodore Roosevelt,[6] and made the famous charge up San Juan Hill; he served in the U.S. Army during the Philippine Insurrection and then as a military aid in Teddy's White House. In 1907, he explored the Orinoco River from its headwaters to its mouth. Fortescue was always game for adventure.

When he arrived in Dinant, the French still held both sides of the river. He found accommodations in a nice hotel, the Tête d'Or, owned by Monsieur Bourgemont, on the right-bank (east-bank) but upon further thought decided to move to a hotel across the river. The German Army was coming from the east — perhaps it would be wiser not to be in its path. "There is an old newspaper axiom that runs — A dead war correspondent is no value to his paper."[7]

Events of the following day confirmed the correctness of his decision. As the Germans fought their way into Dinant, they pushed the French defenders back toward a bridge spanning the Meuse. From across the river, Fortescue watched a group of French soldiers, in a fighting retreat, take shelter near the Tête d'Or. One soldier, hit by a rifle bullet, tried to crawl to safety.

> A grotesque, fattish man in a baggy brown suit, runs out of the hotel. Monsieur Bourgemont! He trots awkwardly down the street amid a rain of bullets. Stooping over the crawling soldier he strives to drag him back to the safety zone. Together they stagger a dozen paces. Then, in that absurd way fat men do, Monsieur Bourgemont falls. The brown body lay limp on the cobbles.[8]

Heroism comes in many guises.

Fortescue witnessed the French defense of Dinant for a couple of days; every German attack failed at great cost. It was a good story, coming at a time when success followed success for the invaders. However, he might never get the story out because French officers staying at his hotel voiced concern as to whether Fortescue was a journalist or a German spy. It was time to leave. Early in the morning, before anyone woke, he made his attempt. "I had the first eyewitness story of the fighting at Dinant. How was I to send that story to my newspaper? Where was the nearest telegraph? I crept over legs and bodies, noiselessly let myself out the door. If I could make my way back to Charleroi?"[9]

Charleroi is a small city 24 miles (38.6 km) west of Dinant. He set out on foot. He was soon under military arrest and sent to Paris. As the arresting officer said, "Correspondents are forbidden to follow the French armies."[10] By the time Fortescue reached Paris, his Dinant story was cold.

Back in Dinant, the Germans were not happy; the French beat back every German attempt to cross the Meuse. On August 21, more German troops arrived and occupied the town; they vented their frustrations over French defense of the left bank on the town's residents. The troops entered as a hoard of barbarians, shooting into houses without provocation, killing unlucky inhabitants who happened to be walking on the streets, and, of course, bursting into cafés where they requisitioned and drank anything containing alcohol. Thoroughly drunk, they began to knock apart the town. "Shouting like savages, smashing street lamps, firing into windows, throwing incendiary bombs into houses, terrorizing the population, ... 'shooting up' the town, as they used to say in the Far West."[11]

Dinant's residents (Dinantais) cowered in their homes, hoping the storm would pass. It did not, the situation only worsened. On August 23, the French blew up the Meuse bridge at Dinant. Since it was Sunday, the Dinantais ventured to their churches for worship, beseeching God with prayers for protection. He must have not heard.

> At half-past six in the morning, the soldiers of the 108th regiment of the line drove the worshippers out of the Premonstratensian Church, separated the men from the women, and shot about fifty of the former through the head. Between seven and nine o'clock there were house-to-house looting and burning by the soldiers, who chased the inhabitants into the street. Those who tried to escape were shot off-hand.[12]
>
> Women and children were forced to stand by and witness the murder of husbands or fathers.[13]

This was just the beginning of the Dinantais' nightmare. Later in the morning, soldiers entered the town in force, driving people from their homes and with blows from rifle-butts herding them like human cattle to the central square and keeping them under guard until six o'clock in the evening. Then an officer separated the men from the women and children — always a bad sign.

> The women were placed behind a line of infantry. The men had to stand alongside a wall; those in the first row were ordered to sit on their haunches, the others to remain standing behind them [as if posing for a photograph]. A platoon took a stand straight opposite the group. The women prayed in vain for mercy for their husbands, their sons, and their brothers; the officer gave the order to fire. He had not made the slightest investigation, pronounced no sentence of any sort.
>
> A score of these men were merely wounded and fell among the dead. For greater certainty the soldiers fired once more into the mass.[14]

Finished with the town for the time being, the soldiers moved the butchery to the suburbs. The random killings continued, all of it senseless. A number of men and women held in the yard of a prison were machine-gunned. When not killing, the soldiers destroyed both the town and suburbs with fire and grenades. And God help the poor souls flushed out of hiding; they were hunted and shot for sport. The soldiers stood by, laughing.

> With wild shouts the soldiers of William the Murderer [Kaiser Wilhelm] chased the people from their houses, and struck down at random those who tried to escape. Soon the soldiers were throwing in hand grenades. Fire shot up and spread with terrible rapidity. Everything was in flames, crackling, splitting, falling. Long clouds of smoke arose from the burning valley and wreathed the surrounding hills. The flames licked the mountain and leapt up to redden the sky.
>
> The valley was filled with awful noise. The sound of the falling houses, the roar of cannon, the crackling of rifles and guns, the hiss of bullets, the shouts of the soldiers, and the cries of the unfortunate inhabitants were all mingled.[15]

By August 25, the French abandoned their positions on the left bank opposite Dinant. The French took about 1,000 casualties defending the river crossing; among the wounded was Lieutenant Charles de Gaulle.[16] The Germans suffered about 1,275 dead and 3,000 wounded at Dinant. Had the Germans forced a crossing of the Meuse south of Dinant instead of wasting days taking and terrorizing the town, they could have perhaps crushed the French Fifth Army in a pincer movement on the left bank south of the fortified city of Namur. The German general in charge of the sack of Dinant "gave away the brilliant prospect of an operational pursuit" of the French Fifth Army in order to "secure the tactical victory" at Dinant.[17]

The pointless "tactical victory" at Dinant left it a smoking ruin; of its 1,400 houses, only 200 remained.[18] "In the center of the town everything, including the large buildings, had been leveled with the ground."[19] In 1914, the town had a population of 7,600; the Germans probably murdered about 10 percent, including 73 women and 39 children between the ages of 6 months and 15 years.[20] The fate of the survivors continued the tragedy. They were either sent to German prison camps or driven into the Belgian countryside to survive as best they could. Those too weak to leave Dinant slowly starved. The only available food was a twice-daily ration of bread from German Army stores. An American reporter visiting Dinant in September 1914 had this to say about what had happened there:

> I do not understand why the contemporary chronicles of events did not give more space to Dinant at the time of its destruction, and why they have not given it more space subsequently.
>
> I presume the reason lies in the fact that the same terrible week which included the burning of Louvain included also the burning of Dinant; and in

the world-wide cry of protestation and distress which arose with the smoke of the greater calamity the smaller voice of grief for little ruined Dinant was almost lost. Yet, area considered, no place in Belgium that I have visited — and this does not exclude Louvain — suffered such wholesale demolition as Dinant.[21]

The Meuse River played a key role in the war, both as a barrier and for transport, the latter role fulfilled by river barges and, more importantly, by a railway system that followed the river valley. From Aachen, the line ran to Liège and at Liège it divided into two trunk lines leading to the French frontier: one, the most direct, went through Louvain, Brussels and ultimately to Paris; the other followed the southerly course of the Meuse River valley to the fortress city of Namur. Located at the confluence where the Sambre River enters the Meuse, Namur was a key railroad junction where the line divided, one line followed the Sambre valley west to the French border and then ultimately to Paris and the other continued south up the Meuse valley to Verdun.

European railways often follow old invasion routes, both seeking the easiest topographic path, and the Sambre/Meuse is such a route. Caesar followed it in 57 BC and the Imperial German Army did so in 1914, the only difference being direction — the Germans followed the rivers upstream from Belgium to France whereas the Romans traveled downstream, from France (Gaul) to Belgium (land of the Belgae). Both armies had to conquer the fortress city of Namur, *Aduaticorum oppidum,* home of the Aduatici in Roman times. After a siege lasting about two weeks, Caesar took the fortified hill (*oppidum*). The Germans took it even faster; Namur fell in two days.

Although significant to the military and under siege numerous times (1692, 1695, 1746, 1792 and 1794),[22] Namur was not recommended as a tourist destination. A European guidebook published in 1876 gives a discouraging description. "Owing to its numerous sieges and bombardments, it possesses few old buildings, except the *belfry tower,* of the end of 14th cent., and it has scarcely any objects of interest."[23]

In 1914, Namur had a population of 32,000 and was becoming known for glass manufacture. Located 14 miles (22.5 km) north of Dinant, it was part of the line of three fortified defensive positions established by the Belgians to guard the Meuse corridor: the first was the fortified city of Liège near the German border, then the fortified city of Namur 38 miles (61.2 km) upstream (south), and half way between sat the river town of Huy, guarded by a small fort. All were significant river crossings, and two, Liège and Namur, were critical railroad junctions. The German Army easily took Huy, encountering practically no resistance.

On August 24, 1914, the intrepid Dutch reporter Lambertus Mokveld entered Huy, only this time he traveled in an automobile rather than on a bicycle as he had in Louvain. "My motor whirled along the gloriously fine road to Huy.... Had the circumstances not been so sad, I should have enjoyed it better."[24]

He saw a town shrouded in clouds of smoke, its houses shot up like sieves; in one street Mokveld counted 28 houses reduced to ashes; it was the same old story, German soldiers running amok. Only this time it was a story with a different ending, and so worth telling before returning to Namur. Mokveld saw the following "order of the day" posted.[25]

> Last night a shooting affray took place. There is no evidence that the inhabitants of the towns had any arms in their houses, nor is there evidence that the people took part in the shooting; on the contrary, it seems that the soldiers were under the influence of alcohol, and began to shoot in a senseless fear of hostile attack.
>
> The behaviour of the soldiers during the night, with very few exceptions, makes a scandalous impression.
>
> It is highly deplorable when officers or non-commissioned officers set houses on fire without the permission or order of the commanding, or, as the case may be, the senior officer, or when by their attitude they encourage the rank and file to burn and plunder.
>
> I require that everywhere a strict investigation shall take place into the conduct of the soldiers with regard to the life and property of the civilian population.
>
> I prohibit all shooting in the towns without the order of an officer.
>
> The miserable behaviour of the men has been the cause that a non-commissioned officer and a private were seriously wounded by German ammunition.
>
> The Commanding Officer,
Major von Bassewitz

Not all Germans were barbarians; some found what was going on in Belgium that August totally repugnant. However, many did not.

The next town that Mokveld passed through on his way to Namur was Andenne, a town of about 8,000 inhabitants. Situated on the right bank of the Meuse, it was about one third of the distance to Namur from Huy. At Andenne, another bridge crossed the river, a bridge the Belgian Army had destroyed as it retreated from the German assault (August 19). The Germans soon constructed a pontoon bridge and began crossing to the left (west) bank in pursuit of the Belgians. In the evening of August 20, a shot rang out, followed by the oft repeated cry, "*Man hat geschossen!*" And all hell broke loose.

> The troops did no longer cross the bridge, but spread themselves in a disorderly manner all over the town, constantly shooting at windows. Even mitrailleuses were brought into action. Those of the inhabitants who could fly did so, but many were killed in the streets and others perished by bullets entering the houses through the windows. Many others were shot in the cellars, for the soldiers forced their way in, in order to loot the bottles of wine and to swallow

PROCLAMATION

A l'avenir les localités situées près de l'endroit où a eu lieu la destruction des chemins de fer et lignes télégraphiques seront punies sans pitié (il n'importe qu'elles soient coupables ou non de ces actes.) Dans ce but des otages ont été pris dans toutes les localités situées près des chemins de fer qui sont menacés de pareilles attaques; et au premier attentat à la destruction des lignes de chemins de fer, de lignes télégraphiques ou lignes téléphoniques, ils seront immédiatement fusillés.

Bruxelles, le 5 Octobre 1914

Le Gouverneur,

VON DER GOLTZ

"PROCLAMATION In future the inhabitants of places situated near railways and telegraph lines which have been destroyed will be punished without mercy (whether they are guilty of this destruction or not). For this purpose, hostages have been taken in all places in the vicinity of railways in danger of similar attacks; and at the first attempt to destroy any railway, telegraph, or telephone line, they will be shot immediately." An example of German terror during the early months of the war. The German Army murdered Belgians at the least provocation, whether they were guilty or innocent of acts of resistance (Klekowski collection).

their fill of liquor, with the result that very soon the whole garrison was a tipsy mob....

The game of shooting and looting went on all through the night of the 20th.[26]

Early that morning, at four o'clock, the soldiers drove all the surviving men, women and children to the town square to continue their macabre game of terror. The soldiers selected about 50 men at random, shot them and tumbled their bodies into the river. And the killing continued. Perhaps as many as 400 civilians perished before the rampage abated. The German officer ultimately in charge, General von Bülow, bragged of the exploit and threatened the same treatment for others.[27]

The next target for the Germans was the fortified city of Namur. However, prior to their arrival an American reporter, Granville Fortescue, traveling just ahead of the leading wave of the invasion, managed to book a train for Namur from Liège, where he had witnessed the start of the German siege. Even though a very experienced war correspondent, what he saw in Namur surprised him.

What struck me most forcibly in Namur was the fact that the citizens seemed indifferent to, or ignorant of, the danger that threatened their city. Outside of the military measures for defense, life went on quite as usual. The shops were open, business was carried on exactly as if no invading army were within a few days' march of the city. Of course soldiers filled the streets, cafés, restaurants. But they went about in a care-free, picnicking manner that astonished me. In my opinion the men of the Fourth Belgian Division were second rate soldiers. My opinion was confirmed when later I heard the Germans took the city with little effort.[28]

A ring of 9 detached forts constructed of concrete and armed with 6-inch guns and 4.7-inch howitzers behind armor-plated turrets defended Namur. The forts were 3,000 to 3,500 m from one another and 7.5 km (4.7 mi) from the city center. Of the 26 bridges that spanned the Meuse River in Belgium, 18 were under fire from Namur's forts. The Allies, with justification, hoped Namur might slow the German juggernaut for weeks, giving them time to assemble a defense of northern France. In contrast to Liège, which had practically no time to prepare for the German attack, the Belgians had 3 weeks to prepare Namur to withstand siege. A garrison of 26,000 men worked to strengthen the place, linking the forts with trenches, covering the front with zones of barbed wire entanglements and minefields. Some barbed wire entanglements, located at critical approaches, carried electrical currents of 1,500 volts. Soldiers dynamited all obstacles obstructing the fields of fire of the guns, barricaded the chief streets of the town in anticipation of defending the place street by street and accumulated immense stores of food and ammunition in preparation for a long siege. "It was confidently anticipated that the siege of Namur would occupy the Germans for weeks and its capture would cost them at least 50,000 men. Instead of that it fell practically at the first attack."[29]

On August 17, a German column cut communications with Brussels[30] and the engagement began. Having learned the hard way at Liège that attacking forts with only infantry assaults was suicidal, the Germans developed a new approach for Namur. The infantry waited for the heavy siege artillery to catch up. Krupp and Škoda heavy mortars, mostly the latter, would destroy Namur, and the infantry would mop up. Although the Krupp 42 cm mortar, known as "big Bertha,"[31] became the legendary "big gun" of the war, big Bertha was just too difficult to transport from place to place. Her name was appropriate; she was big and moved slowly. The Austrian Škoda 30.5 cm was better engineered and the weapon of choice for the forts.

> The effect of its fire was devastating; the Belgian forts were simply blown to atoms. This gun was used against Liége, Namur and Maubeuge,[32] and proved much more serviceable than the "42," around which popular terror spun a legend. These guns could be divided into sections susceptible of motor transport. The motors used were of 100 horsepower, each capable of dragging a weight of

thirty-five metric tons at the rate of ten kilometers an hour. The caterpillar-wheels of these motor-tractors enabled them to travel over ground impassable to ordinary traffic. This comparative mobility, with greater facility in handling and almost equal effectiveness of fire, constituted the superiority of the 305-millimeter gun over the "42" mortar, and permitted use of it in the field.[33]

One battery of 42s and four batteries of 305s destroyed Namur's forts; a battery of heavy mortars consisted of two guns. Of course, a variety of other "conventional" artillery pieces rained shells on Namur's defenders as well. A Reuters correspondent's interview of one of the Belgian survivors gives an inside look at the total collapse of the defenses. The end began on August 21.

> The Germans at first centered their rain of steel upon our intrenchments. For ten hours our men stood this without being able to fire a shot in return. Whole regiments were decimated. The losses among the officers were terrible; and, gradually, the soldiers, unled, became demoralized. With one bound, they at last rose and fled — a general *sauve qui peut* [Run for your life!] Meanwhile, many German guns had been turned on the forts, especially on Maizeret and Marchovelette (which covered the eastern approaches on either side of the Meuse). These could offer but a feeble resistance; and, in fact, Maizeret only fired about ten shots, while it received more than 1,200 shells, fired at the rate of twenty a minute. At Marchovelette, seventy-five men were killed in the batteries, and both forts soon surrendered.... Soldiers declare that officers cried out: "Get out as best you can. The thing is to get to Antwerp." No provision had been made for the destruction of the immense stores; and all these, with the fortress artillery, and most of the field artillery, the horses being killed, fell into the enemy's hands.[34]

The final assault came on the morning of August 23, accompanied by an intensive bombardment. The Germans entered the city that evening. Only six forts still held out, but the heavy siege mortars finished them off in the following couple of days. The relatively easy and quick German success at Namur left the Allies stunned. Nevertheless, the Belgian resistance effectively slowed the invasion through their country.

> This problem may be thus stated: If, against the trivial Belgian Army almost unaided, the invaders could only get from the northern frontiers past the obstacle of Namur in nineteen days (August 4–23), [Aix-la-Chapelle (Aachen) to Namur is ca. 60 miles (97 km)] how was it that they were able, against the French and British armies, to reach the outer forts of Paris [Namur to the Paris forts is ca. 160 miles (258km)] in another thirteen days (August 23–September 5), fighting several big battles, holding Belgium and long lines of communication, and overrunning a large part of eastern France, the while.[35]

Mokveld drove into Namur a few days after its capitulation: "When I drove into Namur, I found the town comparatively quiet; there was some traffic in the streets, and Belgian army surgeons and British nurses in their uniforms walked about freely."[36]

After Namur's surrender, the German Army entered the town in an orderly manner; neither civilians nor property suffered. Then in the evening someone yelled, *"Man hat geschossen!"* and the usual rampage began: about one hundred civilians lost their lives while the crazed soldiers ransacked and then burned large sections of the town. Looting and shooting went on for a couple of days but had quieted down by the time Mokveld arrived.

Three days after Namur fell, the German Army began the investment of Maubeuge, the next, and last, fortified city on the Sambre River. Situated in France about 50 miles (80.5 km) west of Namur and 6 miles from the Belgian frontier, Maubeuge was a critical railway junction for five lines: the line from Cologne, Liège, Namur, Maubeuge to Paris as well as rail lines that would become important in transporting German troops and supplies up and down the Western Front. A ring of six forts, each three to four miles from the city center, defended Maubeuge. The shelling of the forts and the city began on August 27. The Germans surrounded the city with a Reserve Corps and laid siege while the main part of their army continued to attack west into France. Besieged Maubeuge was an island of French and British resistance in a sea of Germans for twelve days before the city finally capitulated. The Germans took approximately 36,000 prisoners and captured 450 guns. However, this prolonged siege deprived the German Army of men who might have helped turn the tide in the Battle of the Marne (September 5 to September 11), a battle the German Army lost and a battle that stopped its drive to take Paris. Trench warfare on the Western Front began after the Marne. It has often been said the Germans lost the First World War that September at the Marne.[37]

The Germans incurred huge losses taking Maubeuge, perhaps suffering as many as 140,000 dead.[38] Among those dead was the Kaiser's nephew, Prince Ernst of Saxe-Meiningen. A French Red Cross nurse tended the badly wounded eighteen-year-old lieutenant after stretcher bearers carried him into the city. When he died, she arranged for a proper funeral and, even though the city was still in French hands, she sent his personal belongings and a letter of condolence to his family in Germany. Because of her kindness to the Kaiser's dying nephew, Maubeuge did not suffer the usual post-capitulation sack.[39]

The American journalist Irvin Cobb visited Maubeuge a couple of weeks after the battle. German officers conducted him on a tour of the remains of Fort Des Sarts and Fort Boussois, forts that once guarded the northern approach to Maubeuge. The officers proudly displayed the effects of their siege mortars, the 42 cm Krupp and the 30.5 cm Škoda. The 42 cm Krupp had Fort Des Sarts as its target. "As a fort Des Sarts dated back to 1883. I speak of it in the past tense, because the Germans had put it in that tense. As a fort, or as anything resembling a fort, it had ceased to be, absolutely."[40]

> Appreciating the impossibility of comprehending the full scope of the disaster which here had befallen, or of putting it concretely in words if I did comprehend it, I sought to pick out small individual details, which was hard to do, too, seeing that all things were jumbled together so. This had been a series of cunningly buried tunnels and arcades, with cozy subterranean dormitories opening off of side passages, and still farther down there had been magazines and storage spaces. Now it was all a hole in the ground, and the force which blasted it out had then pulled the hole in behind itself. We stood on the verge, looking downward into a chasm which seemed to split its way to infinite depths, although in fact it was probably not nearly so deep as it appeared.[41]

The next stop on Cobb's tour was Fort Boussois; here he saw what a Škoda 30.5 cm could achieve when manned by Austrian artillerymen.

> The Austrians must have been first-rate marksmen. One of their shells fell squarely upon the rounded dome of a big armored turret which was sunk in the earth and chipped off the top of it as you would chip your breakfast egg. The men who manned the guns in that revolving turret must all have died in a flash of time. The impact of the blow was such that the leaden solder which filled the interstices of the segments of the turret was squeezed out from between the plates in curly strips, like icing from between the layers of a misused birthday cake.[42]

How did the American journalist Irvin Cobb get a German tour of the ruins of Maubeuge in the fall of 1914? The answer begins in Brussels during the first week of the German occupation. John McCutcheon, Arno Dosch, Will Irwin and Irvin Cobb had just returned from house arrest in Louvain (August 22, see Chapter 2). Not having had enough adventure, the foursome joined Roger Lewis (Associated Press), Harry Hansen (*Chicago Daily News*) and James O'Donnell Bennett (*Chicago Tribune*) the next day to have a go at following the German Army as war correspondents, disregarding German Army policy prohibiting such activity except near Brussels. Authorization papers to travel farther afield posed the first problem, a problem the Americans solved with a small deception. The military governor, Major General Thaddeus von Jarotsky, was in charge of issuing press passes for Brussels and its immediate environs. Details and paperwork were not the general's strong points. He agreed to stamp such documents if the Americans would agree to type them. They did so but left out the qualifier "limited to Brussels and immediate environs." They returned with their fudged documents, von Jarotsky stamped them with the official seal without reading what he stamped[43] and they had their permits to leave Brussels. After a couple of unsuccessful attempts to secure transportation, Dosch and Irwin gave up and returned to Brussels. Undaunted, the remaining five set off; Hugh Gibson remembered their unconventional departure.

> After getting out of their trouble at Louvain, McCutcheon, Cobb and Lewis set forth on another adventure. There are, of course, no motor cars or carriages to

be had for love or money, so they invested in a couple of aged bicycles and a donkey cart. Cobb, who weighs far above standard, perched gracefully on top of the donkey cart, and the other two pedaled alongside on their wheels. They must have been a funny outfit, and at last accounts were getting along in good style.[44]

Another report has Cobb, Bennett, and Lewis in the cart, with McCutcheon and Hansen on the bicycles.[45] Regardless of how the Americans arranged themselves on their transport, one can be sure that Cobb, who was rather portly, did not pedal. By August 27, they were on their way to see the ongoing battle of Maubeuge, approximately 45 miles (72.5 km) south of Brussels. Remarkably, as they wandered around the hills and dales of rural Belgium, members of the German Army were most welcoming. To establish their nationality, they flew an American flag the size of a pocket handkerchief from the whip socket of the cart. A slight blemish, a cigar burn, defaced Old Glory.

The surprising appearance of five Americans traveling in a ramshackle cart pulled by an old nag and accompanied by a couple of ancient bicycles offered comic relief from the war. The fact that Cobb had a sense of humor that crossed the boundary of language gave the five journalists instant friends whenever they stopped. Laughs and gags trumped the lack of valid papers.

> Common soldiers offered repeatedly to share their rye-bread sandwiches and bottled beer with us. Not once, but a dozen times, officers of various ranks let us look at their maps and use their field glasses; and they gave us advice for reaching the zone of actual fighting and swapped gossip with us, and frequently regretted that they had no spare mounts or spare automobiles to loan us.[46]

However, it was not all jokes and camaraderie — what Cobb witnessed made him rethink his view about the so-called glory of war.

> Of the waste and wreckage of war; of desolated homes and shattered villages; of the ruthless, relentless, punitive exactness with which the Germans punished not only those civilians they accused of firing on them but those they suspected of giving harbor or aid to the offenders; of widows and orphans; of families of innocent sufferers...— of all this and more I saw enough to cure any man of the delusion that war is a beautiful, glorious, inspiring thing, and to make him know it for what it is — altogether hideous and unutterably awful.[47]

The Americans blithely blundered along behind the German lines for three days, making friends here and there as they went. They crossed the Meuse River somewhere, missing Dinant, Huy and Namur. Searching for the battle then in progress at Maubeuge, they took a wrong turn and got lost. Eventually they reached the Belgian village of Beaumont, 15 miles (24.2 km) east of Maubeuge but still inside Belgium. There they unwittingly bumped into the temporary headquarters of the Seventh German Army.

Prussian flags decorated Beaumont, giving the place a martial air; a flag even flew from the church steeple, as if the Germans had captured God himself. Long gray war automobiles surrounded the nearby headquarters château, previously the residence of a prince. Prussian officers bustled about importantly in uniforms the height of military fashion. Puffed-up breasts displayed military orders and medals. Orderlies scuttled about carrying messages and tending the needs of officers. A sleek automobile pulled in driven by a soldier chauffeur, out stepped a magnificent example of Prussian pride, a staff officer "all sword and spurs." He saluted smartly and acknowledged an "exalted person" standing on the steps of the château. The "exalted" was none other than the fourth son of the Kaiser, Prince August Wilhelm. A military band serenaded in the background. Everyone and everything was very clean, very crisp, very Prussian. Into this place of Teutonic order and military decorum, like some scene from a Franz Lehár operetta, the American cavalcade entered, feeling VERY out of place. The Americans were definitely not clean or crisp, having been living rough on the road for days. Cobb considered himself the most presentable of the group. He was most concerned about his hair, which was uncombed and sticking straight up through a hole in his straw hat. However, that was the least of his sartorial problems.

> Also, that morning, to save myself from the occasional showers, I had purchased from a wayside butcher his long canvas blouse, which I wore—and so coated over was this garment with suet and tallow and hog grease and other souvenirs of his calling, that had it caught fire I am sure it would have burned for at least half a day with a clear blue flame.
>
> Two days earlier than this I had walked the shoes off my feet and, with the shoes, some tender portions of the feet themselves. So, for this, the occasion of my advent into fashionable military society, I had on a pair of homemade carpet slippers which I had acquired by barter from an elderly Belgian lady. These slippers were gray in color, mottled with white, and of a curious swollen shape, so that they looked rather like a pair of Maltese cats which had died of dropsy and then had been badly embalmed.
>
> I might add that I, probably, was the best dressed person in my crowd; anyhow, I was the one with the most fanciful touches to his wardrobe.[48]

The Germans looked in disbelief as the five hobos entered the courtyard of the château. The band ceased playing; everyone stopped in his tracks. As Cobb put it, "We headed straight into the heart of that sunburst of military grandeur." A colonel approached them and in perfect English asked who they were. Cobb, the designated spokesman, said they were American correspondents. At that point, everyone literally cracked up in laughter. The sight of these insane Americans, in outlandish clothing, traveling as they were, was just too much even for the dour generals. When the chuckles died down, the colonel gave them a hard stare and stated that correspondents were *verboten* in the German Army. Cobb, always quick with a retort, brashly announced that the army now had five.

The colonel disagreed; they were not correspondents, just detainees. He would see them the following morning at 11:00 and arrange transport to Brussels. In the meantime, they should find a place to sleep in the village — if out after dark, sentries might shoot first and question afterward. They found a place to bunk in a schoolhouse and returned the next day for their appointment with the colonel only to find he and most of the headquarters staff had left. A battle south of Maubeuge needed their attention; only a lieutenant remained with orders "to do something with the Americans." He did; he locked them in a jail cell near an improvised powder magazine. In the distance, artillery fire droned as thunder in the background, causing the five to worry about a stray shell reaching Beaumont.

The cell, a filthy hole, housed eighteen French and Belgian prisoners of war. At the far end, Cobb saw acquaintances from Brussels: Maurice Gerbeault, a Frenchman living in Brussels and employed as a correspondent for a Chicago paper; his Belgian photographer Victor Hennebert;[49] and Lawrence Stein Stevens, a young American artist from Michigan enrolled in the Royal Academy of Fine Arts in Antwerp. The three had left Brussels in an automobile in search of a story behind German lines, the American evidently tagging along for the adventure. Since their auto carried a Red Cross pennant without authority to do so, they soon faced arrest. When the Germans discovered a camera, the trio came under suspicion as spies and received rough treatment, especially the American.[50]

Eventually the lieutenant released the five American correspondents plus Gerbeault, Stevens and the Belgian photographer, housing them as guests of the German Army in a *taverne*. He noted that they were guests, not prisoners, but should they try to leave he would order them to be shot. At least they were no longer in the filthy cell. Two days of house arrest in the *taverne* followed; all Cobb records in his journal is the lack of enough to eat. Finally, they were to leave by train, not back to Brussels but to Aachen (Aix-la-Chapelle), Germany. Before starting out, a German captain came into the *taverne* for a drink; recognizing the Americans, he became chatty. Cobb asked where he learned English. "'I suppose I come by it naturally,' he said. 'I call myself a German, but I was born in Nashville, Tennessee, and partly reared in New Jersey, and educated at Princeton; and at this moment I am a member of the New York Cotton Exchange.'"[51]

American journalists repeatedly encountered fellow citizens of German extraction who had flocked to the Kaiser's colors. Although much has been written about the thousands of Americans who volunteered to help the French, the story of the Americans serving in the German Army is yet to be told.

After two days of confinement in the *taverne,* in the dark of the night the eight detainees[52] joined British, French and Belgian prisoners of war for a mile-long march to a railway siding where they boarded a train with many German wounded. After two days of very slow travel, the train reached Aachen (Aix-la-Chapelle), where the eight got off, free once again. Holland was only twenty minutes away by tram and Belgium less than an hour away by automobile. Aachen was remarkably calm considering there was a war going on not far away.

> When we landed in Aix-la-Chapelle, coming out of the heart of the late August hostilities in Belgium, we marveled; for, behold, here was a clean, white city that, so far as the look of it and the feel of it went, might have been a thousand miles from the sound of gunfire. On that Sabbath morning [August 31, 1914] of our arrival an air of everlasting peace abode with it.[53]
>
> To-night the cafés will be open and the moving-picture places will run full blast;... The cafés that had English names when the war began have German ones now. Thus the Bristol has become the Crown Prince Café, and the Piccadilly is the Germania.[54]

With time on their hands and isolated from the war zone in Aachen, John McCutcheon, Irvin S. Cobb, Harry Hansen, James O'Donnell Bennett and Roger Lewis collaborated on a remarkable article whose thesis was the rumors of German atrocities in Belgium were groundless. They argued that in all their travels in Belgium with the German Army (100 miles [161 km] in two weeks), "We are also unable to confirm rumors of mistreatment of prisoners or non-combatants with the German columns."[55] Fearing British censorship if the text went by cable from London, they sent it to Berlin for wireless transmission to the United States. The article reached the delighted Kaiser who instructed his Reichskanzler to write a letter of thanks to the Americans. Being quick off the mark, McCutcheon, Cobb and Bennett (Lewis and Hansen traveled to London) immediately wrote a letter to the Kaiser directly in which they implied they might write more favorable press if allowed to go to the front with the German Army. Remarkably, the Kaiser acceded to their brash request in the interest of "unbiased reporting."[56] "For three days they heard nothing; then a resplendent staff colonel arrived with parchment documents, decorated with seals and ribbons and signed by the Kaiser himself, allowing them to go and do practically as they pleased in Germany and behind German lines."[57]

The three Americans, as foreign correspondents embedded with the German Army, received royal treatment. That was how Cobb managed to visit the ruined forts at Maubeuge; he was on a tour sanctioned by the Kaiser — a point he omits from his war memoir.[58] McCutcheon, Cobb and Bennett paid back their debt to their Hohenzollern patron in articles extolling the German Army for being "polite and kindly" in Belgium.[59] So the question is how did three well-respected American journalists come to this conclusion? The probable answer is because they were embedded with the German Army, with soldiers who essentially became their comrades and from whom they eventually accepted the German angst about *francs-tireurs,* civilian snipers. Once accepting the assumption that civilian snipers were nearly everywhere, it was an easy step to condone war and terror against civilians.[60] Consequently, these Americans acceded to the German doctrine of "the punishment for hostile acts falls not only on the guilty but on the innocent as well."[61] Events western eyes deemed atrocities and crimes against innocent civilians, the Germans considered as the cost of total war. McCutcheon, Cobb and Bennett agreed with the German view and thus saw nothing they called an atrocity, seeing only acceptable wartime behavior. Atrocities for them were Allied claims of German soldiers bayoneting babies, raping nuns, and mutilating captives, claims impossible to substantiate. Therefore, by tightly defining what constituted an atrocity, they could honestly say they saw none.

Historians have not agreed with this tight definition. The 1907 Hague Convention on Land Warfare, which Germany signed, placed the German actions against civilians in Belgium in the category of war crimes or atrocities.[62] The German Army killed 5,521 civilians in Belgium in August and September of 1914, claiming the killings were in response to a large-scale campaign of terror by civilians (or civilian snipers) against German soldiers. Essentially the Germans believed a "People's War" was being fought against them in Belgium.[63] The American reporters embedded with the German Army believed this as well.[64] Historical research does not substantiate this belief, in fact demonstrates just the opposite. There is no evidence to support the claim that *francs-tireurs* were everywhere — there was no "People's War." The historians John Horne and Alan Kramer, after analyzing both German and Belgian sources, reached the conclusion that "organized civilian resistance on a scale commensurate with German reactions in August 1914 is an historical impossibility." The German soldier's angst over *francs-tireurs* was, according to Horne and Kramer, a fantasy, "a massive case of collective self-suggestion." "A million men were swept by a delusion which mistook the fantasy of the franc-tireur war for reality. The German atrocities were the symptomatic result of the mobilizing power of the fantasy."[65]

Chapter 4

Besieged Antwerp

> If one had been asked to name a city which was a shrine of peace and a citadel of that bourgeoise civilization which it was fondly hoped had made war impossible, the odds are that Antwerp would have been chosen.[1]— Francis Whiting Halsey, 1919

On the evening of August 17, 1914, the Belgian government and the army abandoned Brussels and moved to Antwerp, a city with the most robust defenses in Europe. Antwerp would serve as the capital of free Belgium. Led by King Albert, a greater part of the Belgian Army reached Antwerp on August 20.

In the latter part of the nineteenth century, the Belgians had embarked upon a fortress-based strategy to defend their country in the event of invasion. Three cities formed the crux of the defense: Liège near the German border, Namur near the French border and Antwerp near the Dutch border. A ring of forts defended each city. Evidently, the Belgian plan was as follows: if the Germans attacked, then Liège would hold them until the French arrived; if the French attacked, then Namur would hold them until the Germans arrived; if all failed, the Belgians would retreat to Antwerp, await the British and hope for the best.[2] The downside of Fortress Antwerp was it did not control its own access to the North Sea. Located on the right bank of the River Scheldt (Schelde), the fortress stood about 17 miles (27.4 km) upstream (south) of the Dutch border; in other words, the river's mouth was in Holland. All shipping had to pass through neutral Holland to reach Antwerp and the Dutch took their neutrality very seriously. British warships could not enter the Scheldt. Consequently, British warships had no role in the defense of Antwerp in 1914, despite its being a deep-water harbor. To aid Antwerp, British troops needed to land at another port and travel overland. For the British, Antwerp was essentially a land-locked city difficult to reach.[3]

For the Germans, Antwerp was also a major headache. Again geography played a role; from Antwerp, Belgian troops could strike out and disrupt those

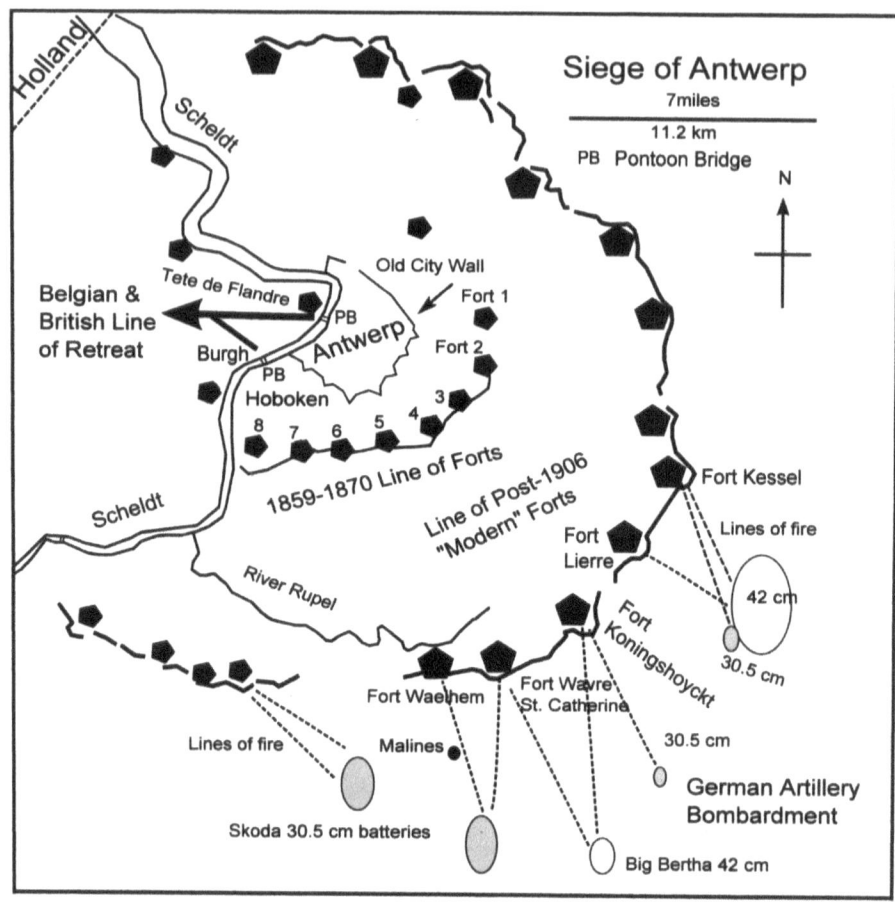

railways from Aachen (Aix-la-Chapelle) that supplied the German armies operating in western Belgium and eastern France.

> A bunch of railway lines stretch to half dozen points of the compass east of Aix-la-Chapelle like the extended fingers of a hand. They link Aix with eastern, northern, and southern Germany. Now Aix is no commercial centre. There is no more reason why Aix should be a huge railway-centre with vast sidings and miles of platforms than, say, Wiesbaden. But these are not commercial sidings. The railways are military and strategical.[4]

To sustain the invasion of Belgium and France in 1914, an umbilical cord began in Aix-la-Chapelle (Aachen) and stretched across Belgium — a knife from Antwerp could sever that umbilicus. German anxiety heightened when the Belgians launched an attack from Antwerp on a broad front in the vicinity of Louvain; this action possibly was the catalyst for the sack of Louvain.[5] Although German reprisals in towns where the Belgian sorties had success were often draconian, occasionally there was a touch of mercy. "Over a small group of houses in the poorer section of the city, where the prostitutes were quartered, grim Prussian humor, or perhaps a sense of value received, had prompted the conquerors to write in white chalk marks in German script, 'Gute Leute. Nicht brennen!' (Good people. Do not burn!)"[6]

To cover Antwerp and its 100,000-man Belgian garrison, the Germans detached two Reserve Corps[7] from their First Army, substantially weakening it.[8] The First Army missed those men in the Battle of the Marne; their presence might have helped turn the battle in Germany's favor. Although Belgian resistance at Liège was decisive in the early days of the war, the tying up of German troops around Antwerp probably proved equally as important.

From August 20 until September 26, the German Army slowly invested Antwerp in preparation for the siege against the city's forts. Nevertheless, during that month, the city was readily accessible from Holland. American reporters who for one reason or another started late for the European war skipped German-occupied Brussels in favor of Antwerp. From Antwerp, stories still could be sent to American editors through the cable to England and then via the transatlantic telegraph cable to America, whereas German-occupied Brussels was cut off. However, not all visitors to Antwerp were bona fide journalists; many were "war as a sport" buffs. A couple of Harvard men, Willard Luther, a Boston lawyer, and Horace Green, a correspondent for the *New York Evening Post,* were among the "war tourists" to reach the city.[9] Their motivation was adventure rather than reporting. A Dutch border official described the pair as "An amateur correspondent and a slow correspondent."[10] Which was which remained unsaid. From Holland, they traveled to the environs of Antwerp and finally saw the war firsthand.

> Judging from the looks of the country and the burning villages, we were on the heels of a devastating Army. For three, four, and five miles on either side of the road beautiful trees lay flat upon the ground. It was not until we saw groups of Belgian soldiers tearing down their own walls and hedges and applying match and gasoline to those which still stood, that we realized that this was a case of self-inflicted destruction. Farmhouses, stores, churches, old Belgian mansions, and windmills were either in flames or smouldering ruins.[11]

What the Americans encountered was the Belgian Army clearing a free-fire zone from the city's ramparts to the ring of forts so an investing force would have no cover. The Belgians destroyed property worth $80,000,000 in the suburbs of Antwerp that August and September, probably doing more damage than the Germans did during the actual siege. Trenches, machine gun emplacements, minefields and barbed wire entanglements filled the new open spaces, some of the barbed wire being grounded and connected to the city's electrical grid; when turned on, a lethal electrical shield protected the city. As it turned out the destruction of the city's suburbs was pointless because the Germans never attempted a ground assault, having learned the folly of that at Liège. German siege artillery sited a dozen miles away destroyed the forts and forced the city's capitulation. The trenches, machine gun emplacements, minefields and electrified barbed wire entanglements were for nothing. However, in September 1914, that would have been hard to predict.

Upon entering the Antwerp military zone, Luther and Green encountered a new obstacle; did they know the password? Bored sentries bounced the pair about like a couple of marbles in a pinball machine. "We were stopped, questioned, and searched by thirteen different groups of soldiers. There were many occasions where, after one pair of stupid sentries had put us through the grill, a second pair, watching from a distance of thirty yards or so, promptly repeated the entire performance."[12]

They heard the word *Spion* (spy) muttered by the sentries and the pair got very anxious; "sooner or later a wool-witted sentry would shoot first and investigate later."[13] Since it was their maiden war-time adventure, the pair arrived in the city proper quite rattled. Once within the city gates they headed for the Hôtel St. Antoine near the cathedral. At the time, the St. Antoine was the residence of the foreign diplomatic corps who had evacuated Brussels on August 17. The Hôtel St. Antoine, standing 300 m from the Royal Palace and across the street from the headquarters of the Belgian General Staff,[14] became the heart of war-time Antwerp. Consequently, nearly all the foreign correspondents stayed there. The role the Palace Hotel played in Brussels, the St. Antoine filled in Antwerp.

Exploring the city, Green and Luther found it quaint, sleepy, and very dull — not what they had expected. At the St. Antoine, a journalist remembered someone who may have been Willard Luther.

> One youth, who in his busy moments practiced law in Boston, though quite frankly admitting that he was only actuated by curiosity, was exceedingly angry with me because I declined to take him to the firing-line. He seemed to regard the desperate battle which was then in progress for the possession of Antwerp very much as though it was a football game in the Harvard stadium; he seemed to think that he had the *right* to see it.[15]
>
> Now you must bear in mind that although one could get into Antwerp with comparative ease, it by no means followed that one could get out to the firing-line. A long procession of correspondents came to Antwerp and remained a day or so and then went away again without once getting beyond the city gates.[16]

There was evidence of war in Antwerp, of course, with wounded soldiers and hordes of refugees wandering about, but no action. Bored and seeing no story in Antwerp, Green and Luther left the city in search of war adventures elsewhere, traveling to Ghent and then Brussels. They got their adventure: the

German Army arrested the pair on the outskirts of Brussels, held them for two weeks, and then shipped them to Aachen. From there they crossed into neutral Holland and, undaunted, Green later slipped back into Antwerp.

However, not all correspondents received equal treatment. E. Alexander Powell, a correspondent for *The New York World* on special assignment with the Belgian Army, had access to the Antwerp front line. Staying at the fashionable Hôtel St. Antoine, he commuted 20 or 30 miles (32.2 or 48.3 km) over stone-paved roads in a powerful and comfortable chauffeured automobile to witness the fighting. In the afternoon he returned to the St. Antoine after a "tough day at the office" to dress for dinner.

> Imagine leaving a line of battle, where shells were shrieking overhead and musketry was crackling along the trenches, and moaning, blood-smeared figures were being placed in ambulances and other blood-smeared figures who no longer moaned were sprawled in strange attitudes upon the ground — imagine leaving such a scene, I say, and in an hour, or even less, finding oneself in a hotel where men and women in evening dress were dining by the light of pink-shaded candles, or in the marble-paved palm court were sipping coffee and liqueurs to the sound of water splashing gently in a fountain.[17]

Powell's partner for these jaunts was his photographer, Donald Thompson. From Kansas, thirty years old, and of slight build (five feet four inches tall and weighing 120 pounds), Thompson shot still photographs and motion pictures—the latter required lugging a camera the size of a "parlor phonograph." Powell described him as "hard as nails, tough as raw-hide," and on the battlefield Thompson had "more chilled steel nerve than any man I know."[18] Powell had met Thompson during a short visit to Ostend (then still in Belgian hands) on the Belgian coast; together they traveled to Antwerp to report on, and film, the siege.

When the war began, Thompson, in Canada at the time, secured permission to film the Canadian Army for a Montreal newspaper and sailed to England aboard a troop ship. His luggage consisted of an overcoat, a toothbrush, two clean handkerchiefs, and three large motion picture cameras. He left two of the cameras in England as a reserve and traveled to Paris with one. However, neither the British nor the French permitted free-lance photographers at the front. Thompson made nine attempts to reach the front from Paris, eight of which resulted in arrest; finally, the French decided to deport him to England. He escaped from the train taking him to the Channel coast and boarded a British troop train heading for Mons in southern Belgium.[19] He filmed parts of the battle with the British Army until the fighting became too dangerous. He then moved to the French line for safety, a mistake as it turned out because the French again deported him. On board another train heading for the coast, he realized French customs officials would confiscate his films. Meeting a

Russian princess on board, he convinced her to hide the films on her person. She agreed to do so — for a thousand francs.[20] The princess, the films and Thompson reached England.[21] In London, Thompson sold his still pictures for $5,000 to a newspaper syndicate, which then hired him at the exorbitant salary of $800 per week plus expenses for more war pictures. He returned to Belgium, landing at Ostend where he cached a reserve camera. He boarded a train and got to within 25 miles (40.3 km) of Brussels; then he began walking, carrying his camera, field glasses, a revolver, and 300 films. On this second attempt, the German Army arrested him, smashed his camera and destroyed his films. Deported once more, he somehow reached Ostend, retrieved his cached camera and met E. Alexander Powell. The two of them traveled to Antwerp[22] where Thompson learned Belgian authorities banned photographers from the front lines. Thompson, being Thompson, set out to change their minds, by going over their heads. "He sought an audience with King Albert of Belgium; after roughing up a guard and arguing with a private secretary, he got his way. Perhaps the King realized Thompson would cause even more trouble if he refused; he gave him an unlimited pass to work at the front."[23]

Only once did the King's *laissez-passer* fail. Thompson and Powell, along with an American military observer, Captain Raymond Briggs, U.S. Army, drove out to the fighting line near an outer fort. Belgian soldiers, weary of visitors, arrested the Americans. Taken to division headquarters and confronted by a very irate staff major, Thompson did his best to provoke the man. Thompson ambled into the major's office smoking a very large and very fat black cigar. Powell remembered the insane confrontation:

"Take that cigar out of your mouth!" snapped the major in French. "How dare you smoke in my presence?"

"Sorry, major," said Thompson, grinning broadly, "but you'll have to talk American. I don't understand French."

"Stop smiling!" roared the now infuriated officer. "How dare you smile when I address you? This is no time for smiling, sir! This is a time of war!"[24]

One can empathize with the Belgian officer, who, after all, had more important things at hand than dealing with the juvenile antics of a noncombatant; he probably agreed with the German officer who said, "You see, we were prepared for everything — except ze invasion of ze American newspaperman."[25] Thompson returned to Antwerp under arrest, charged with insubordination. Saner heads quashed the charge.

Over Antwerp, the siege became airborne. In the early hours of August 25, a gigantic black cigar, accompanied by a loud buzzing sound similar to a swarm of angry bees, slowly passed over the city. Objects resembling falling stars curved downward across the sky followed by tremendous explosions. It was a German Zeppelin on its maiden bombing run; the buzzing sound came from its engines. The brainchild of Count Ferdinand von Zeppelin, the military dirigible was another German first. The count had once served as a German military observer with the Union Army of the Potomac during the American Civil War. While in Virginia, he took a ride in a tethered observation balloon. This experience supposedly was the inspiration that ultimately led to the airship bombing Antwerp that morning. The bombing run achieved little militarily, killing about a dozen civilians and wounding forty others (see Chapter 2 for a description).

Remarkably, there is an account of the Zeppelin attack from the German side. The Zeppelin was the *Sachsen* under the command of Captain Ernst Lehmann.[26] Manned by a crew of 3 officers and 15 men, she was a commercial passenger airship before the war. Late August 24, on a moonlit night, the *Sachsen* drifted from her Cologne hanger and followed the railroad line to Aix-la-Chapelle, carrying 1,800 pounds of crude bombs. Because of the heavy load, the airship had difficulty maintaining an altitude of 6,000 feet (1,864 m) and thus was within the range of ground fire. For defense, the crew had only rifles and pistols.

> Out of Liege we penetrated a cloud bank and rode above it, the throbbing engines and whirring propellers making the ship a vibrant thing moving over a veritable sea of silvery mist, for such the thick clouds appeared from above them, bathed in the clear rays of the moon. It was difficult for me to realize the serious nature of our mission, that this was to be part of a bitter war.[27]

The clouds disappeared as the *Sachsen* reached the vicinity of Antwerp. A much-too-easy target in the moonlight, the *Sachsen* cruised around neutral Holland for an hour waiting for the moon to set. As the morning progressed, the air warmed and the aircraft became difficult to control. In order to maintain an altitude of at least 5,500 feet (1,692 m), it was necessary to point her nose up at a sharp angle. Inside the control gondola suspended beneath the Zeppelin, everyone slipped and scrambled as the ship became unmanageable and nearly out of control. As Captain Lehmann understatedly noted, "It wasn't exactly the proper way to begin an air raid."

The *Sachsen* approached the outer ring of forts with engines screaming at full throttle while Lehmann tried to control the up-tilted ship. Everyone on the ground heard her coming and prepared a welcome. Searchlights attempted to find her, but they were too weak. Belgian artillery fired blindly at the sound. Soldiers in the trenches between the forts fired thousands of rounds from rifles and machine guns at the dark monster, probably doing some damage to themselves as the hail of bullets fell to earth. A big searchlight locked on to the ship and the artillery fire became a real menace. In the dark control gondola, the crew silently waited with bombs to hurl by hand; the searchlight was their first target and after a couple of tries, it went out. The *Sachsen* drifted over Antwerp, the crew hurling bombs. In twenty minutes, the airship passed from one side of the city to the other.[28] Without bombs, and thus with a lighter load, the Zeppelin became more manageable and turned for home, reaching Cologne after twelve hours in the air (Cologne-Antwerp-Cologne). Militarily, the entire adventure achieved nothing substantial, although it did throw the burgers of Antwerp into a panic. "As a result of the precautionary measures which were taken, Antwerp, with its four hundred thousand inhabitants, became about as cheerful a place of residence as a country cemetery on a rainy night. At eight o'clock every street light was turned off, every shop and restaurant and café closed, every window darkened."[29]

Since Zeppelins attacked only under the cover of darkness, the diplomats and many correspondents moved to the cellars of the Hôtel St. Antoine. The building sat upon the ruins of an old monastery, thus damp, dank cells awaited the new residents. While Antwerp prepared for the next Zeppelin attack with high intensity searchlights and more high-angle guns, Powell decided to take his chances in his above ground accommodation.

A Zeppelin was basically an aluminum girder frame covered in a tough fabric that gave aerodynamic stability to the airship. The fabric-covered, cigar-shaped exterior housed gas cells, huge non-rigid bags of rubber or fabric that contained hydrogen gas. These gas cells, held in place by cables and netting, had valves to control the flow and release of gas. Because hydrogen gas is lighter than the atmosphere, fourteen times less dense than air, a Zeppelin literally floats in the air, the motors giving it horizontal and lateral movement. Zeppelins were vulnerable to attack in two ways: puncturing the gas cells caused leakage and loss of lift, bringing the craft to earth; or incendiary bullets or rockets fired into the gas cells ignited the flammable hydrogen gas, turning the airship into an inferno from which there was little chance of escape. The only protection was stealth and flying at an altitude beyond the range of ground fire. The second Zeppelin attack took place in September from high altitude over a totally dark city; the bombs fell in the outskirts doing little damage.[30]

> Though the Zeppelin raids proved wholly ineffective, so far as their effects on troops and fortifications were concerned, the German aviators introduced some novel tricks in aerial warfare which were as practical as they were ingenious ... throughout the attacks on the Antwerp forts, German dirigibles hovered at a safe height over the Belgian positions and directed the fire of the German gunners with remarkable success. The aerial observers watched, through powerful glasses, the effect of the German shells and then, by means of a large disk which was swung at the end of a line and could be raised or lowered at will, signaled as need be in code "higher — lower — right — left" and thus guided the gunners — who were, of course, unable to see their mark or the effect of their fire — until almost every shot was a hit.[31]

During the first year of the war, Zeppelins turned out to be disappointing as far as the German war effort. Repeated bombing raids against London and other Allied targets achieved little, at a very high cost. That year German Headquarters reported the loss of forty airships, most due to Allied guns.[32] It was time to innovate — and German engineers innovated; they came up with the "cloud car," a bomb-shaped single passenger vehicle attached to the mother ship, the Zeppelin, by a strong cable. Carrying a very brave, or insane, observer, the cloud car hovered as much as half a mile below the mother ship. The mother ship cruised above the range of ground fire, hiding in the clouds if there were any, while the observer down below in the cloud car guided the mother ship to its target through telephone communication. After ordering "bombs away," the observer waited anxiously, hoping none would hit his cloud car. The cloud car attached to a long cable caused considerable drag on the mother ship, much like towing a sea anchor. There are a number of odd stories about the cloud car. In one case the cloud car hit a cliff that was not supposed to be there, killing the observer; in another, a hawk-like bird attacked the observer — the cloud car evidently threatened its nest. The German Army favored the device whereas the Germany Navy thought it useless.[33] Nevertheless, there were some in the high command who concluded that Zeppelins, with or without a cloud car, were counterproductive, especially when used to bomb English cities.

> Only because there is no military advantage in Zeppelining that it is stupid and the men who order it are stupid pigs. We don't blow up any munition factories, and for every miserable woman killed, hundreds, aye, thousands of Englishmen rush into the army to come over to the front to fight us. We are doing their recruiting for them ... and I repeat: Zeppelining is bad, and it is bad simply and entirely because it has no military advantage.[34]

Throughout most of September 1914, the German Army tightened the noose around Antwerp, all the while transporting its siege artillery from the French fortress at Maubeuge. A September 24 report in the *New York Times* stated that two big Berthas (42 cm mortars) were on the road through Brussels for Antwerp and that the guns had come from Maubeuge.

> For their hauling the two guns need no fewer than twenty-six traction engines. Each gun is in four pieces, and each piece is drawn by three traction engines, the spare engines going on ahead to be used as helpers uphill.
> The engines appear to be in the nature of steam rollers, and all but two bore the name plate of an English firm.[35]

Although invested by the German Army, Antwerp still had telegraphic cable links with England, and thus to the transatlantic cable. The American Consul-General at Antwerp received frantic requests from the U.S. Department of State concerning Brand Whitlock in Brussels, there having been no word from the American Legation for three weeks. Since Brussels was under German occupation, there was understandable anxiety. Unanswered communiqués were piling up in Antwerp. E. Alexander Powell and M. Manly Whedbee volunteered to try to establish contact with Brussels. Both men were Americans and therefore should be able to pass through German lines unmolested, especially since Powell, an accredited correspondent with the Belgian Army, had an automobile at his disposal and Whedbee, the director of the Belgian branch of the British-American Tobacco Company, had an endless supply of cigarettes. Powell prepared the auto for the trip with "two American flags mounted on the windshield, and the explanatory legends *"Service Consulaire des Etats-Unis d'Amérique"* and *"Amerikanischer Consulardienst"* painted in staring letters on the hood, we hoped, however, to make it quite clear to Germans and Belgians alike that we were protected by the international game-laws so far as shooting us was concerned."[36]

Whedbee did something that was even more important in assuring the trip's success; he stuffed the auto with a huge quantity of cigarettes. Although the men had official permits from the American Consul-General and the Belgian Military Governor of Antwerp, their endless packs of cigarettes got them through German checkpoints; the permits usually went unnoted.

They drove very slowly, always on the lookout for German sentries, not wanting to surprise them. Their first contact occurred on the outskirts of the town of Aerschot (Aarschot) where about one hundred Germans lay in ambush behind a hedge. Fortunately, sunlight glinting off rifle barrels alerted the Americans who immediately jammed on the brakes. Just ahead of the auto, a taut wire stretched across the road at chin height, an unpleasant surprise for anyone in an open touring car. An officer ordered them out with their hands up. He was hostile and gruff at first. As soon as he found out they were Americans, he thawed. He had been to America and had visited Atlantic City, Niagara Falls, and Coney Island. Moreover, he wanted to reminisce about his trip. "Imagine, if you please, standing in the middle of a Belgian highway, surrounded by German soldiers who looked as though they would rather shoot you than not, discussing the relative merits of the hotels at Atlantic City, and which had the best dining-car service, the Pennsylvania or the New York Central!"[37]

Finally, the reminiscences ended and the Americans proceeded to Aerschot — or what was left of Aerschot. What they saw was a heap of smoking ruins inhabited by "half a hundred white-faced women." A town of 7,600 when the war began, it was here the German Army literally went crazy, shooting up the town and murdering many of its inhabitants. Brand Whitlock learned of what happened in the small town from Madame Tielemans, the wife (widow) of the Burgomaster (mayor) of Aerschot — who with his fifteen-year-old son was among the murder victims.[38]

At eight o'clock in the morning of August 19, 1914, the German Army

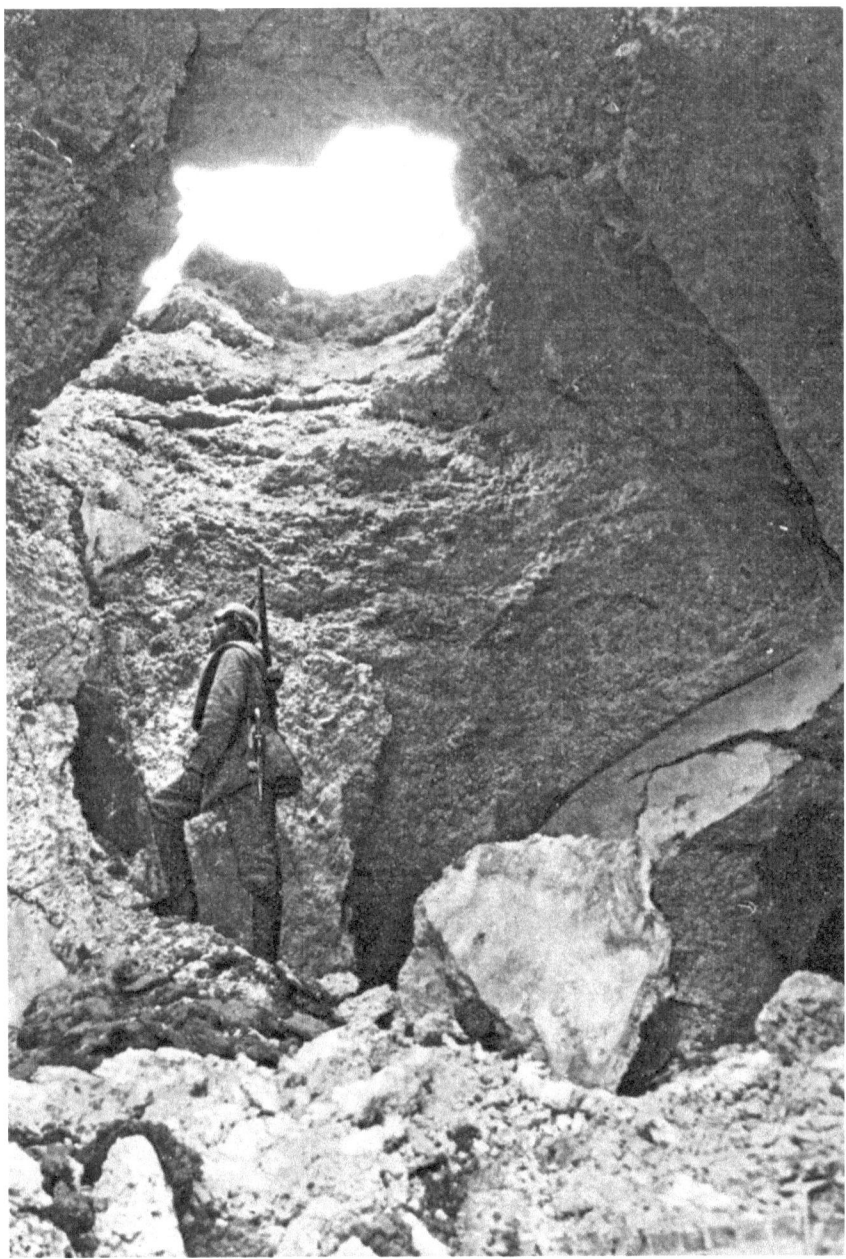

Inside an Antwerp fort. A heavy mortar shell, either 42 cm or 30.5 cm, literally punched its way through the concrete carapace before exploding inside the fort. Against such mortars the forts were simply indefensible death traps (*Hamburger Fremdenblatt*, 1914).

seized Aerschot. German officers commandeered choice rooms in the Burgomaster's house facing the Grand Place; a balcony overlooked the square and from it Colonel Stenger, commander of the 8th Brigade, and two aides watched their troops resting. Suddenly there was smoke and a number of rifle shots. The usual mêlée ensued; soldiers went mad, firing like lunatics. The Tielemans family sought refuge in the cellar. "After a few moments of indescribable anguish, one of the aides-de-camp came downstairs shouting: 'The general [Colonel Stenger] is dead, I want the mayor.' The general had been struck by a German bullet as he stood on the balcony."[39]

Unable to accept responsibility, the army took its vengeance out on the town — a Belgian guerrilla (*franc-tireur*) *must* have been responsible for the colonel's death. Separating out the men, the Germans executed 76 on August 19, and the following day they executed every third man and deported the survivors to Germany. Burning and looting continued for several days and nights; on August 28, the Germans marched 1,000 of the remaining residents, including the old and infirm as well as women and children, to Louvain, 10 miles (16 km) distant, for more brutality. Estimates are that 156 civilians perished to avenge Colonel Stenger's accidental death.[40]

What Powell and Whedbee saw as their auto rolled into Aerschot stunned them. Although an experienced war correspondent, Powell could not believe his eyes.

> In many parts of the world I have seen many terrible and revolting things, but nothing so ghastly, so horrifying as Aerschot.... It needed no one to tell us the details of that orgy of blood and lust. The story was so plainly written that any one could read it.
>
> For a mile we drove the car slowly between the blackened walls of fire-gutted buildings.
>
> We passed a little girl of nine or ten and I stopped the car to ask the way. Instantly she held up both hands above her head and began to scream for mercy.... That little child, with her fright-wide eyes and her hands raised in supplication, was in herself a terrible indictment of the Germans.[41]

After Aerschot, the Americans passed through Louvain, or what was left of Louvain, and then on to Brussels. In the city their first destination was, of course, the Palace Hotel for lunch and news. After dropping off diplomatic communiqués at the American Legation and picking up some for Washington, they applied to German authorities for a permit to pass through German lines and return to Antwerp. The German commander refused; the Americans must remain in Brussels. Telling him they would return the next day to pursue the matter further, they climbed into their car and stealthily fled town, following the same route used the preceding day. Again, Whedbee's cigarettes did the trick. "All along the road we found soldiers smoking the cigarettes we had distributed to them. Instead of stopping us and demanding to see our papers they waved their hands cheerily and called, '*Auf wiedersehen!*'"⁴²

At Aerschot, the officer who had been to Atlantic City, Niagara Falls and Coney Island detained them an hour so they all could chat with a fellow German officer who once had lived in Chicago. This officer finally returned from checking the outposts. For this chubby fellow, who must have put on his uniform with a shoe horn, meeting the Americans was like old home week. He had been an assistant manager at an Armour meat-packing plant in the city for twenty years. After reminiscing about restaurants, the theater, and American *wiener schnitzel*, he finally let them go. As they left he said, "Well, so long boys. If you get back to the States before I do, give my regards to Broadway."⁴³ All the while, the pair nervously waited, fearing a phone call from the German commander in Brussels ordering their arrest. It never came and they made it back to Antwerp.

In Antwerp, the German Army went from investing the city to besieging it. The fortified camp of Antwerp presented three lines of defenses to an attacker. Old fortifications dating from the sixteenth century, and of dubious value against "modern" weapons, immediately surrounded the city. About four miles from there stood the second line of defenses, a ring of some twenty obsolete forts dating from the eighteen sixties but robust nevertheless.

> At a distance of five miles from the second line — i.e., nine or ten from the city — we reach the first line of defence. This consists of about twenty cupola forts strongly constructed of armour-plated concrete, and half concealed below the surface of the ground. The cupolas, which contain the most modern guns of large calibre, are actuated by electricity. Several of these forts have a smaller fort in front of them, built in the same fashion.⁴⁴

On September 25, a large number of German troops, eventually numbering two hundred thousand, arrived as well as heavy Škoda and Krupp siege artillery. Positioning the Škoda 30.5 cm mortars and Krupp 42 cm big Berthas took about forty-eight hours. On September 28, the mortars began their bombardment of the two principal forts on the south side, Forts Waelhem and Wavre St. Catherine. The forts were about nine miles from the city center and guarded one of the main roads into Antwerp. "These forts were much damaged on the first day, and more or less destroyed on the second. It became clear that the defense of Antwerp could not be protracted any more than had proved to be the case at Namur, Maubeuge, and other French fortresses."⁴⁵

> Behind Fort Waelhem, where a 12 inch [30.5 cm Škoda] shell penetrated the magazine, a heavy steam engine which furnished power for the light plant was blown 20 yards from its base. The entire top of the fort here was torn off and 60 men of the garrison are said to have been buried underneath the debris.⁴⁶

As the siege mortars reduced Fort Waelhem to a smoking crater filled with shattered masonry and broken bodies, a big gray Minerva touring car sped out of Antwerp. Traversing a road swept by artillery fire, the sleek auto shot down the road toward the fort. A slender, fair-haired woman in a khaki uniform, Mrs. Gladys Winterbottom, was at the wheel; beside her sat the American photographer Donald Thompson. Originally from Boston, a graduate of the MacDuffie School in Springfield, Massachusetts, Gladys had married an English officer,[47] and when he came to the front in France, she traveled to Antwerp and joined the Belgian Field Hospital. Now she was on her way to bring in the wounded.

> Though shells were shrieking and howling overhead, Thompson tells us that Mrs. Winterbottom was as cool as though she were driving down Commonwealth av [Boston's main avenue] on a Sunday morning. When they reached the fort shells were falling all about them, but the men filled the car with wounded and Mrs. Winterbottom started back with them for the Belgian lines.[48] [see book cover]

Thompson remained at Fort Waelhem to take photographs. After her first trip, Gladys Winterbottom returned to the fort to pick up the remaining wounded.

German and Austrian gunners turned their attentions to an adjacent fort, but first they needed to reposition their mortars. German strategy was to destroy a sufficient number of adjacent forts in the southern arc of the first line of defenses to permit an army to pass.

> I was present at the destruction of one of our forts and was amazed at the rapidity, nay, the simplicity of the procedure. A German captive balloon in the air gave telephonic directions to the gunners. Off goes a shot! It falls two to three hundred meters in front of the fort, and the whole earth quakes as though the end of the world were come. The balloon telephones that the shot has fallen short. Five minutes later another projectile — this time 100 meters in rear. Once more the German observers correct the aim, with the result that at the third shot the shell falls right at the principal cupola of the fort, totally destroying it, exploding the magazine, and, alas, killing tens or hundreds of our comrades within. A few rounds more and the fort has ceased to exist.[49]

> On the 1st, 2nd, and 3rd of October the principal fortresses of Wavre, Waelhem, Kessel and Broechem were finally reduced to silence, the result of which was that a breach was effected large enough to permit the German armies to pass *without danger*.[50]

The city's defenses crumbled. However, because the German focus was on the southern part of the first line of forts, Antwerp still was not cut off from the outside. One could travel west to and from Ghent and Ostend and also to Holland in the north. Bridges crossing the Scheldt stayed open. Railways to Ostend and Holland were working. The Belgian Army began to move supplies and stores to Ostend, anticipating having to evacuate Antwerp. The exodus from the city was beginning, but not everyone was leaving. The American correspondent Horace Green[51] entered the city from Holland aboard a river boat on October 4. He had been there in early September but departed seeking war adventures elsewhere, Antwerp being too dull. In October 1914, Antwerp was anything but dull. He booked a room at his old haunt, the Hôtel St. Antoine, but found there had been a change during his absence; the hotel was now British Staff Headquarters. "Charging down the Avenue de Keyser came a hundred London motor-busses, Piccadilly signs and all, some filled, some half filled, with a wet-looking [probably a reference to their youth and inexperience] bunch of Tommies, followed by armored mitrailleuses, a few 6.7 naval guns, officer's machines, commissary and ammunition carriages."[52]

On October 3, a brigade of British Royal Marines, perhaps 2,000 men, arrived by special train from the port of Dunkerque. Well-armed and well trained, they immediately marched to the trenches south of the city to relieve the battle-weary Belgians. Over the next couple of days approximately 6,000 more men of the Royal Navy Volunteer Reserve arrived by train, with their ammunition and supplies traveling in London

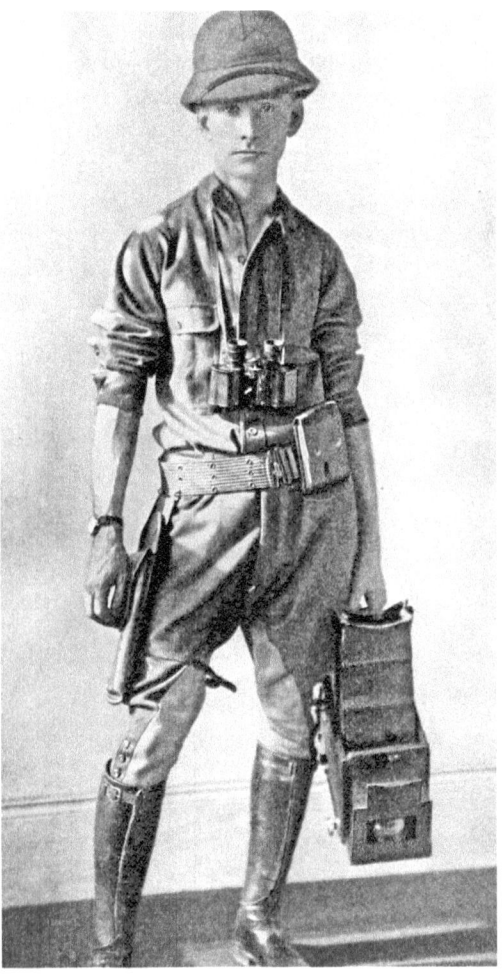

Donald Thompson, fearless combat photographer. When the war began, he was 30, a Kansas native who spoke neither French nor German, yet single-mindedly determined to record the war on film. He filmed the British retreat at Mons, was at the siege of Antwerp shooting both still and motion pictures, and was with the German Army at Dixmude where his luck ran out. Badly wounded, he eventually returned to the United States to promote his 90-minute film *Somewhere in France*, an epic shot mostly in Belgium (*Leslie's Photographic Review of the Great War*, 1920).

motor-buses at Dunkirk. The reservists were not "first-class fighting men" but were courageous and determined, although poorly trained, poorly equipped and poorly led. The poet Rupert Brooke was one of these reservists. The American correspondent E. Alexander Powell described them, "They were, in fact, equipped very much as many of the American militia organizations were equipped when suddenly called out for strike duty in the days before the reorganization of the National Guard."[53] The reservists joined the Royal Marines defending the trenches south of the city. Their leader, the First Lord of the Admiralty, entered Antwerp with a theatrical flourish on October 3.

> At one o'clock that afternoon a big drab-colored touring-car filled with British naval officers tore up the Place de Meir, its horn sounding a hoarse warning, took the turn into the narrow Marché aux Souliers on two wheels, and drew up in front of the hotel [Hôtel St. Antoine]. Before the car had fairly come to a stop the door of the tonneau was thrown violently open and out jumped a smooth-faced, sandy-haired, stoop-shouldered youthful-looking man in the undress Trinity House uniform. There was no mistaking who it was. It was the Right Hon. Winston Churchill.[54]

Churchill bolted into the crowded hotel lobby, rushing past everyone toward the stairs to his room. Meeting Antwerp's Burgomaster, Churchill slowed and shouted, "I think everything will be all right now, Mr. Burgomaster. You needn't worry. We're going to save the city."[55] And he disappeared up the stairs. It was a spectacular entrance, leaving the crowd in the lobby stunned. Energetic, impetuous, and without doubt brave, Churchill spent four days in Antwerp racing around inspecting the front lines, coming under fire, and conducting long meetings with King Albert and military officials at the St. Antoine. However, it was all for naught; he arrived with too little too late to affect the city's fate. Churchill was aware that the only way to save Antwerp was for it to have free and uninterrupted communications with the sea. British ships must have free passage up the Scheldt. He pushed his government to negotiate such a passage, but nothing happened.[56] Many considered the British naval expedition a fiasco that caused more harm than good.[57] It gave a false sense of hope that delayed the city's evacuation. What could have been a more orderly exodus spread out over days became at the end a time-pressured crush to escape.

> It was due to his arrival with the Naval Division, and to his optimistic view of the situation, that the civil population were not informed of the true state of affairs, but, on the contrary, were led through the Press to take a cheerful view of the situation when it was really critical. It was certainly due to the optimistic promises made by Mr. Winston Churchill to the Belgian authorities, that the proclamations telling the people to leave the city at once, were not posted.[58]

On the evening of October 6, Churchill departed for the coast in a fast car under convoy of an armored motor car. The majority of Antwerp's inhabitants were still unaware of the real danger to themselves and their city. On October 6 and 7, the Belgian Army moved to the left or west bank of the Scheldt, beginning its retreat from the city. Mrs. Winterbottom traveled along with the retreating army as did the diplomats and Belgian King and Queen. Three lines of fortifications guarded the city: the old city wall, the middle ring of forts, and the outer ring of forts. The enemy breached the outer ring and turned its attentions to the middle ring. British marines and naval reservists held the trenches between the middle ring forts. An American correspondent visited these slipshod defenses. "The trenches were hasty affairs, narrow and shoulder-deep, very much like trenches for gas or water pipes, and reasonably safe except when a shell burst directly overhead."[59] Guided by observation balloons, German artillery pulverized the forts and their nearby trenches. The British retreated into the city. The bombardment of the city proper began on the evening of October 7. Through the efforts of the American Legation, the Germans obtained maps marked with the location of the cathedral and other important buildings.[60] "By an express order of the Emperor all buildings of great historic and art value, such as the cathedral, the other churches, the town hall, museums, etc., were to be spared. The zoological gardens were also on the list of items which were not to be bombarded."[61]

After the public relations fiasco resulting from the senseless destruction of Louvain, the Kaiser now presented himself as the savior of Europe's art and culture. German artillerists attempted to protect Antwerp's historical and cultural heritage by primarily using antipersonnel shrapnel shells,[62] although high explosive and incendiary shells also hit the city.[63] "The Germans did not bring up their heaviest guns against the city itself. From the beginning until the end when high-explosive shells were employed, the great majority of the projectiles used were shrapnel, which generally burst above the roofs. The actual destruction of the fabric of buildings, therefore, was at no time large in proportion to the severity of the bombardment. The object of the attacking force was evidently to terrorize and kill, rather than to destroy buildings."[64]

The following day, the Hôtel St. Antoine closed and its guests moved to safer accommodations. Most of the Americans moved to the Queen's Hotel along the Scheldt, believing it might be easier to escape the city by being near the river. However, not all the Americans resided at the St. Antoine that October. Donald Thompson, the idiosyncratic photographer from Kansas, rented a house from a wealthy Antwerp family who had opted to escape the city early in the siege. Since there were not many takers, the rent was cheap. Located in the southeastern quarter of the city on a tree-lined boulevard, the beautiful three-story house was finely furnished. Thompson invited several friends to join him in his palatial abode: Edwin F. Weigle of the *Chicago Tribune*, Edward Eyre Hunt of *Collier's Weekly*, and D.H. de Meister, Dutch Vice-Consul at Antwerp.

Weigle was a young cinematographer shooting footage for a war documentary. He had struck a deal with the Belgians to donate half the proceeds from the *Tribune* film to the Belgian Red Cross. The Red Cross furnished him with an automobile and a driver and *carte blanche* to shoot still or motion pictures anywhere in Belgium. The resulting documentary earned $20,540 for the Belgian Red Cross.[65] On October 3, the undeveloped film left Antwerp on its way to Chicago for processing and editing. Probably Weigle moved in with Thompson and the others on October 4 or 5. Each occupied a floor; the consul had the top floor; Weigle, the second; and Hunt and Thompson each took a room on the first floor. Unfortunately, the southeastern quarter of Antwerp was a prime German artillery target. One night, with everyone tucked in, the shelling began in earnest. "At 12 o'clock I was awakened by the most horrifying shots I have ever heard. Four loud 'booms' followed in rapid succession. They were accompanied by the crumbling of buildings, the breaking of hundreds of panes of window glass, a general disorder that seemed only comparable to an earthquake. The entire house quivered like a leaf in the wind."[66]

In total panic, and so frightened they could hardly speak, all ran for the basement. Thompson pointed to a small door leading to a sub-cellar used for coal storage, a dingy hole, only eight feet long, four feet wide and four feet high. Everyone crawled into it. However, was it safe enough? They scuttled out, returning with mattresses and boards to barricade the coal cellar's door. "Just as we were about to shut ourselves into the sub-cellar, a shell struck the building across the street from us. It made a terrific noise. An entire row of buildings across the street was leveled. Every window in our house shattered like fine china dropping on the floor. The shell was so powerful that the concussion rocked our house, and broke every window in it. We locked ourselves in the dingy sub-cellar and decided to await death."[67]

Huddled in the light of a flickering candle, the four waited for the projectile inscribed with their names. Each contemplated death differently: Hunt did not care, his life meant nothing since the death of his sweetheart in America; Weigle and Thompson stoically accepted their fates — over which they had no control; the Dutchman prayed and pleaded with God to save him. The Americans began to scratch in their names on the cement cellar wall. Learning their motive was for identification should they perish, the Dutchman became even more anxious.[68] During a lull in the bombardment, Horace Green visited and left a description of the American outpost.

> Two doors from the corner of a narrow street covered with bricks and mortar fluttered a United States flag, and beneath it the door of 74 Rue de Péage. This place was later spoken of as "Thompson's fort," because Donald C. Thompson, a Kansas photographer, took possession of it after the Belgium family fled, and plundered the neighborhood for coffee, rolls, and meat, with which he stocked

his little cellar. The house next door had already been struck, and shattered glass littered the pavement. The doorstep of 74 was covered by a couple of mattresses and sand-bags. Beneath this, in a dingy sort of coal-bin, heaped with straw, I found crouching the tenant of "Thompson's fort."[69]

Besides Thompson, Horace Green met the other tenants of the fort: Edwin Weigle, Edward Eyre Hunt, and the Dutch Vice-Consul. After his visit, Green returned to the Queen's Hotel.

About half an hour later, when we were sitting in the Queen's, Thompson, pale as a sheet, staggered into the deserted lobby closely followed by Weigle and Hunt and the Dutch Vice-Consul, the latter somewhat out of his head. Just after I left 74 Rue de Peage, a 32 c.m. shell burst on the roof, tearing off the two top floors of the house, throwing Thompson's bed into the street, and setting the place on fire. At sundown the house was in ashes. Somehow or other the men all got out, rescuing a portion of their paraphernalia.[70]

On October 8, Churchill's men, those not killed or too severely wounded, began their exodus from Antwerp. There were two ways open, crossing the Scheldt on military pontoon bridges and heading west to Ostend or going north down river to Holland. The inhabitants of Antwerp, finally learning that the German Army would soon take the city, stampeded to get away. Nearly a half million terror-stricken people sought to leave the doomed city — the exodus included refugees from the nearby countryside. A British nurse traveling aboard a London bus with her charges recalled the scene:

The only way to get out of Antwerp was across the Scheldt by a pontoon-bridge made of barges with planks between. It would not bear too much traffic, so the authorities let people and vehicles cross one by one, still looking at passports.
For one and a half hours we stood there waiting for our turn to come. Just after we were safely over a shell struck the bridge and it broke in half.[71]

The Belgian Army soon repaired the bridge.

A crush of people descended upon the pontoon bridge, perhaps two hundred thousand managing to cross before the Belgian Army blew it up to deny the Germans. The remaining refugees escaped by river to Holland. "Anything that could float was pressed into service — merchant steamers, ferry-boats, dredges, scows, lighters, barges, canal-boats, tugs, fishing schooners, yachts, launches, skiffs, canoes, and even extemporized rafts. There was no attempt to enforce order. The fear-frantic fugitives piled aboard until the gunwales were almost level with the water."[72]

Refugees jammed every road and lane leading to Holland. Anything with wheels was a luxury, whether it was a car, truck, bicycle, horse carriage, farm cart or wheelbarrow. The majority walked with what they could carry. "The confusion was beyond all imagination, the tumult deafening — the rattle of

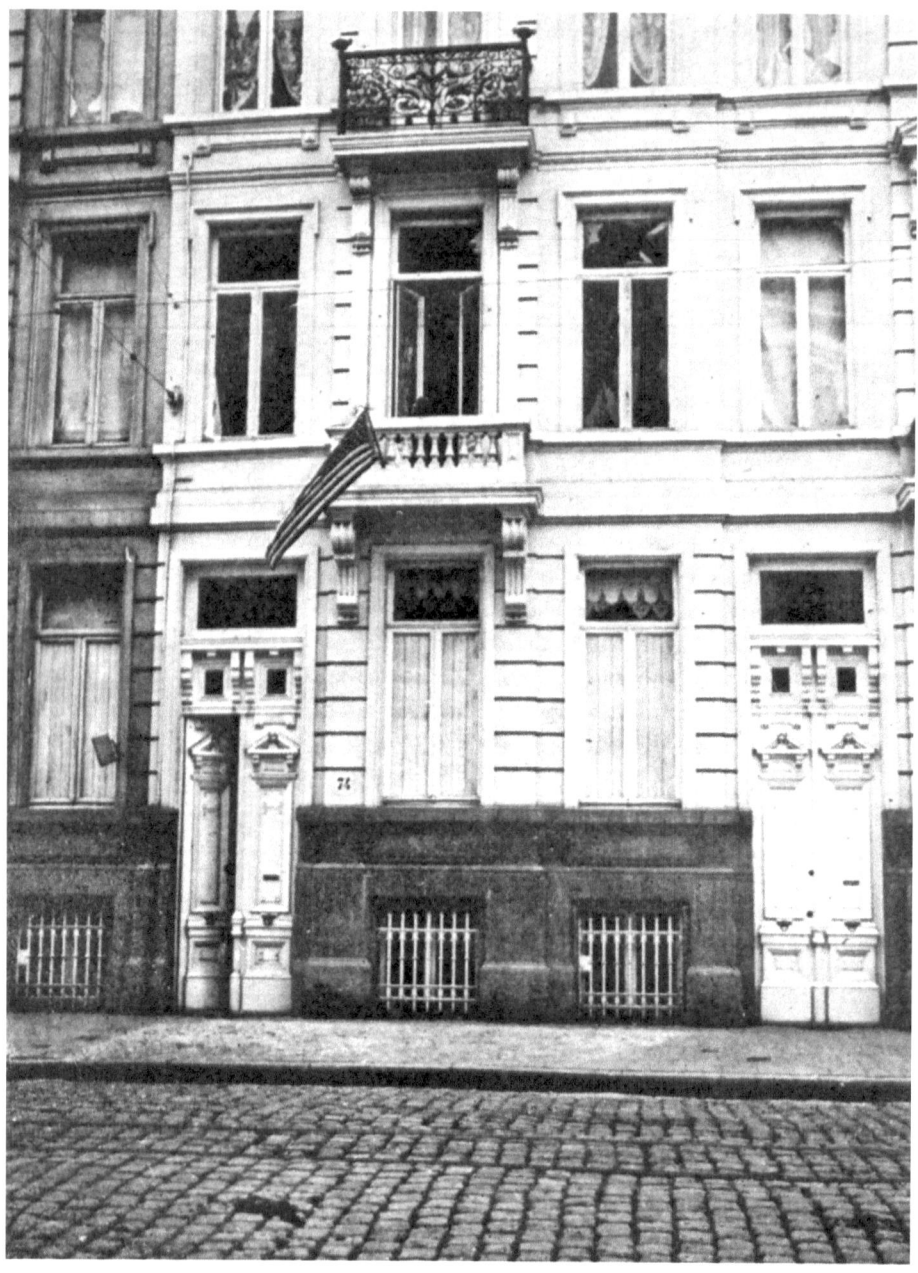

Thompson's Fort, 74 Rue du Péage (now renamed Tolstraat), Antwerp, before the bombardment when it served as a refuge for Donald Thompson, Edwin F. Weigle, Edward Eyre Hunt, and D.H. de Meister, Dutch vice-consul at Antwerp. The building, though damaged, survived the war (Edward Eyre Hunt, *War Bread*, 1916).

wheels, the clatter of hoofs, the throbbing of motors, the cracking of whips, the groans of the wounded, the cries of women, the whimpering of children, threats, pleadings, oaths, and always the monotonous shuffle, shuffle, shuffle of countless weary feet."[73]

The American Horace Green escaped into Holland along with the refugees. Hundreds of thousands of panicked civilians overwhelmed border crossings and flooded into neutral Holland. The Dutch responded with a generosity that was astounding.

> The kindness of the Dutch — as yet personal, unorganized endeavor — was beyond conception.
>
> Churches, houses, public halls, stations were thrown open to the multitude. You saw hundreds of Dutch soldiers join in the procession, lift babies and bundles, and walk with them for miles. At Dordrecht, when the trains came through, peasants passed scores of babies' milk-bottles into the cars. When a jolly-looking Dutch girl, with a great big gleaming smile that reminded me of someone, gave me milk and chocolate, the tears began to trickle down my cheeks. I suppose it was the reaction, or because I was tired, or, perhaps, because the crowd was cheering and waving at us. For the others there were piles of bread, Dutch cake, and, best of all, some good, long drinks of water. For ten days Antwerp's water supply had been cut off.[74]

After October 7, Antwerp no longer had telegraphic links with the outside world. The nearest links were in Ghent or Holland. E. Alexander Powell drove 40 miles to Ghent, had his story telegraphed to London and New York, and got back to Antwerp in the early hours of October 8. He managed to talk his way into the closed Hôtel St. Antoine. After a brief sleep in the hotel's bombproof cellar, he wrote an eyewitness account of the city's bombardment and traveled to Holland to telegraph the story to his editors. Returning to Antwerp by boat, he spotted two ferry-boats loaded with British soldiers coming down the Scheldt, escaping from Antwerp. He managed to stop them and informed the supercilious lieutenant colonel in charge that the boats would soon be in Holland and that the Dutch would intern the Brits for neutrality violation. Squinting to hold his monocle in place, the officer drawled, "How extraordinary," and the ferries continued downstream. "There was no use arguing with someone as dumb as that, so I dropped down to the deck of my own boat and headed at full speed for Antwerp. As I looked back I saw the two troop-laden steamers continuing steadily toward Holland. Just as I predicted, the entire brigade [2,000 men] was interned upon reaching Terneuzen and spent the next four years in a Dutch internment camp."[75]

Late afternoon of October 8, Powell got back to the Hôtel St. Antoine and collapsed from exhaustion. The bombardment of the city ceased the following day; German officers met with the burgomaster and city council that afternoon and negotiated Antwerp's surrender. Almost immediately, the first

German soldiers arrived. "The initial phase of the German occupation of Antwerp resembled a bicycle club meet rather than a great military triumph, for the first troops to enter the city consisted of a battalion of cyclists. They came pedaling in silently, through the Porte de Malines, and in an astonishingly short time the entire city was being patrolled by helmeted wheelmen with rifles slung across their shoulders."[76]

The city itself was a filthy hole, having been without municipal water for a week. When Fort Waelhem capitulated, the nearby reservoir supplying the city with water fell into German hands. Cut off from water, the city's sewage disposal system failed. Unflushed drains and sewers emitted an overpowering stench that mingled with pungent odors from piles of rotting garbage on the streets and the nauseating reek of decomposing bodies (mostly horses, but a few humans) left in the byways. Immediately the Germans set detachments of sanitary corps to clean the place up and make it habitable again. While this cleaning and disinfecting was going on, Powell visited the American Consulate. He found the building closed. Evidently, Consul General Diederich fled the city early in the bombardment — almost the only neutral diplomat to do so. Thoroughly embarrassed by his compatriot's fear, Powell opened the building and ordered the American flag hoisted.[77] The flag became a rallying point for those members of the American colony still in Antwerp. Even the American photographer Donald Thompson showed up. The following day the Imperial German Army staged its triumphal march into the very empty and still pungent city. It was the usual ostentatious affair with blasts of trumpets, the crash of kettle drums, a parade of beautiful uniforms, mighty horses, endless batteries of artillery, a torrent of marching men singing in chorus "Deutschland über Alles," ending with the Austrian artillerymen and their Škoda 30.5 cm mortars — the weapons that made the taking of Antwerp relatively easy. Watching the parade from the balcony of the American Consulate with his friend Powell, Thompson remarked, "It reminds me of a circus that's come to town the day before it was expected."[78] The Germans goose-stepped down empty boulevards and avenues, their triumph unacknowledged.

Powell now had to get the story of Antwerp's final days to a telegraph office for transmission to New York and London. The trip would nearly kill him. He set out on October 11, without German authorization to leave Antwerp, on a decrepit bicycle pedaling for Holland. In addition to his story, he carried a money belt containing $2,000 in gold coin and British notes. As the day progressed, he became weaker and weaker, suffering from a neck wound he received during the bombardment that had become infected. Finally unable to pedal, he managed to purchase a very old and infirm horse and an ancient carriage for $90 and employ a driver. With Powell nearly delirious from fever in the rear seat, the horse, a reject from both the Belgian and German armies, pulled very slowly for Holland. Twelve miles short of the telegraph office, the horse rolled over dead. Powell now set off on foot; four hours later, he staggered into the telegraph office, only to hear that his message was too long to send! After much yelling and threats, Powell managed to negotiate a special charge (bribe?) of $800 to transmit the five thousand-word message. Feeling weaker, with his wound greatly inflamed and swollen, he made it to a pharmacist for help. Out of dressings except for a used cotton gauze on the floor, the pharmacist soaked this makeshift dressing in iodine and slapped it on Powell's neck.

With the help of many good Samaritans, Powell eventually reached England, showing up at his paper's London bureau. "I hadn't shaved for three days, my clothes were stained and dusty, there was a gaping hole in the knee of my breeches as a result of the fall from the bicycle, and the bandage about my neck was caked with blood."[79]

He spent the next ten days in a private hospital at his paper's expense. While in hospital, a publisher approached Powell for a book about his experiences. From his bed, he dictated the tale to a stenographer in eleven days, and *Fighting in Flanders* went on sale less than two weeks later. The book became a war-time best seller in England, France (there was a French translation) and the United States. Germany banned it.[80]

A couple of weeks after the German triumphal march, an American correspondent, George Porter of *Harper's Weekly*, crossed over from Holland to Belgium in a decrepit automobile chauffeured by an equally rough looking driver.[81] After a perfunctory check of papers, the pair drove into German-occupied Antwerp. Except for a few soldiers lounging in the streets, he saw an essentially empty, desolate, deserted city. The shutters of every shop were down, the houses, except for those torn open by shells, appeared shut-up and empty. Antwerp was a ghost city. As so many foreign correspondents did before him, Porter stopped at the *Hôtel St. Antoine* for a room. However, the hotel was now German Headquarters and barred to foreigners.

Although the Germans closed the hotel, the Dutch closed the port. Napoleon once described the great port of Antwerp as "a pistol pointed at the heart of England." In 1914, owing to the neutrality of the Scheldt, the pistol was empty. German naval attacks upon England could not originate from Antwerp nor could German submarines operate out of this port. Should Germany disregard the neutrality of the Scheldt, there was the threat of a fully mobilized Dutch Army and the possibility of a third front in Germany's backyard.[82] Consequently, Germany honored Dutch neutrality throughout the war.

> But now the harbour, usually so teeming with life and filled with a roar and bustle unequalled by almost any other seaport town, lies still and silent. Huge sheds were filled with railway wagons, with and without valuable loads. A whole trainful of petrol in tanks was a find which particularly gratified the

German officers. Another train had brought in colossal piles of compressed hay, covered with tarpaulins. A warehouse had been found to contain considerable stocks of colonial produce, oats, flour, coffee and other supplies, which in due course would be examined and made use of.[83]

This unexpected loot helped sustain the German pursuit of the Belgian Army. However, Antwerp was not a cornucopia, the retreating Anglo-Belgian Army destroyed about a thousand abandoned motor vehicles as well as setting alight huge petroleum storage tanks, letting loose an inferno of flames and clouds of black smoke that filled the sky.

> They were a wonderful sight, these jet-black, weltering, rolling clouds with their rims of grey and brown, writhing and whirling up into the sky. We could hear the hissing and seething inside, and now and again the blood-red flames succeeded in forcing their way through the smoke. Occasionally there was an explosion. It was clearly not advisable to go too near this inferno. At one or two points, wreathed in smoke, we caught sight of the American flag still flying on its pole, soon to be reached and devoured by the flames.[84]

The flag probably marked an American business.

Chapter 5

The Last Ditch in Belgium

> Engulfed in a torrent of refugees, the Army of Belgium had degenerated into an uncontrollable mob which had to be extricated with all speed to some place of safety where it could be rallied, sorted out, rested and reformed.[1]— Lieutenant-General Galet, chief of staff of the Belgian Army

The main body of the Army of Belgium crossed to the left bank of the Scheldt during the night of October 6–7. King Albert and Queen Elizabeth followed the army that afternoon. On October 8, the civilian exodus went into full swing. The bombardment ended late on October 9, and Antwerp officially capitulated the following day. Having lost the city, the Belgians now attempted to save the army — no easy task. Safety lay somewhere to the west but where and how to get there? The first stepping-stone was to reach the city of Ghent, 32 miles (51.5 km) west of Antwerp. The problem was how to move seventy thousand soldiers through a sea of hundreds of thousands of refugees also fleeing in the same direction.

> It was a general sauve qui peut [every man for himself]. The refugees carried with them their precious belongings, the men keeping pace with the exhausted women and children who again and again were compelled to rest. Their carts obstructed the progress of the troops, which were thrown into the wildest disorder.[2]

Five London double-decker buses packed with wounded added to the congestion. Traveling very slowly and with numerous delays, the buses covered the 32 miles (51.5 km) from Antwerp to Ghent in fourteen and a half hours.

> Have you ever ridden in a London bus? If not, I can give a little idea of what our poor men suffered. To begin with, even traversing the smooth London streets these vehicles jolt you to bits, whilst inside the smell of burnt gasoline is often stifling, so just imagine these unwieldy things bumping along over cobble stones and the loose sandy ruts of rough tracks among the sand-dunes, which constantly necessitated every one who could, dismounting and pushing behind

and pulling by ropes in front, to get the vehicle into an upright position again, out of the ruts. When you have the picture of this before you, just think of the passengers — not healthy people on a penny bus ride, but wounded soldiers and sailors.[3]

The corridor available for travel was about 20 miles (32 km) wide, bordered in the north by Holland and in the south by the Imperial German Army. Should the Belgian Army stray into Holland it would face internment for the war's duration; should the Germans close the corridor before the Belgians passed through it, the Belgians would need to fight their way out. "This dismal crowd, moving under lowering skies, during long days and longer nights, without food, without shelter, was thrown from time to time into a state of panic by rumours that 'the Germans were there.' There were spasmodic halts, making confusion worse confounded. The retreat had become a rout."[4]

A number of Americans traveled west from Antwerp that autumn: the photographer Donald Thompson was with the German Army in pursuit of the Belgians; Gladys Winterbottom, the woman who fetched wounded from one of Antwerp's outer forts in her grey Minerva, was among the pursued since she traveled with the Belgian Army. A British nurse aboard one of the London buses spotted Winterbottom (identified as Mrs. W—) in Ghent. "Down a little street I suddenly spied a familiar war-grey motor car with a big Red Cross on the back. 'Why, there is Mrs. W—'s motor car!' I cried. We concluded the chauffeur had put up there for the night, for over the door was a lamp proclaiming 'Night Watchman.' Imagine my surprise at finding both Mrs. W— and my friend, G—, cozily tucked up in a four poster bed, and quite amused at our anxiety!"[5]

Mrs. Winterbottom remained with the Belgian Army throughout the great retreat from Antwerp; she was there when the Belgians made their final stand in the fall of 1914 and was still with her Belgians in 1916. May Sinclair, British novelist, described Mrs. Winterbottom as, "of all the women I met 'at the front' she was, by a long way, the most attractive."[6] Belgian soldiers agreed.

> She lives in a one-room shack which the soldiers have built her immediately in the rear of the trenches and within range of the enemy's guns. Her only companion is a dog, yet she is as safe as though she were on Beacon Hill, for she is the idol of the soldiers. She has a large recreation tent, like the side-show tent of a circus, but painted green to escape the attention of the German airmen, and in this tent she entertains the men during their brief periods of leave from the trenches. She gives them coffee, cocoa, milk, and biscuits; she provides them with writing materials.... Three times a week she gives "her boys" a phonograph concert in the first-line trenches.[7]

Winterbottom funded the entire enterprise personally. In 1916, when her friend E. Alexander Powell visited her "one-room shack" and asked what she most needed, her list included a small metal portable phonograph as her wooden model was warping from the Flemish dampness. When Powell last saw her, "she was wading through a sea of mud, in rubber boots and a rubber coat and a sou'wester, to carry her 'canned music' to the men on the firing line."[8]

Edgar Allen Cantrell, a banjo player originally from Kentucky, also traveled with the Belgians. Having lived in Antwerp since 1894, Cantrell played banjo as part of the Ragtime Duo in London music halls in the early nineteen hundreds. By the time war broke out, Cantrell was a businessman living in Brussels. He and his wife managed to escape the city, reaching London at the end of September.[9] Then, for reasons unclear but perhaps a need for adventure, Cantrell decided to return to German-occupied Brussels to save his household effects. Entering Belgium at Ostend, Cantrell met a colleague who persuaded him to make a detour through Antwerp to deliver a message to the colleague's wife. Part of the persuasion was a very handsome fee.

> I got to Antwerp with my passports without any trouble, but the first man I ran into was an old friend from Brussels. He greeted me like a lost friend. He took me to the commandant in the garrison and introduced me to a lot of officers. "This fellow is one of us," he said to the commandant. "We enlisted about the same time." There I was, and I was in for it.[10]

Fourteen years earlier, feeling that he owed a debt to Belgium since he made his money there, Cantrell joined the Garde Civique, the national civil guard. Cantrell attended a few drills and then forgot about the organization. However, the Garde Civique did not forget about him. Less than twenty-four hours after entering Antwerp that fall, Cantrell was in the trenches defending the city; in his words, "fighting like a madman." "I saw a Belgian soldier shot down beside his wife and baby. I saw the baby killed by another shot, and then I saw the woman take up her husband's rifle and empty it at the Germans."[11]

Cantrell could have escaped the trenches by asserting his American citizenship; however, seeing what was going on around him, he stayed, fought and was part of the exodus from Antwerp that October. Once outside Antwerp, his commandant released him from the Garde Civique. Cantrell made his way to Ostend, crossed to England, found his wife and they sailed to New York, their ultimate destination being Cantrel's hometown, Newport, Kentucky.[12]

Near Ghent, another American joined the Belgian exodus; her name was Mrs. Helen Hayes Gleason. In the summer of 1914, she was studying music in Paris and living in the American Art Students' Club. Her music studies ended when the Germans invaded Belgium. Rather than returning to America as did most of her fellow students, she traveled to England and volunteered.

> I crossed in late September to Ostend as a member of the Hector Munro Ambulance Corps. With us were two women, Elsie Knocker, an English trained nurse, and Mairi Chisholm Gooden-Chisholm, a Scotch girl. There

were a round dozen of us, doctors, chauffeurs, stretcher bearers. Our idea of what was to be required of women at the front was vague.... What we were to do with the wounded wasn't clear, even in our own minds. We bought funny little tents and had tent practice in a vacant yard. The motor drive from Ostend to Ghent was through autumn sunshine and beauty of field flowers. It was like a dream, and the dream continued in Ghent, where we were tumbled into the Flandria Palace Hotel, with a suite of rooms and bath, and two convalescing soldiers to care for us. We looked at ourselves and smiled and wondered if this was war.[13]

Gleason had no idea what to expect; she even worried that she might faint if she saw blood. The road to Damascus for her came just outside Ghent, where she saw her first casualties. Here was war, "red in tooth and claw." Assigned to a Convent Hospital, she found the wounded lay so packed one literally stepped over stretchers to move about, and everywhere smelled of foul blood, malodorous medicines, the stench of trench clothes, and the mangled bodies. While assisting in her first operation, simply holding a lamp over a man "with a yawning hole in his abdomen," she became light headed. Giving the lamp to another nurse, Gleason rushed into the courtyard and fainted. The plight of the war wounded affected nearly all the volunteers; a male stretcher-bearer with the Munro reported exactly the same feelings.

> The smell of wet and muddy clothes, coagulated blood and gangrened limbs, of iodine and chloroform, sickness and sweat of agony, made a stench which struck one's senses with a foul blow. I used to try to close my nostrils to it, holding my breath lest I should vomit. I used to try to keep my eyes upon the ground, to avoid the sight of those smashed faces, and blinded eyes, and tattered bodies, lying each side of me in the hospital cots, or in the stretchers set upon the floor between them.[14]

A doctor found Gleason in the courtyard and comforted her; he said it was a matter of stomach, not nerve, so she must just steel herself. Recovering, she returned to her ward and stayed with her wounded. For the year that she spent at the Belgian front, she never faltered again. However, the wounded always affected her more than the dead. The writhing and moaning of the wounded communicated their pain to her; she never got over it. "I had no fear of dying, but I had a fear of being mangled." Gleason summarized her feelings this way, "A red quiver is worse than a red calm."

> Antwerp fell. The retreating Belgian Army swarmed around us, passed us. In the excitement every one lost her kit and before two days of actual warfare were over we had completely forgotten those little tents that we had practiced pitching so carefully, and that had meant to sleep in at night. Little, dirty, unkempt, broken-hearted men came shuffling in the dust of the road by day, shambling along the road at night. Thousands of them passed. No sound, save the fall of footsteps.... We picked up the wounded. There was no time for the dead.[15]

Gleason and her compatriots joined the soldiers and refugees heading toward Ostend. At Ostend there was the possibility of a ship to England. However, the Munro Ambulance Corps did not cross the Channel; instead, it became part of the Belgian Army.

King Albert arrived in Ostend on October 10 and conferred with his British and French allies — the key issues, where to draw the line; where to halt the retreat, stand and fight? It would be safer to make the stand in front of Dunkirk, close to the British supply port. However, that was in France, and Albert determined to make the stand in Belgium. But where? The German Army was advancing very quickly, taking Ghent on October 12 and the following day, Bruges. Ostend was obviously the next target. It fell into German hands on October 15.

In contrast to Britain where the king was not in charge of the army nor involved in substantive military decisions, Albert, King of the Belgians, was both King and Commander-in-Chief of the Army; all responsibility was his — and all mistakes. His only true confidant was his Bavarian wife, Queen Elizabeth. "The Commander-in-Chief witnessed the disorganization and demoralization of the small army which he had done so much to strengthen, to spare and to encourage. The King was brought into close contact with the spiritual and physical sufferings inflicted by the War on his people, especially on the ruined peasants clinging desperately to their last possessions. He was almost alone."[16]

After three days in Ostend and in consultation with senior officers of his army as well as his allies the King reached a decision.[17] The Belgians would make their stand at the canalized Yser (Ijzer) River, a small tidal river that emptied into the North Sea at Nieuport Bains (Nieuwpoort-Bad). The army would still be in Belgium, but only just, being only 15 km (9.3 mi) from the French frontier. An order went out to the Belgian Army, signed by the King: "The line of the Yser is our last line of defence in Belgium, and its retention is essential for the general plan of operations. This line must therefore be held at all costs."[18]

The Yser was the last ditch in Belgium. The defensive line (the Yser Front) began in the sand dunes along the North Sea near the mouth of the Yser River, followed the river south (4 km) to the town of Nieuport (Nieuwpoort), and then followed the canalized Yser River to the town of Dixmude (Diksmuide), on to the juncture with the Ypres Canal and to the small city of Ypres (Iper), the total length from the North Sea to Ypres measuring 43 km (ca. 26.7 mi). This was the northern most stretch of the Western Front. King Albert had 75,000 men to hold the Yser Front, including a 6,000 man French Naval Brigade defending a salient around Dixmude. The key bridgeheads were at Nieuport and Dixmude, about 10 miles apart. For the German Army, attacking the Yser Front was an aquatic nightmare; the landscape where the fighting took place was essentially reclaimed wetland. Albert had made a good choice for his last stand.

> The country on both sides of the canal is flat, and difficult for observation purposes. The high level of the water necessitates drainage of the meadows, which for this are intersected by deep dykes which have muddy bottoms.... The country is densely populated and is consequently well provided with roads. But these are only good when they have been made on embankments and are paved. The frequent rains, which begin towards the end of October, rapidly turn the other roads into mere mud tracks and in many cases make them useless for long columns of traffic.
>
> The digging of trenches was greatly complicated by rain and surface water.... It was only on the high ground that trenches could be dug deep enough to give sufficient cover against the enemy's artillery fire; on the flat low-lying ground they could not in many cases be made more than two feet deep.[19]

The British Navy also contributed to the defense. To deal with the shallow waters of the North Sea in this area of the coast, it deployed three strange vessels (monitors).[20] Originally built for the Brazilian government and designed as armed patrol craft for the Amazon River, the ships were broad in beam and shallow of draught, needing only six feet of water. They could move in shoal water where an ordinary warship would run aground. The monitors were floating artillery batteries. When the Brazilians were unable to pay for the ships, they put them up for sale in early 1914.[21]

> In August, 1914, the British Admiralty purchased these craft, which appeared in the Navy List as the *Humber*, *Severn*, and *Mersey*. They were heavily armored and carried each two 6-inch guns forward in an armored barbettes, and two 4.7-inch howitzers aft, while four 3-pounder guns were carried amidships.... German big guns could not reach the British, and their submarines could not maneuver in shallow water. The torpedoes which they fired, having been set for much greater depth than the monitors' draught, passed harmlessly beneath their hulls. British guns swept the country for about six miles (9.6 km) inland.[22]

British naval fire was effective against targets near the shore, essentially denying it as an invasion route; however, beyond the dunes it did not much impress the German Army.

> Battleships, cruisers and torpedo-boats worried the rear and flank of the 4th *Ersatz* Division[23] with their fire, and the British had even brought heavy artillery on flat-bottomed boats close inshore. They used a great quantity of ammunition, but the effect of it all was only slight, for the fire of the naval guns was much dispersed and indicated bad observation. It became still more erratic when our long-range guns were brought into action against the British fleet.[24]

For German strategists, breaking through the Yser Front was critical in their drive to capture the Channel ports. Two French ports on the English Channel, Dunkerque and Calais, linked the British forces in France with England. Taking these ports could change the course of the war. Dunkerque is only 18 miles (29 km) west of Nieuport, whereas Calais, situated at the narrowest part of the Channel, is 23 miles (37 km) west of Dunkerque. The barrier standing between the Germans and success was the Belgian Army, an army that, at least so far, was only good at retreating. The Germans attacked on October 16; the Amazon River monitors left Dover for the Flemish coast on the following day. Thus began the Battle of the Yser.

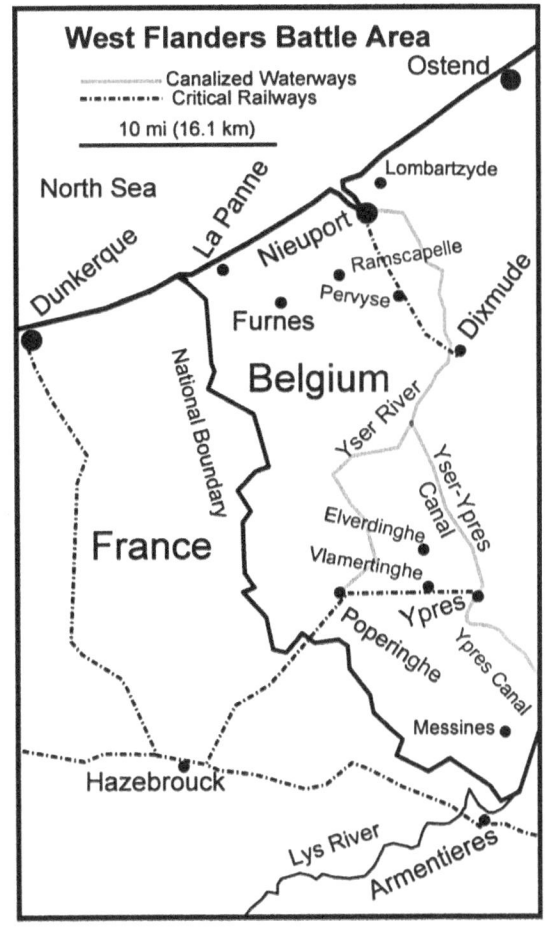

The town of Dixmude came under attack on October 16. A pre-war *Baedeker Handbook for Travellers* described Dixmude as a quiet little town on the Yser. Of interest to visitors was the parish church of St. Nicholas, a seventeenth century edifice containing a "fine Rood Loft in the richest Flamboyant style." By November 10, the Rood Loft, the church and the rest of the "quiet town" no longer existed. Only charred wood and piles of masonry marked the location of Dixmude.

Dixmude's difficulties stemmed from its location on the wrong side of the Yser. The town lay on the east bank and the main Belgian defenses were on the west bank, leaving Dixmude as a salient into the German lines.

> The opposing sides lay within a hundred yards of each other. Artillery preparation, attack and counter attack went on incessantly. Our [German] artillery did fearful havoc and DIXMUDE was in flames. The Franco-Belgian garrison was, however, constantly reinforced, and conducted itself most gallantly.[25]

> Down in their ditches by Dixmude, 5,000 Belgians under General Meyser and 6,000 French Marines under Admiral Ronarc'h, held out against three corps of the Duke of Würtemberg's army from October 16 to November 10, in torrents of rain hardly less painful than the fire of German guns.[26]

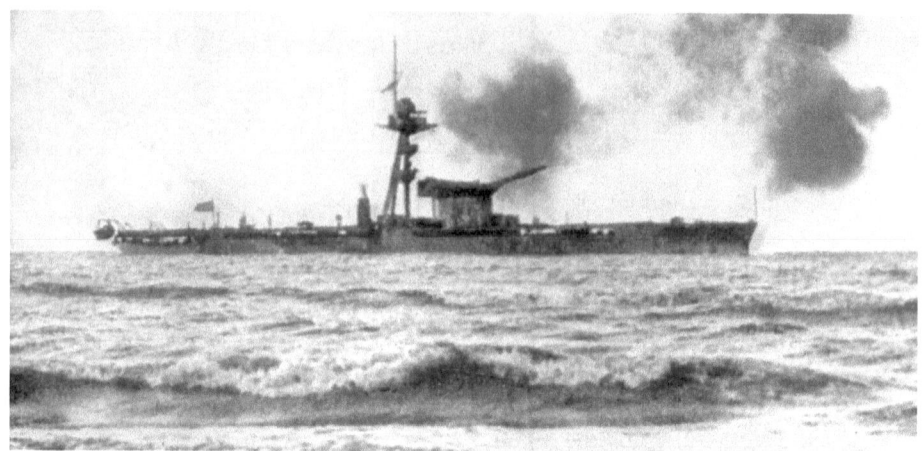

A British monitor shelling the Belgian coast near Ostend, probably one of the Amazon River vessels. Being broad abeam and having a shallow draft for operating in the Amazon, monitors worked close to the shore, preventing the German Army from using the beachfront as an invasion path in 1914. However, since designed for tropical rivers, the ships were nearly unmanageable in heavy seas (*Collier's Photographic History of the European War*, 1917).

The American photographer Donald C. Thompson, reporting for *The New York World*, was with the German forces attacking Dixmude. After the fall of Antwerp, Thompson followed the German Army to the Yser Front. In Dixmude, he found himself with six German officers in a ruined house taking shelter from incoming artillery fire. There his luck ran out; a shell exploding close by wounded him in the face and back.

> I felt as though I had been struck by a thunderbolt, he said, and that I was being whisked into the air. Then I knew no more until I found myself in a field hospital, lying among a batch of German wounded with a bandage strapped across my face and my whole body a mass of bruises. I guess I have had enough of the show for a spell, and am getting across to England as quick as I can for a rest.[27]

At the same time, on the other side of the line, an American volunteer stretcher-bearer moved Belgian and French wounded to safety from the ruins of Dixmude. Arthur H. Gleason, former associate editor at *Collier's Magazine*, (1908–1913), was a member of the Munro Ambulance Corps. Both he and his wife Helen Hayes Gleason, as volunteers in the Corps, traveled with the Belgian Army as it retreated through Ghent. Now Mr. and Mrs. Gleason were on the Yser Front where the Munro Ambulance Corps would serve a military hospital housed in a convent located in Furnes (Veurne), a small town about 10 miles (16.1 km) northwest of Dixmude. They called their convoy of motor ambulances

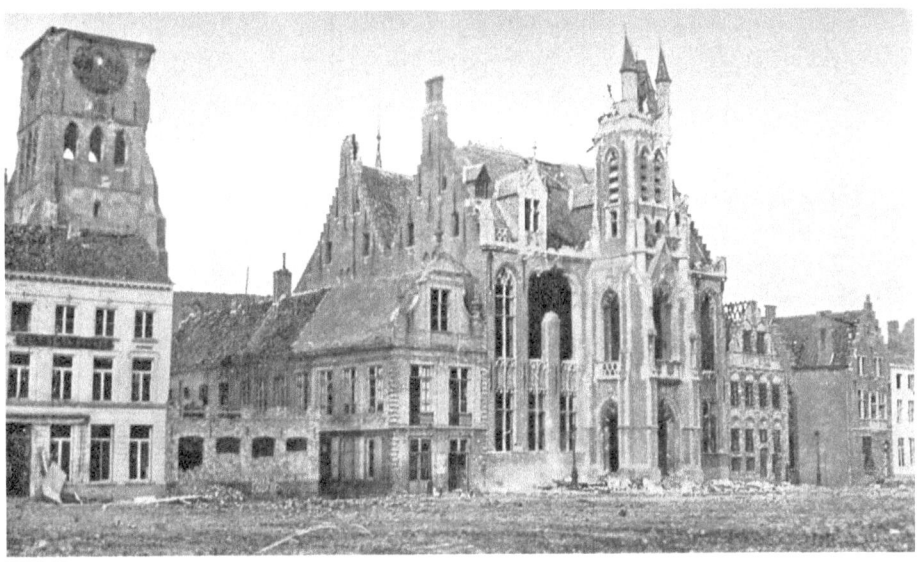

Dixmude's Hôtel de Ville (town hall) and nearby buildings on the market square at the beginning of the battle for possession of the town. Some damage from artillery fire is evident. The cellar of the town hall served as refuge when the shelling became very intense and it was here the Munro Ambulance Corps picked up wounded (Charles Le Goffic, *Dixmude*, 1916).

the "flying column" because it entered the fighting area quickly and without hesitation, picked up its wounded and left in a hurry. Men and women staffed the "flying column," working as physicians, nurses, stretcher-bearers and drivers. The officer in command was Lieutenant de Broqueville, son of Baron de Broqueville, Belgian Minister of Defense. The lieutenant, along with Dr. Munro, planned the flying column's missions, directing it to places of greatest immediate need. A British journalist, Philip Gibbs, briefly served with the flying column and later wrote one of the best descriptions of a day at Dixmude. The day began waiting for orders in the convent yard in Furnes. On that particular day, the flying column consisted of three ambulances and two motor cars.

> Three ladies in field kit stood by their cars waiting for the day's commands, and there were four stretcher-bearers, of whom I was the newest recruit. Among them was an American journalist named Gleason, who had put aside his pen for a while to do manual work in fields of agony, proving himself to be a man of calm and quiet courage, always ready to take great risks in order to bring in a stricken soldier.[28]

They heard Dixmude before they saw it, the explosions sounding like a continuous roll of thunder in the distance. Then, on the horizon, a great pall of black smoke billowed above jabs of red-yellow flames, white puffs of shrapnel shells burst almost continually above and through the smoke. Clouds of particles raised by the almost never-ending hammering of high explosive shells against brick masonry marked the reduction of man-made structures to dust. It seemed as if the portal to hell opened in this "quiet little town on the Yser." Philip Gibbs looked in awe as they drove closer and closer, "I watched how the flames rose, and became great glowing furnaces, terribly beautiful." About a mile from the town, near where a Belgian soldier lay dead, cut in half by a steel fragment from a burst German shell, the ambulance convoy pulled over. Nearby, a Belgian artillery battery fired salvo after salvo. Return fire from the Germans targeted the battery. "We were between two fires, and the Belgian and German shells came screeching across our heads. The enemy's shells were dropping close to us, plowing up the fields with great pits. We could hear them burst and scatter, and could see them burrow."[29]

Here the party divided; the three women and the motor cars were to wait while the rest of the convoy entered Dixmude. The women would transport wounded retrieved from Dixmude to the Furnes hospital while the ambulances returned to get more injured men. Arthur Gleason and Philip Gibbs were among those making the return trip to Dixmude.

> I was in one of the ambulances and Mr. Gleason sat behind me in the narrow space between the stretchers. Over his shoulder he talked in a quiet voice of the job that lay before us. I was glad of that quiet voice, so placid in its courage. We went forward at what seemed to me a crawl, though I think it was a fair pace, shells bursting around us now on all sides, while shrapnel bullets sprayed the earth about us. It appeared to me an odd thing that we were still alive. Then we came into Dixmude.[30]

High-explosive shells poured into Dixmude, seemingly from every direction. Explosions brought down walls, gutted houses, and set fires; the town center was a roaring furnace. Shell splinters burst from points of impact into fountain-like sprays of deadly red-hot steel that scythed through the air and inflicted horrible wounds. Shrapnel shells exploding above the streets fired hails of lethal lead bullets, puncturing man and beast. To be in the open was to be almost immediately dead or seriously wounded, to survive one had to go underground.

The wounded were in the cellar of the town hall on the market square. The brick structure was rapidly decomposing to rubble under the incessant bombardment; the wooden beams of the upper floor were blazing furiously and would soon reach the lower floors and then the flaming mass would crash into the cellar. Next to the town hall and also engulfed in flames stood the seventeenth century parish church of St. Nicholas with its "fine Rood Loft in the richest Flamboyant style"; it would soon be only a memory. The ambulances

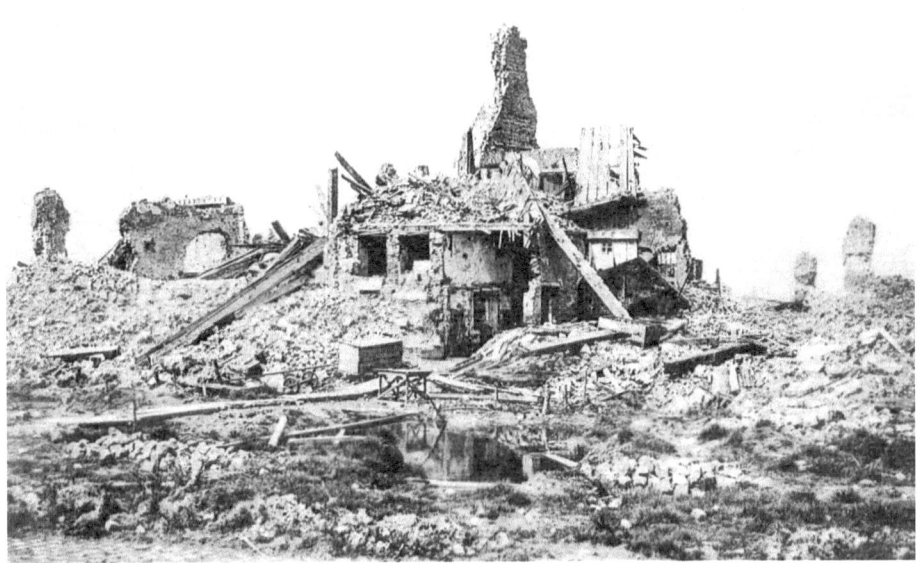

Dixmude after the battle ended. The large ruin in the center is town hall. When the Germans finally took the town there was nothing left standing (Klekowski collection).

cautiously entered the square and the stretcher-bearers ran, dodging shot and shell, for the entrance of the town hall.

> Inside the town hall were piles of bicycles, loaves of bread, and dead soldiers, all in gruesome confusion. In the cellar dead and wounded were lying together. The wounded had all to be carried on stretchers, for everyone who could crawl had fled from that ghastly inferno, and only those who have shifted wounded on stretchers can appreciate the courage it requires to do it under shell fire. At last they were all packed into the ambulances, and even as they left the building with the last, a shell struck it overhead and demolished one of the walls. How they ever got out of Dixmude alive is beyond the ken of a mere mortal.[31]

Arthur Gleason made many ambulance runs from Furnes to Dixmude in October 1914, and survived. During that time, Helen Hayes Gleason was nearby, under fire in Pervyse (Pervyzje), a small town about 5 miles (8.1 km) north of Dixmude on the steam-tram line that connected Nieuport and Dixmude. The tram ran upon a low embankment just above the flat landscape of open fields.[32] Pervyse was about 2.5 miles (4 km) west of the defensive line established by the Belgians on the canalized Yser River and served as a dressing station for that part of the front. From Pervyse ambulances carried wounded to the hospitals in Furnes.

Pervyse was within range of German artillery and repeatedly hit. The railway station resembled a sieve, most of the houses were absolutely destroyed and only a few battered walls and heaps of stone and brick marked the location of the parish church. Craters in the churchyard exposed shattered coffins and brought the long dead to light. The dressing station was just behind the railway station in the house of the village chemist. The house retained a roof and portions of walls. It had plenty of ventilation, of course, where shells had blown holes in the structure or just passed clean through it without exploding. Its most important attribute was its cellar, which served as a bomb shelter. Helen Hayes Gleason was among the first women at the Pervyse dressing station.

> The soldiers needed a dressing station somewhere along the front from Nieuport to Dixmude. Mrs. Knocker established one thirty yards behind the front line of trenches at Pervyse. Miss Chisolm and I [Mrs. Gleason] joined her. In its cellar we found a rough bedstead of two pieces of unplaned lumber, with clean straw for a mattress, awaiting us.... The two soldiers who had been living in our room had given it up cheerily. They had searched the village for a clean sheet, and showed it to us with pride. They lumped the straw for our pillows, and stood outside through the night, guarding our home with fixed bayonets.[33]

The room above the cellar functioned as the surgery; it was here wounded soldiers were brought from the nearby lines. The room also functioned as a daytime living room, allowing the staff an airy escape from the musty cellar. Every day a six-cylinder Daimler ambulance arrived from Furnes to pick up a cargo of wounded. Bullet holes from shrapnel shells and large and small dings from shell splinters enhanced the big car's bodywork, with each trip adding a few more scars. Often the ambulance men joined the Munro Corps women for tea before returning to Furnes. It was all very civilized.

> They seemed to be in particularly good spirits, and they told us that the house had just been struck by a shell, that the big Daimler ambulance had been standing outside, and that its bonnet had been riddled by shrapnel bullets. We went outside to see for ourselves, and there we found a large hole in the side of the house, through which a shell had entered a room across the passage from that occupied by the Corps.[34]

Although she dealt with the dead and dying almost every day and was continually in danger, it was the "dreariness of war" behind the trenches that most affected Gleason. She hated sleeping in one's clothes for weeks, washing in cold water before dawn, having hair uncombed and dirty, and always the feeling of "personal mussiness." Nevertheless, she stuck it out for a year. For her work at the front, King Albert decorated Gleason with the Order of Leopold II, the highest Belgian honor for valiant service.[35] However, let us return to the "mussiness" of trench life. "The toothbrush was the one article of decency clung to. I seemed never to go into the back garden to clean my teeth without bringing on shell-fire. I got a sense of there being a connection between brushing the teeth and the enemy's guns."[36]

> The mornings were bitterly cold. Very early in my career as a nurse, I rid myself of skirts. Boots, covered with rubber boots to the knees in wet weather, or bound with puttees in warm; breeches; a leather coat and as many jerseys as I could walk in — these were my clothes.[37]

On October 22, under the cover of darkness, two battalions of German infantry managed to sneak across the Yser River at a bend about 5 km east of Pervyse. The following day more Germans crossed and established a bridgehead in the center of the Belgian Yser defensive line. As the bridgehead expanded, the Belgians fell back toward Pervyse, establishing a new defensive line at the railway embankment.

> The Germans, having crossed the river where it makes a great bend in the neighborhood of Tervaete, almost opposite Pervyse, had pushed on to the railway. If they had crossed that, the Belgian front was pierced, and they must retreat to the shelter of the guns of Dunkirk. But by a fierce bayonet charge they re-established their position. In revenge the Germans rained shells upon Pervyse until it was a heap of ruins.[38]

Nearly every day the women collected wounded from some "tight angle" with their ambulance, brought them to the dressing station to wash off the mud and apply simple first aids, and prepared the men for the journey to hospital in Furnes. Every day the Munro volunteers had narrow escapes. Every day Gleason worried that finally she might be wounded, or to use her words, "get pinked." "Shells dropped every day, some days all day."[39] "If shells came no nearer than four hundred yards, we considered it a quiet day."[40]

Things were not going so well for the Belgians at the northern end of the Yser either. By October 22, Nieuport was under unceasing bombardment. Key villages and farm strong points around the besieged town fell to the enemy by the following week. Newly established German long-range coastal artillery positions kept British warships from close-to-shore bombardment; consequently, there was little help from the sea for the beleaguered Belgians. What with the breakthrough near Pervyse and the anticipated collapse at Nieuport, all seemed lost. It was time to consider retreating from the Yser to Dunkirk. The army headquarters and medical facilities prepared to abandon Furnes. Plans were made to move the Belgian royals to England. The German Army could taste victory. "The resistance of the enemy was broken, and when the 33rd *Ersatz* Brigade on the northern wing advanced from the north-east against NIEUPORT, the enemy retired. Airmen reported enemy's columns retreating toward FURNES. Nothing could stop the victorious advance."[41]

However, there was still one option that might save the day. Just as Moses

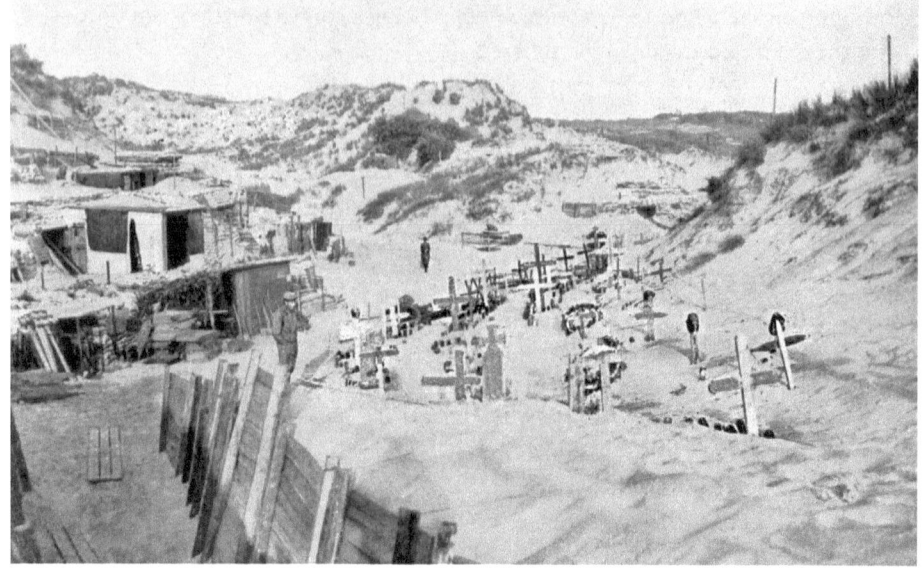

German dugouts in the dunes along the North Sea near Ostend. Beach life was not without its dangers, as evidenced by the many graves in the foreground (*Kriegs-Album des Marinekorps Flandern 1914–1917, 1918*).

parted the sea to escape his enemy, perhaps the Belgians could reverse the procedure, i.e., use the sea to protect them from theirs. The land east of the railway embankment running between Nieuport and Dixmude was below sea level at high tide by as much as three to five feet. The water table was only a foot or so below the surface. The weather in Flanders is wet, often raining for three out of four days at a stretch, thus there is water in abundance. Ditches crisscross the landscape draining excess water into the Yser River, small streams and canals. These larger waterways carry the water to locks just outside Nieuport. Beyond the locks, the water drains into the tidal part of the Yser River and flows into the North Sea. The land stays dry because of the locks — closing the locks at high tide keeps the sea out and opening them at low tide lets the land drain. However, what if one did the reverse? Open the locks at high tide letting the sea flood inland and close them when the tide was out to lock in the seawater and any freshwater accumulation from rainfall. If one repeated this maneuver every twelve-hour tidal cycle for a few days, a flood of water would slowly flow inland, inundating the German positions between the railway embankment and the canalized Yser River — at least that was the hope! To implement the inundation, one had to know which locks to open and close; it would be just as easy to flood the Belgian positions, or both the German and Belgian positions, or simply have the water drain away to someplace else.[42]

On October 21, 1914, members of a Belgian Army engineering unit received orders to try a limited inundation. Advised by Nieuport bargeman Henry Geeraert about which gate to open and how to channel the water, the operation was successful. A small area near Nieuport was flooded. On October 25, King Albert ordered a major inundation to try to stop the German drive opposite Pervyse and the Belgian line along the railway embankment. Charles Cogge, supervisor of the Furnes North Water Authority, was the technical advisor for this inundation. He not only identified the key lock, he toured the active front with the army, pointing out which ditches to dam and culverts to block in order to guarantee the water flooded only German positions. However, since the lock was between the lines and in view of German observers,

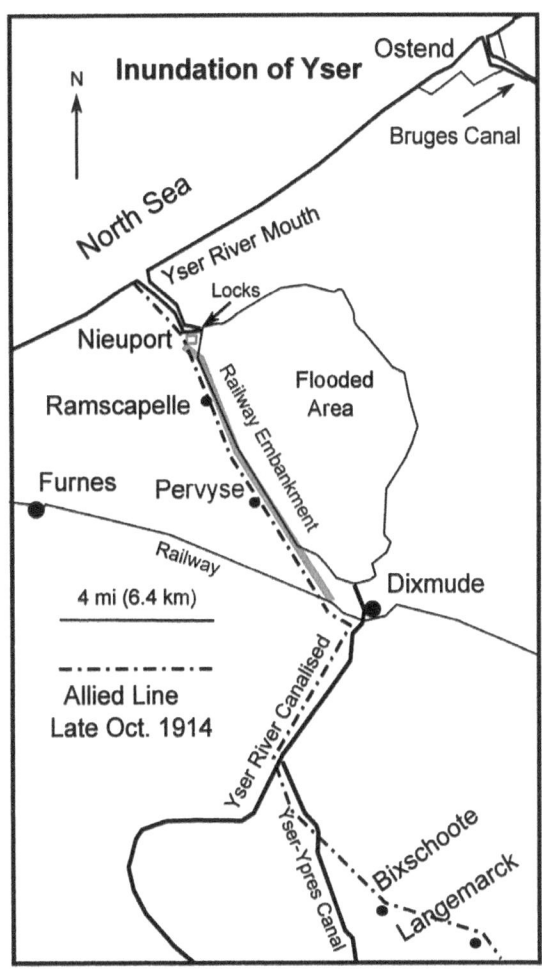

some brave souls had to sneak out to it every twelve hours to open and close the lock doors manually. King Albert had almost waited too long before ordering the inundation, giving time for the German lines to advance close to Nieuport and its locks. Remarkably, German observers failed to realize the significance of the activity at the lock during the six tidal cycles (three days) required to flood the land between the railway embankment and the canalized Yser. The 20.5 miles (33 km)-long embankment with its plugged culverts became a long dam. This dam was the limit of German advancement in this area of Belgium for the rest of the war. The Belgians had finally stopped retreating![43]

On October 29, German commanders noted that something was amiss, normally wet Flanders was getting wetter:

At 11:30 p.m., however, a General Staff officer of the 6th Reserve Division reported that the attack could be continued no further owing to the constant rising of the water. What had happened? On the morning of the 30th the advancing troops had been up to their ankles in water; then it had gradually risen until they were now wading up to their knees, and they could scarcely drag their feet out of the clayey soil. If any one lay down for a moment under the heavy artillery, machine gun and rifle fire, he was lost. The rise of the waters was attributed to the torrential rain of the previous few days, and it was hoped that on the approach of dry weather the excellent system of canals would soon drain it off. But the rising flood soon prevented the movement of wagons with ammunition and supplies, and when the attackers looked back from the railway embankment, it seemed to them as if the whole country had sunk behind them: the green meadows were covered with dirty, yellow water.[44]

To burden the reader with another biblical reference, what the German Army now needed was an Ark. The inundation ended the Battle of the Yser. Nevertheless, the killing continued, just at a slower rate. One of the first American journalists to visit the now somewhat becalmed Yser Front was Arno Dosch.

A little piece of the Low Countries, so small I walked across it in two hours, was all that remained of Belgium in the last days of October [1914]. A tidewater stream, the Yser, ebbed and flowed through the sunken fields, and there King Albert with his remnant of an army stopped the German military machine in its advance on Calais.... The Yser was the last ditch in Belgium.[45]

Dosch stayed at a hotel in La Panne (De Panne), a pretty seaside village just inside Belgium, about four miles from France. The royal couple, King Albert and Queen Elizabeth, lived nearby in an unheated modest house on the seashore. It was so modest it lacked indoor plumbing.[46] Dosch often saw Albert in the village or walking on the beach, "It seemed to be a point of courtesy on the part of the Belgians not to bother their king with ceremony at this trying time."[47] Dosch visited the front along the seashore near Nieuport where he found Belgian cavalry riding naked into the sea and frolicking while out at sea English and French ships fired upon German positions on the distant sand dunes.

We climbed the sand dunes and there we came suddenly upon a perfect panoramic view of the battle all the way from the dunes across the inundated fields to Dixmude in the distance.... At two points we could see the Yser Canal and at one of these the Germans were trying to throw across a pontoon bridge.

We could see it only through the smoke of breaking shells, but it was the most exciting event I have ever witnessed. At three miles or more, though, the figures of the men were so small, it was hard to keep the fact in mind that those who dropped were not merely stooping, but had been shot.[48]

He tried to visit Ramscapelle, a village on the famed railway embankment just south of Nieuport. He got within a hundred yards and witnessed a German artillery barrage pound the small hamlet. Understandably, Dosch opted to return to the peace of La Panne. Besides safety and a pleasant beach to stroll on, La Panne had another attraction; a submarine cable connection to Dover.[49] Presumably, Dosch used it to file his story.

In early 1915, Mary Roberts Rinehart, an American mystery writer,[50] made the Yser junket. She arrived in London in January and visited the Belgian Red Cross. There she met its founder and president Dr. Antoine Depage.[51] Learning that Rinehart had graduated from the Pittsburg Training School for Nurses in 1896, Dr. Depage organized a tour of Belgian medical facilities. Her mission was to publicize their needs to American benefactors. She would publish her experiences in a series of articles in *The Saturday Evening Post* and then pull the articles together into a book.[52] With an assortment of letters of introduction to important people, she crossed the English Channel to Boulogne in January and then traveled by hospital train to Calais where she stayed in a large and very cold house belonging to the Belgian Red Cross. From there a Belgian Red Cross open touring car took her to Dunkirk and then to La Panne. Two weeks and four days after she left America, Rinehart was in Belgium beginning her Yser junket. Her first official stop was a tour of a military hospital established by Dr. Depage, the *Ambulance de l'Océan* at La Panne, *ambulance* being the word for military hospital in French.

> This is the base hospital for the Belgian lines. The men come here with the most frightful injuries. As I entered the building to-night the long tiled corridor was filled with the patient and quiet figures that are the first fruits of war. They lay on portable cots, waiting their turn in the operating rooms, the white coverings and bandages not whiter than their faces.
>
> The Night Superintendent has just been in to see me. She says there is a baby here from Furnes with both legs off, and a nun who lost an arm as she was praying in the garden of her convent. The baby will live, but the nun is dying.[53]

Rinehart made many visits to the *Ambulance de l'Océan* and what she saw there sickened her; she came to view the patients as "pawns in the great chess game of empires." "It makes one wonder," she wrote, "if the result of this war will not be a great and overwhelming individualism, a protest of the unit against the mass."[54] She underestimated the need of most to be part of a human herd, to be one of the masses, not to stick out.

Rinehart's Yser tour included the usual places: the trenches at Nieuport and Dixmude, the Munro dressing station at Pervyse, the railway embankment defenses, and the Belgian headquarters at Furnes where she had an audience with King Albert. Everywhere she heard of instances of bravery, self-sacrifice, heroism and glory. However, she drew a different conclusion. Instead of the glory of holy war, "I can see only greed and lust of battle and ambition."[55]

Probably the high point of her stay in Belgium was an invitation to visit with Elizabeth, Queen of the Belgians, at the royal villa in La Panne. After worrying about what to wear since her wardrobe was a bit shabby, she decided, "furs would cover some of the deficiencies." She soon discovered the royal villa was also a bit shabby.

> The villa itself is small and ugly. The furnishing is the furnishing of a summer seaside cottage. The windows fit badly and rattle in the gale. In the long drawing room — really a living room — in which I waited for the Queen, a heavy red curtain had been hung across the lower part of the long French windows that face the sea, to keep out the draft.
> On a center table were books — H.G. Wells' The War in the Air; two American books written by correspondents who had witnessed the invasion of Belgium; and several newspapers.[56]

Rinehart described Elizabeth as small, slender and strikingly beautiful. She spoke English with a continental inflection that charmed Rinehart. Elizabeth spoke highly of Brand Whitlock and his efforts on behalf of the Belgians. She was a patron of the nearby *Ambulance de l'Océan* and visited it daily. She knew the wounded by name, whether Belgian, French or German, who all adored her. The brutality of the war horrified her. She wondered why — how men could do such terrible things? Perhaps Rinehart had the answer: the masses were pawns, and pawns followed orders and were expendable. Making her point, Rinehart titled the book she wrote about her experiences, *Kings, Queens and Pawns*.

On November 10, 1914, Dixmude finally fell to the Germans. One of the final assaults occurred through a cemetery just outside the town. The French held a trench line that incorporated the cemetery wall, with the cellars of the caretaker's house being a strong point.

> In his invariable fashion, the enemy was preparing his attacks by a systematic clearing of the ground; shrapnel and *marmites* [high explosive shells] were smashing the tombstones, decapitating the crosses, breaking up the iron grilles, the crowns of *immortelles*, and the coffins themselves. The Flemish subsoil is so permeable that coffins are not sunk more than a couple of feet below the surface, so that their occupants were strewn about in a frightful way. Several [French] Marines were wounded by splinters of bone from these mobilized corpses.... In the fogs of Flanders, when the mystery of night and the great disc of the moon added their phantasmagoria to the scene, all this surpassed in *macabre* horror the most ghastly inventions of romantic fiction and legend.[57]

After suffering about 10,000 casualties, the Germans took possession of a town reduced to smoking heaps of rubbish backed by an impregnable line beyond. The heavily fortified left bank of the canalized Yser just to the west of the town was impassable. The drive to the channel ports through the Yser was a failure.

However, perhaps there was another way. It might be possible to reach the channel ports through Ypres, a town 32 miles (51 km) south of Dixmude.

Wartime Belgium became a "must see destination" for certain peculiar types of American tourists. Especially in 1914 and early 1915, with the country still in flux and restrictions for travel lax, Americans wanting to see the war first hand usually included Brussels, Antwerp, the Yser Front and Ypres in their war-travel itinerary. A book based upon your exciting adventures would help off-set the cost of travel. Americans were very keen on first-hand accounts, especially about Belgium. Walter Austin of Boston was such a war voyeur; he styled himself as a "War Zone Gadabout." For him war was a grand sport, a sporting event that he must see. Without objection from his wife, so he said, Walter sailed from New York on October 14, 1914, aboard *Lusitania* bound for Liverpool. Besides his passport, the fifty-year-old gadabout carried only a single credential, a business card indicating that he was a "special correspondent" for the *Dedham Transcript*, a Boston suburb newspaper. Walter had the card specially printed; it was his cover. From England, he crossed to Holland and took a train to Antwerp. Presenting his American passport at the train station, the German passport officer waved him through with the comment, "Welcome to our city." It had been "theirs" for about two weeks. Antwerp was not to Walter's liking. "Antwerp was like a morgue, swarming with hostile officials in gray uniforms and spiked helmets. All hotels, shops, and places of amusements were closed. The resident population had practically disappeared."[58]

From Antwerp, he traveled to Berlin, which he also did not like, before returning to England. There he met Edwin B. Hotchkiss, a fellow war gadabout. An engineer, Hotchkiss had been in business in Brussels for twenty-five years, knew the country and had connections. The pair teamed up with J.A. Allen, another war adventurer. A Londoner, about thirty-five years old, Allen owned a Mercedes limousine. Austin and Hotchkiss rented the Mercedes with Allen as driver.

> On the 12th of November [1914] three men in a motor-car bowled on to the deck of the Channel steamer. Two minutes later, the ship being under way, the Three Musketeers repaired to the smoking room, where they drank success to their new Goddess, La Belle France, their forty-horse-power machine, "The Dreadnaught," and to the Great Adventure ... we adorned the front of the "Dreadnaught" with a Belgian flag on the right side and the American flag on the left.[59]

Arriving in the port of Boulogne, they pointed the nose of the Mercedes east for the Belgian frontier. In addition to official documents, they carried a bushel and a half of cigarettes as "gifts" to ease their way with officials. In Calais, they met Edwin Hotchkiss's son Harold, who not only joined the party but brought along George Milner, the sixteen-year-old son of the American consul at Calais. Now a fivesome, the war tourists arrived in Dunkirk on

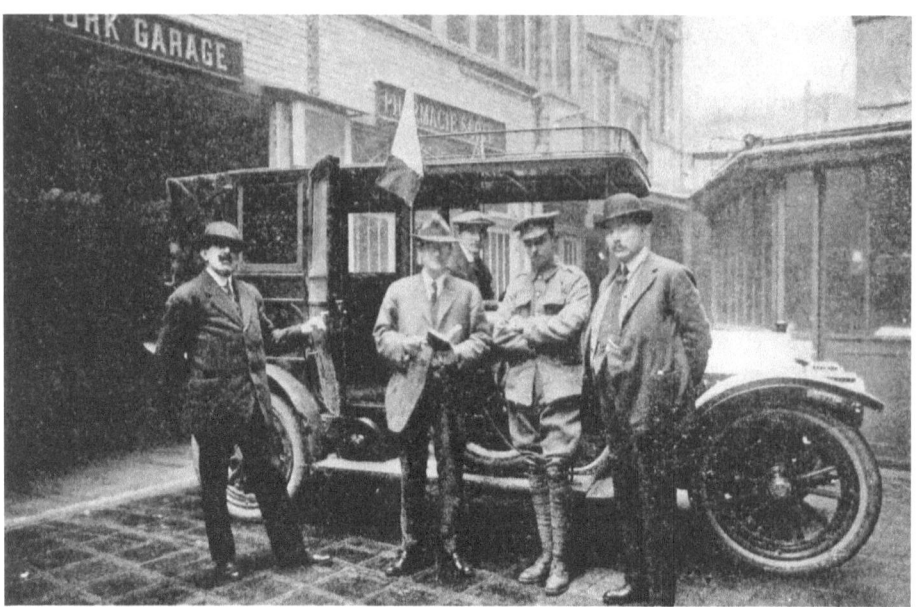

Probably the most madcap tourists of the war, they called themselves the "war zone gadabouts." Led by a middle-aged American from Boston, Walter Austin, posed with the book, the trio included Edwin Hotchkiss, on the left holding the door, and J.A. Allen, behind the Mercedes. Hotchkiss had lived in Brussels for 25 years and knew his way around and knew people. Allen, a Londoner, owned the Mercedes, which the trio christened the "Dreadnaught." Walter Austin recorded their adventures in a published memoir; reading it makes one question their good sense (Walter Austin, *A War Zone Gadabout*, 1917).

November 19. They were getting closer to the action; they could hear the muffled roar of artillery in the east. Although their travel *permis* limited them to Dunkirk, Edwin Hotchkiss hoped to extend this permission to include Furnes and Ypres because of his friendship with the commandant in charge of the city. In spite of this friendship, he was unable to get the *permis* officially extended but did receive oral permission to continue east. On November 20, they reached Furnes. There the commandant, another Hotchkiss friend, issued the necessary *permis,* again only orally, so they could continue their insane journey seeking war and gore. No one wanted to leave a paper trail condoning this foolish trip. Prohibited from visiting Nieuport or Dixmude because of the heavy fighting there, the gadabouts headed for Ypres. But first they gassed-up, "So we fed the insatiable 'Dreadnaught' with ten gallons of petrol, at three dollars and ten cents a gallon, and at half-past ten pointed her nose south-east towards Ypres." On their arrival, they entered a city under bombardment and got their first taste of real danger.

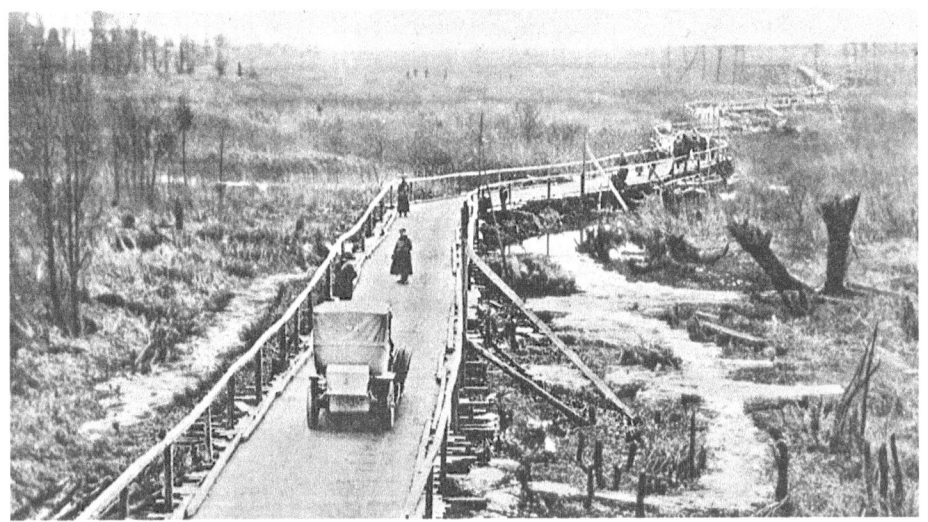

A bridge constructed by the German Army over part of the flooded Yser district. The inundation of the area between railway embankment and the Yser River turned much of the surrounding landscape into a swamp, so that for the Germans even reaching their new lines was difficult (*Hamburger Fremdenblatt*, 1915).

> When the shell struck, there was a deafening roar—like a thousand tons of coal being shot all at once down a gigantic iron chute. We saw smoke and falling masonry. Our car was slewed violently to one side. Dense smoke and clouds of dust rose from the ruins. Allen shut off the engine and applied the brakes. The car was dead.[60]

Allen managed to start the motor and they made a brief tour. In the fall of 1914, Ypres was in the initial stage of its destruction; although punctured by shells, its buildings were mostly still standing. Thus, there was much to see. In a couple of years that would not be the case. Zigzagging from side to side to avoid shell craters, the Dreadnaught left the city at mid-day and headed northeast toward Roulers (Roeselare), then on the front line. The action in Ypres was still too mild for the gadabouts; they wanted to see the front lines. They drove for about six and a half miles while artillery batteries on each side of the road "volleyed and thundered." They passed houses shattered by gunfire, trees splintered and broken. Trenches paralleled the road, their occupants staring in disbelief as the Dreadnaught rolled by full of wide-eyed tourists. "Not one of us had the remotest idea where we were going. Yet we all seemed bent on keeping on until something—we knew not what—should stop us. No one spoke. But all our faculties were keenly alive. Nothing that could be seen or heard escaped us."[61]

Finally, a French soldier with fixed bayonet stopped them. Did they know they were beyond the advanced trenches of the French, and that the German trenches were only half a kilometer distant? Ludicrously, the gadabouts viewed this as "cheering news!" They were actually in No Man's Land — what great luck. What a tale to tell at home. What a story to write. Anti-personnel shrapnel shells exploded above them, sending down hails of lead balls, while high-explosive shells exploded in the distance. "There were moments that were almost deafening when, all at once, we could hear the scream of flying projectiles, the explosions of shrapnel and the deep booming of howitzers."[62]

The gadabouts milled about in the open near the car, as if viewing Fourth of July fireworks. Their nonchalant behavior was beyond foolish; it was insane.

> Presently from the direction of Ypres came sounds of hard riding. We turned and saw a French cavalry captain. He dismounted and approached us. But although he was French, he was not polite. Neither was he pleasant.
> "What are you doing here?" he roared.
> Harold Hotchkiss, who spoke French as well as his father, replied: "We're merely sightseers."
> "Well, you're a pack of damned fools," roared the captain, or words to that effect. "Get back into that automobile!"[63]

Feeling like intruders, like lame-brained tourists, they meekly climbed into their car. Where men were dying, they were touring! It was so insensitively stupid. Ordered back to Ypres under guard, the gadabout tour of Belgium came to an ignominious end.[64]

What Walter and his friends had blundered into was the First Battle of Ypres (October 29–November 15, 1914). The French line circumscribed an arc northeast of Ypres linking to the British line near the road to Roulers, presumably the road on which the Dreadnaught traveled. The combined French and British defenses formed a semicircle or salient pushing east into the German line. The Ypres Salient was yet another hazard blocking the German drive for the Channel ports. In the First Battle of Ypres, the Germans managed, at great human cost, to reduce the radius of the semicircle, bringing Ypres within range of their artillery.

> Our semicircle around the town became so reduced that it was brought within range of our artillery from three sides, and there could be no more threats of a big hostile offensive based on the YPRES district. The fact that neither the enemy's commanders nor their troops gave way under the strong pressure we put on them, but continued to fight the battle round YPRES, though their situation was most perilous, gives us an opportunity to acknowledge that there were men of real worth opposed to us who did their duty thoroughly.[65]

The British held the Ypres Salient for the entire war although German artillery bombardment essentially erased much of the town.

Chapter 6

Prussian Belgium

It is a matter of course that the military administration of Belgium, so far as its needs are concerned, holds the country in an iron grip, guarding the conquered territory in every way.[1]— Baron Adolf von Bachofen

Most of the industry in the country is paralyzed and there are thousands out of work.[2]— Ernesta Drinker Bullitt

With the stalemates on the Yser Front and Ypres Salient in the fall and early winter of 1914, the boundary between free and occupied Belgium stabilized on the north south line of trenches separating the opponents. Nevertheless, for much of the war the boundary remained fluid around the salient and to the south as each contestant captured or lost small pieces of over-valued real estate. To administer subjugated Belgium, the occupiers divided the country into three zones reflecting military needs. The westernmost part of the country, a strip of territory a few miles wide following the front line, was the zone of military operations or *Operationsgebiet*. This zone reflected the fortunes of war and thus could shift east or west. East of the *Operationsgebiet* was the zone of depots and communications, the *Etappengebiet*. Both of these zones were under military jurisdiction, which imposed harsh conditions on Belgians who lived there. Belgian citizens could not buy, sell or barter without official permission; they endured frequent house searches; and, especially in the *Operationsgebiet*, they could be drafted to dig trenches, fill sandbags, and build bridges or other construction tasks directly helping the war effort.[3] Fortunately, the majority of Belgians resided under the relatively more liberal *General-Gouvernement* where the military at least paid lip service to civilian law. A governor-general, who answered directly to Kaiser Wilhelm, commanded the *General-Gouvernement*. During the first months of occupation, Baron von der Goltz was governor-general. At the end of 1914, Kaiser Wilhelm reassigned Baron von der Goltz to the Turkish military and Baron von Bissing became governor-general. Based in Brussels, the governor-general was at the head of a Byzantine constellation of overlapping German military and civilian administrators who controlled, or attempted to control, all aspects of Belgian life. Ranging from the improvement of coal mines to social planning, German ministries tried to make Belgium more like Germany. "A big step toward improving social conditions was taken in Brussels when some 3,000 disorderly girls were forced to go to work under the threat of deportation in case they refused."[4]

However, using threats to promote social change, even though sometimes positive, did not go down well with the Belgians. The governor-general and his minions could not make the Belgians into Germans, no matter what. The German high command lamented this failure and sought an explanation.

> To people like the Belgians, who have grown up under the protection of neutrality, and in whom the sense of individual freedom has been developed to a remarkable degree, the thought of being joined to Germany, with its subjection of individual interests to those of the community, with its military service and social provisions, must be infinitely unsympathetic.[5]

> But we dare not cherish expectations that the rapprochement will become genuinely deep and hearty, because, aside from their history and development, the inhabitants of Belgium, be they Walloons or Flemish, have been impressed with customs and ideas that lead them into entirely different ways from those which are natural and right to Germans.[6]

German authorities greatly restricted travel both within and outside of Belgium. No Belgian male of military age could leave the country under any circumstance, a restriction designed to prevent him joining the Belgian Army. One of the missions of German guards posted on the Dutch frontier was to prevent Belgian men from crossing into neutral Holland. There is a story of a clever ruse devised by a group of Belgian sportsmen to cross *en masse*. A German bureaucrat, presumably in charge of an office fostering good relations with the locals, gave permission for a group of Belgians to organize a bicycle race from some point in Belgium to a finish line near the Dutch border at Maastricht. They obtained this permission on condition that each bicycle must prominently fly a small German flag. With feigned reluctance, the Belgians agreed. "The race was held; but, instead of stopping at the finish line, all the contestants kept on at full speed over the boundary into Holland, and, as they had the German flag on their bicycles, they were not arrested by the sentries, and thus escaped."[7]

Presumably, the sentries, seeing the mass of bicycles with German flags approaching the border, assumed it was some kind of official bicycle tour. Of course, the ruse only worked once!

Everyday life in occupied Belgium was not without its humorous moments — and often those moments dealt with time and money. The Germans

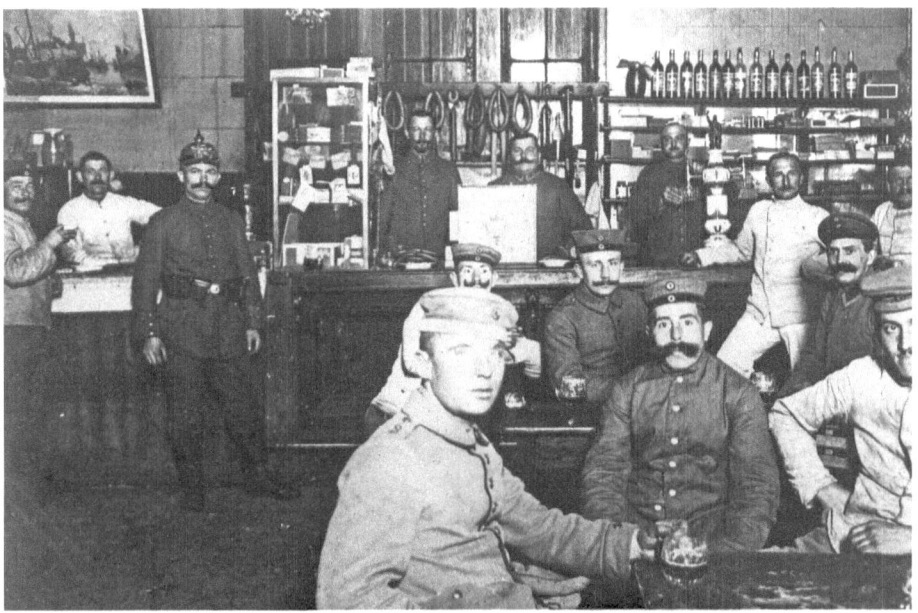

German soldiers relax in a Brussels *Kneipe* (bar). After the horrors of the Western Front in Belgium and Northern France, soldiers on furlough in the city flocked to its restaurants, bars and other entertainments (Rainer Hiltermann collection).

set their clocks and watches to Berlin time (European Central Time), while the Belgians set theirs to Belgian time (Greenwich Mean Time), one hour behind Berlin, e.g., 12 noon German time was really 11:00 a.m. Belgian time, conveniently providing Belgians a patriotic reason for always being late. Important appointments usually stated both times. "Clocks on church towers and in all public places were obliged to keep German time, or those responsible for their upkeep were fined.... Many clocks in public places were allowed to run down as a patriotic protest."[8]

Money was another source of confusion as both German marks and Belgian francs were in circulation. Of course, shops and restaurants posted their prices in francs while Germans usually had only marks. In 1914, the exchange rate was 1 mark equal to 1 franc 25 centimes. If you paid in marks, you received your change in both currencies — you needed considerable mathematical dexterity to keep it all straight. A *New York Times* correspondent observed the following incident in the restaurant of the Palace Hotel in Brussels. A German general finished his meal and received a bill from his waiter for 7 francs; in payment, the general tendered a 100 mark note and received the following baffling heap of change, "including 1 and 2 franc Belgium paper notes, 5 and 10 mark German bills, Belgian and German silver, and Belgian nickel coins with holes punched in the centres. The General takes out his pencil and begins elaborate calculations on the menu — then sends for the head waiter. It takes some time and much talk to convince him that he is not being 'short-changed.'"[9]

The influx of thousands of German soldiers with marks in their pockets enlivened Belgian cities. For example, in Brussels, crowds filled the principal shopping area, overflowing the sidewalks into the street; soldiers crowded the cafés and other places of amusement.

> Orders have been issued to the German soldiers never to go about the streets without a rifle, on the ground that "an ounce of prevention is worth a pound of cure." On a busy evening at the famous "Princess Café" which is now monopolized by the German private, one may see the rifles stacked in the aisles while the soldiers are having their Munich beer — which, by the way, is brought fresh from Germany every twenty-four hours.[10]

Hundreds of military automobiles loaded with officers sped on joy rides about the city. For German officers and enlisted men, Brussels was their ersatz Paris, a place where every day seemed a holiday.[11] "They use Brussels as a sort of pleasure city, where those soldiers who cannot reach Berlin may take their holiday from the trenches."[12]

Young men, with time and money on their hands, away from girlfriends, wives or mothers, in a city where they were acknowledged conquerors, sought more than Belgian chocolates or even Belgian beer to satisfy their wants.

> Many women sold their bodies to Germans. And no wonder, for the lower classes in the city were very miserable. Begging on the streets continually increased. This explains why prostitution grew so enormously. Aside from the numerous cocottes of an earlier day, of whom the better class had fled to London or Paris, the great majority of these *femmes entretenues* were girls whose cavaliers had gone into service or skipped, so that the poor creatures, unable to earn a penny, saw themselves compelled to sell their bodies to the hated Germans. Thus the bars, cinemas, cafés, etc., were overrun by girls; and by noon the merry chase after the man was on, only in a more discrete way among the Germans. But after the closing of the cafés at eleven o'clock, a great stream of girls poured out into the streets and accosted soldiers and civilians alike with the greatest freedom.[13]

The occupiers called Brussels "The Love Station" with due cause. However, it was not the only Belgian city known for a seedy good time; Antwerp, Ghent and Liège were also notorious.[14] Ghent, which served as the center of German operations and thus had hundreds of thousands of soldiers passing through it, documented the cost of this seldom-mentioned dark side of the war. More than 80 percent of the city's part-time prostitutes were married mothers with from three to eight children whose husbands were at the front, dead, or in captivity. These women supported their families the only way they

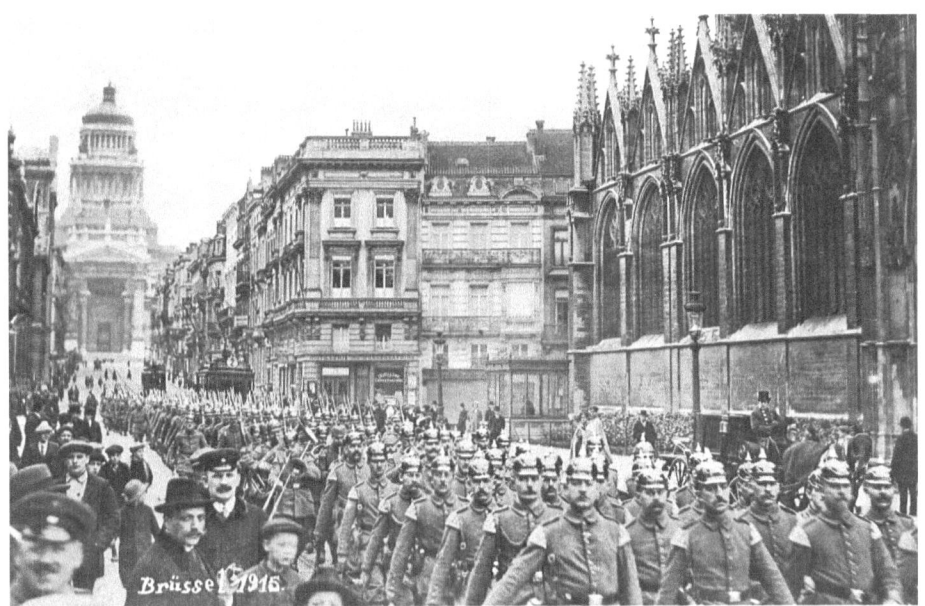

German troops parade down the Rue de la Régence in Brussels in 1916. The large building with a dome at the far end of the street is the Palais de Justice, the high court; since there was little litigation and thus no need for courts in occupied Brussels, this building served as a very large barracks (Rainer Hiltermann collection).

could, by selling their bodies. Many of these women contracted venereal disease, which was rampant among the soldiers.

Remarkably, considering the many American visitors to Belgium, none commented upon the degradation of women through prostitution during the German occupation. Why? Perhaps they were too prudish to discuss the subject or, more likely, they did not want to comment on anything that might cast the Belgians in a negative light. However, there was one American visitor, a Congregational minister and radical social reformer, who no doubt would have said something about the evils of prostitution under the occupation. Unfortunately, not long after his arrival in Brussels he did something foolish and was soon under arrest as a spy.

> Minister Whitlock also feels vastly relieved that he has got practically all non-official Americans out of Belgium, the two score still here being mostly resident business men, with a sprinkling of the boldest tourists, who are staying "to see the fun," in spite of Ministerial warnings.[15]

Horace Green (see Chapter 4) and Walter Austin (see Chapter 5) were among those Americans staying "to see the fun" in 1914. Another "fun-seeker" was Albert Rhys Williams, a graduate of Hartford Theological Seminary who also studied at Cambridge University in England and Marburg University in Germany. A socialist and labor-organizer, Williams' passion was the welfare of the working class. While a Congregational minister in Boston, he raised money to help striking textile workers. When the war began, he took leave from his church to see the conflict first hand, eventually obtaining an appointment as a journalist for *The Outlook,* a ranking weekly magazine of news and opinion published in New York City. Theodore Roosevelt was an associate editor.

> The outbreak of the Great War found me in Europe as a general tourist, and not in the capacity of war-correspondent. Hitherto I had essayed a much less romantic role in life, belonging rather to the crowd of uplifters who conduct the drab and dreary battle with the slums. The futility of most of these schemes for badgering the poor makes one feel at times that these battles are shams and unavailing. This is depressing.[16]

Burned out social worker and fledgling war correspondent, Williams traveled to Holland and crossed into Belgium, arriving too late to see any fighting. Eventually Williams found his way to Brussels where he stayed at the Hôtel Métropole, which boasted a bar américain — perhaps the hotel's attraction to Americans. Williams was in his room on September 28, 1914, when the hotel porter knocked and announced an American guest. The guest turned out to be not an American but a member of the German counterespionage service who arrested Williams on a charge of spying for the Allies.

According to Williams, a Dutchman had approached him the day before on the street-car, saying he was taking people on an automobile tour through the countryside between Brussels and Holland; it would be a unique opportunity to see German soldiers in the field and visit ruined villages. As a novice war correspondent, Williams saw the trip as the basis of his first war story and agreed to invest money in the trip, giving his hotel address for further contact. Alas, what was one man's war story was another man's espionage. The Dutchman was a German agent trolling for Allied spies. Brand Whitlock learned of William's plight the following day.

> Brussels, 29 September 1914
>
> Excellency,
>
> I just learned that Mr. Williams, American citizen, staying at Hôtel Métropole, is said to have been arrested by the German authorities.
>
> Should he not have been released in the meantime, I would appreciate if you could let me know the reason for his arrest and enable me to communicate with him as soon as possible so as to give him all the protection he might need.
>
> Yours Faithfully,
> Brand Whitlock
>
> His Excellency Baron von der Lancken
> Brussels[17]

German authorities kept Williams locked up for a few days before giving him his day in court. The American Legation lawyer defended him, successfully. Released under the condition that he must leave Belgium, he was soon on his way to his room at the Hôtel Métropole. On the street, temptation surfaced — three different shady-looking individuals offered him prohibited Antwerp papers and a woman with an English accent offered to drive him through the German lines to Ghent. He refused all propositions; he was absolutely neurotic about speaking with strangers, saying, "I wouldn't have talked to my own mother without a written permit from the military governor."[18]

> One of Whitlock's great worries is the insistence of American tourists, who do not find it very difficult to get into Brussels, but who, once they are there, find it a very difficult matter to get out again.[19]

Williams wrote a successful book, melodramatically titled *In the Claws of the German Eagle*, describing his few days of incarceration in Brussels. He never returned to the ministry, becoming a journalist (*New York Post*) and writer. In 1917, he covered and participated in the Russian Revolution. Williams wrote propaganda for Leon Trotsky and became a friend of Lenin, thus returning to his left-wing roots.

Some American visitors to Belgium came as guests of the German government and consequently had little need of the services of the American Legation. Ernesta Drinker Bullitt and her husband William were newly married. The adventurous couple decided to honeymoon in Europe. At the height of the war in the summer of 1916, while the Battle of Verdun was ongoing and U-boats stalked the seas, they sailed across the Atlantic. This was at a time when bookings to Europe were down more than 70 percent compared to pre-war.[20] Their ultimate destination was Berlin. William, who spoke German, was a journalist with the Philadelphia paper *The Public Ledger*. He interviewed German officials while Ernesta, who could not speak German, toured women's help organizations with an English-speaking guide.[21] Left to her own devices, she spent much of her time visiting with, and collecting gossip about, American women married to German nobles.

> Heard a delightful story about Mr. Gerard from Mrs. —. She said that to tease Countess B — he asked her why she hadn't married some nice stockbroker in New York, who could have provided her with much better-looking clothes, and more of them, than Count B —. She went home in a rage and told the Count, who also became furious and they both told all Berlin that Mr. Gerard was so anti–German that he disapproved of German-American marriages. Mrs. Gerard implores her husband to save his jokes for those who have a sense of humor.[22]

James W. Gerard, American Ambassador to the German Imperial Court, was known for his irreverent and sometimes outrageous wit.

The Bullitts made a two-week visit to Belgium as guests of the German government. Their guide and travel facilitator, resplendent in dress uniform, was Excellenz Coates who made sure his charges saw only that which reflected well upon the German occupation. He also made sure that their experience was one of luxurious isolation. In Brussels, the Bullitts were given a suite at the Hotel Astoria rather than the Palace Hotel, thus reducing their chances of chatting with the journalistic and diplomatic riffraff that frequented the latter. They dined and toured only with German barons and counts. "The Germans told us quite frankly that they had not brought us here to talk to Belgians."[23] They obtained permission to go to tea with Minister and Mrs. Whitlock at the American Legation only after appealing to their German controller.

On their last night in Brussels, they dined with Baron von Bissing, the governor-general, at his château outside town. A gray automobile adorned with the German coat of arms picked them up at the Astoria. Ernesta, who was a beautiful woman, charmed the seventy-two-year old baron. However, since he did not speak English and she spoke no German, they conversed in rudimentary French. They mostly chatted about the positive achievements of the occupation under von Bissing's leadership. After returning to the Astoria, Ernesta's husband asked if she had a good time. "'Yes,' I said, and with true regard for the important things in life, I added: 'But I had on the most dreadful dress I own.'"[24]

This adventurous couple divorced seven years later; Ernesta changed her name to Ernesta Drinker Beaux, taking her mother's maiden name.[25] Her aunt, Cecilia Beaux, the noted American artist, painted her niece's portrait in 1914, *Girl in White, Ernesta,* (Metropolitan Museum of Art). Ernesta became a noted interior decorator and socialite in New York City. During World War Two, Ernesta was on the radio as Commando Mary. William Bullitt viewed the Russian Revolution and Communist take-over positively. He was President Wilson's emissary to Lenin (1919). President Franklin D. Roosevelt appointed him American Ambassador to the Soviet Union (1933–1936). His relationships with both presidents ended badly, as did his love affair with Communism. William Bullitt was a romantic idealist who could be both charming and brilliant and also "offensive and ridiculous to a good many people of importance."[26]

However, back to the summer of 1914 — after a Belgian sojourn of two weeks, the Bullitts returned to Germany having learned very little about life in occupied Belgium. "As for Brussels itself, it seemed to us, who had been in Berlin for six weeks, a gay and cheerful place."[27]

Brand Whitlock saw Brussels differently; it was anything but gay. Often in the late afternoon, he strolled alone about the city as a way of fleeing the responsibilities of the Legation or as he said, "To forget for a while." He remembered a city that before the war was gay, a Belgian Paris, and now was a city

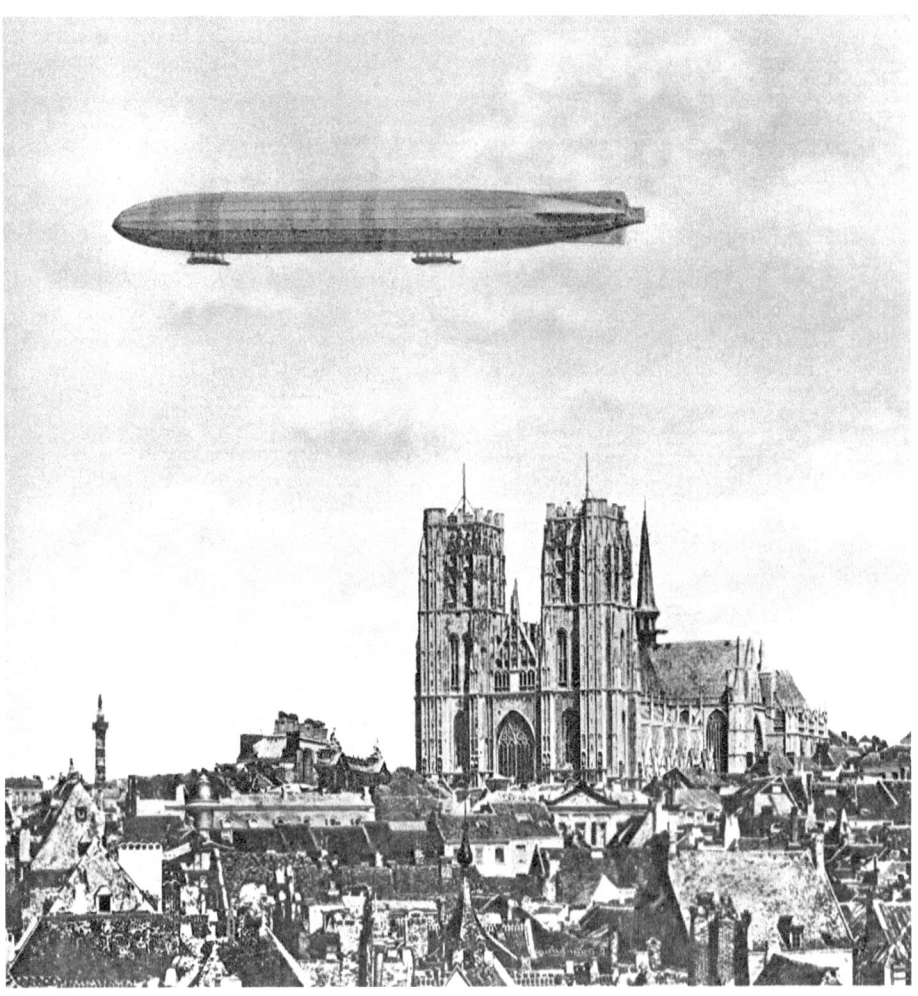

A German Zeppelin flies serenely over the Cathedral of St. Michael and St. Gudule in Brussels. A Zeppelin base was outside the city; the American writer Julia Twells lived nearby and remembered Allied planes attacking the large hangar (*Illustré*, 1914).

of closed houses and deserted streets. Prussian Brussels was a city of idle, unemployed and indolent soldiers, a city without gaiety, a city of melancholy streets.

> And there, not far away, the long waiting line at a soup kitchen, shivering in its rags, stretched in woe and misery and hunger far down the street.
> No, there was no escape. One could not banish from the mind that line of pinched, pathetic faces, those huddled forms in old clothes.[28]

Brand Whitlock's Brussels was not the one Ernesta Bullitt visited.

Although the Dutch and Spanish legations also remained in Brussels during the German occupation, it was Brand Whitlock and the American Legation who won the hearts of the Belgians. This was in great part due to the food assistance sent to Belgium from the United States (see Chapter 7). This generosity literally kept the Belgians from starving. However, as visitors noted, it was more than the food aid; Belgians revered Whitlock almost as much as they did their king.

> Whitlock's influence with the Belgians is so great that he, more than any other living man, is able to keep them out of trouble. On more than one occasion it has been the advice and influence of the American Minister that has prevented deplorable conflicts and avoided additional bloodshed in that unhappy country.[29]

On New Year's Day 1915, only four months into the occupation, crowds thronged the American Legation to say thank you. Over 3,000 Belgians signed the guest book and left cards. From nobles with high titles to the poorest slum dweller, all came to offer their gratitude to the Whitlocks and the United States.[30] Washington's Birthday, February 22, 1915, saw another pro–America celebration in Brussels. Schoolchildren had a holiday, the citizens wore their best clothes, and every Belgian had an American flag (or what passed for one) in his/her buttonhole. Post cards symbolizing American/Belgian friendship sold by the thousands.[31] Baron von Bissing realized that the Belgians celebrated things American as a way to protest things German, but because America was a powerful neutral, he tolerated the Belgian antics. However, in 1915 an act of war nearly ended that neutrality. That act of war did not occur in Belgium, nor did it even occur in Europe; it occurred on the high seas.

On May 1, 1915, the shipping news section of the *New York Times* ran an advertisement for the British Cunard Line. *Lusitania*, described as the "fastest and largest steamer now in Atlantic service," would sail from New York to Liverpool that day at 10 a.m., and after returning from Liverpool would again depart on May 29, also at 10 a.m. On the same page, and only inches away, was another advertisement.

> Notice!
> Travellers intending to embark on the Atlantic voyage are reminded that a state of war exists between Germany and her allies and Great Britain and her allies; that the zone of war includes the waters adjacent to the British Isles; that, in accordance with formal notice given by the Imperial German Government, vessels flying the flag of Great Britain, or of any of her allies, are liable to destruction in those waters and that travellers sailing in the war zone on ships of Great Britain do so at their own risk.
> Imperial German Embassy
> Washington, D.C.
> April 22, 1915[32]

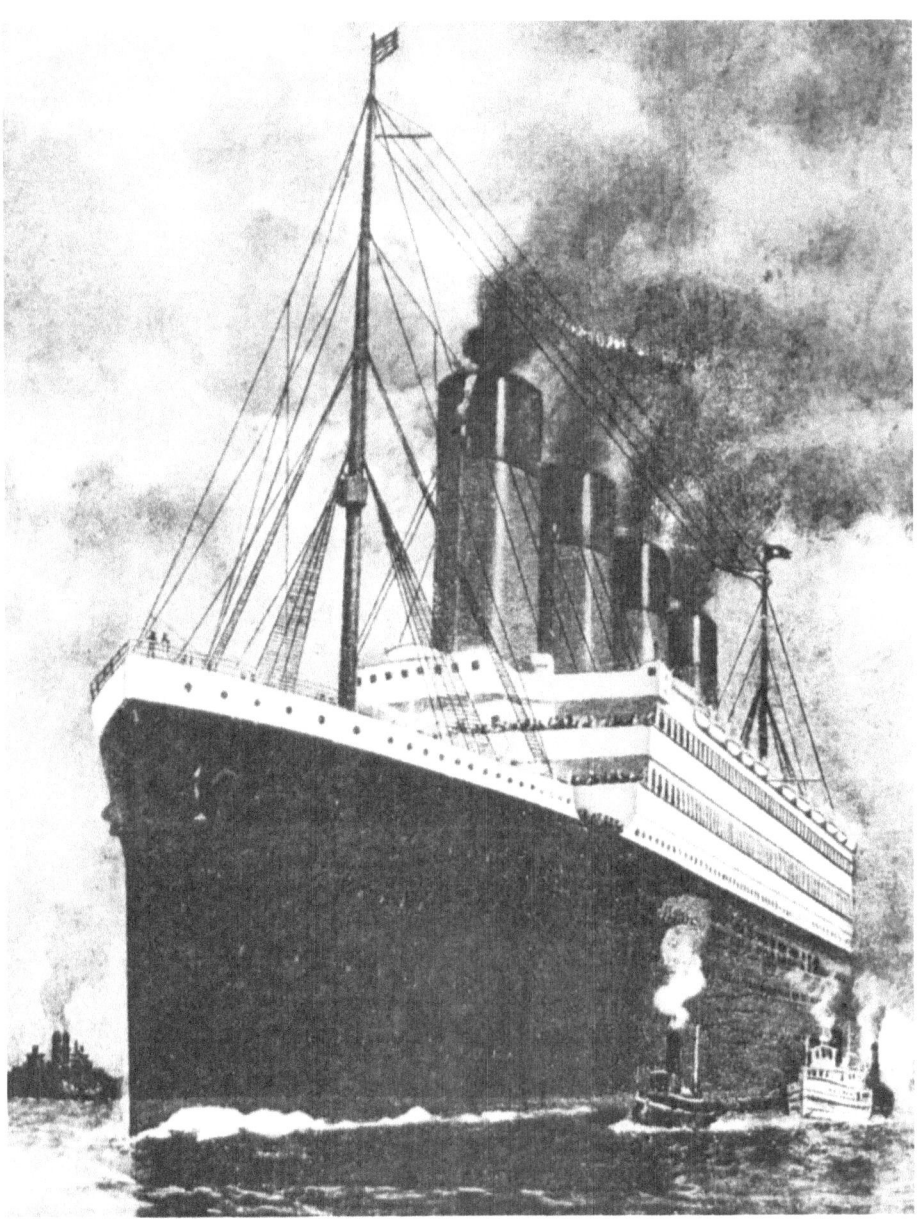

The Cunard liner *Lusitania* was the most luxurious liner on the Atlantic run in 1914. Known for her lavish first-class staterooms and cabins, she held the speed record for the Liverpool to New York run with a crossing time of four days, 19 hours, 52 minutes. Considerable social prestige accrued from traveling aboard *Lusitania*. Not generally known to her socially aware passengers was that *Lusitania* also carried American-made munitions for the Allies, and thus from the German view, was a legitimate target. She made the run to and from New York about every four weeks until sunk by a German U-boat on May 7, 1915 (*Illustré*, 1914).

Directly below the Cunard Line advertisement was one for the American Line whose ships sailed under the American flag and therefore not targeted by German U-boats. The American Line also had a ship, *New York,* leaving New York for Liverpool on May 1, but at noon. Presumably, *New York* was not as luxurious or as fast as *Lusitania*; however, she was definitely safer. As with all trans–Atlantic liners at the time, she was under booked.

On May 1, the *New York Times* contacted the Cunard Line about the warning. The Line's New York agent, Charles P. Sumner, first dismissed the warning as a fraud or prank to destroy Cunard's business. "'The Germans,' said Mr. Sumner, 'have been trying to spoil our trade for some time. I anticipate that from this time on every German method that can be devised will be used to keep people from traveling on our ships.'"[33]

When pressed as to the possible danger, especially from submarine attack, Sumner said, "Yes; as for submarines, I have no fear of them whatever."[34] Of course, he was in a safe office in New York and not aboard the ship.

Lusitania slipped out of New York harbor at noon on May 1, 1915. Captain William Turner was in charge. She carried 1,257 passengers (including 129 children) and was only a little over half full. Most of the passengers initially learned of the German warning either dockside or aboard the ship. Practically no one cancelled, very probably because of the timing of the warning, coming as it did only hours before scheduled departure. There was simply insufficient time for most to react. At sea, some passengers sensed something amiss. Captain Turner refused to order lifeboat drill for the passengers, and many never learned how to put on their buoyant lifebelts. The captain's excuse for this omission was that it might cause panic and worry among his travelers. The passengers observed that the crew never had any actual practice in launching a lifeboat. The lackadaisical attitude of the captain to the danger of submarine attack seemed insane to some.[35] It was as if he relished thumbing his nose at the German warning.

On May 6, *Lusitania* reached the war zone, at the southern end of the Irish Sea, and began to turn north for the run to Liverpool. Here the German submarine U-20 waited for its prey, having already sunk three British ships in the previous few days. The British Navy knew of the U-20 and radioed a warning to *Lusitania*.[36] That evening, nervous passengers formed a committee to instruct all, especially the children, how to put on lifebelts. Captain Turner approved of the committee's agenda but cautioned them not to imply that the safety measure was at all urgent.[37] He evidently believed that because of its speed, *Lusitania* was submarine proof; she could out run the danger. Men who risked their lives in trans–Atlantic shipping strongly disagreed. "A torpedo, they said, could travel faster than any ship, and should the Lusitania or any other liner pass within short range of a submarine all the speed in the world could not get those ships out of the way of a properly aimed Whitehead torpedo."[38]

A submarine making a torpedo attack had to lead its target, much as a sportsman does when shooting birds, i.e., the bird literally flies into the shotgun pellets. Thus, the target ship should be on a steady straight course to facilitate the estimation of the lead by the U-boat, i.e., the U-boat captain aimed the torpedo to a spot slightly ahead of the ship. Just as a bird flying erratically decreases its chance of being hit, a ship zigzagging is also harder to hit. On May 7, on a sunny morning with a flat sea and the Irish coast in view, Captain Turner ordered a straight course at a constant speed for 12 miles (19.3 km) and then left the bridge for his cabin.[39] Turner's order doomed *Lusitania*. He did not know that all morning a U-boat had been stalking him, trying to get close enough to try a shot. Then, in disbelief, the U-boat captain watched as the great ship turned toward him and began her straight 12 miles (19.3 km) run. He aligned his boat to be at a right angle to the ship as it passed.

On board the ship, the passengers were at luncheon or ambling around the deck looking at the Irish coast. There seemed to be no official concern that the ship was in a war zone and that a U-boat was close by despite a second and more urgent warning sent by the British Navy. Lifebelts remained stowed in staterooms below decks. Captain Turner seemed oblivious to the danger. Just after noon, at a distance of about 800 yards, the U-20 launched a single torpedo. The torpedo measured 20 feet in length, weighed 3,000 pounds and had a warhead of 350 pounds of explosive; it took 35 seconds to reach *Lusitania*, during which time the ship traveled forward 1,200 feet. The torpedo struck the ship on the starboard side approximately 180 feet aft of the bow, 10 feet below the water.[40] It was a near perfect shot. An explosion and then a second explosion (cause of which is a mystery)—the torpedo tore open a 5,000 square foot hole in the hull and the secondary explosion opened another 5,000 square feet to the sea.[41] The forward momentum of the ship increased the rate of water entry, much like a scoop, causing *Lusitania* to ship over 800 tons of water per minute from the torpedo damage. Although Captain Turner ordered the portholes closed, as required in a war zone, he sent no one to check. Because many portholes were open, they accounted for another 375 tons per minute as the ship listed.[42]

On board, there was chaos as people fled to their staterooms below decks for lifebelts. Many took the elevators. Unfortunately, the ship's electrical power system failed four minutes after the torpedo struck. The elevators stopped, trapping people between floors, the elevator cars with their elegant grills became cages for the doomed.[43] On deck, people fought for lifebelts and places on lifeboats. It was everyone for himself, rather than women and children first.[44] *Lusitania* sank in 18 minutes. Among those on board, passengers and crew,

1,198 perished including 128 Americans. Of the 129 children on board, 94 died.[45] Captain Turner did not go down with his ship; he survived.

Initially Kaiser Wilhelm and his officials viewed the sinking as a great victory; however, once the allied and neutral press began portraying him as a barbarian killing innocent women and children, the victory became a public relations disaster. It was another Louvain. Excuses and explanations could not erase the senseless slaughter of civilians; even the feeble justification that a warning had been published went nowhere. William Gerard, the outspoken American ambassador in Berlin, put it this way to the German Chancellor, "Your argument about the *Lusitania* amounts to just this. If I were to write a note to your sister and say: 'If you go out on the Wilhelm Platz, I will shoot you' and if she did go out on the Wilhelm Platz and I shot her — that would be her fault, wouldn't it?"[46]

A few days before *Lusitania* sailed on May 1, the *New York Times* ran the following story: "Mme. Marie Depage, wife of Dr. Antoine Depage, surgeon to King Albert, who is in charge of the entire field force of the Belgian Red Cross will sail for home on Saturday on the Lusitania. She has been in this country soliciting subscriptions for the Belgian Red Cross and has succeeded in collecting $100,000 in money and $50,000 of supplies."[47]

Mme. Marie Depage was among those who perished. She was in the United States raising funds for the *Ambulance de l'Océan* at La Panne (see Chapter 5). Earlier that year she was in Brussels working at the Ecole d'Infirmières Diplômées, a nursing school established by her husband. From Brussels, she managed somehow to cross into neutral Holland and from there, she traveled to the United States.

Marie Depage's close friend in Brussels was the English nurse Edith Cavell. In 1907, Edith Cavell came to Brussels from England to establish and run a nursing school. Dr. Antione Depage, professor of medicine at the University of Brussels and head of a surgical institute, invited her to teach modern English nursing practices in Belgium, where, according to Depage, nursing had not progressed beyond the days of the Napoleonic Wars. In Belgium at that time most nurses were nuns; they were caring but untrained in modern nursing practices. Dr. Depage's hope was to establish a secular nursing school, an idea not popular with Church authorities. Depage appointed Edith Cavell Directress of the Ecole d'Infirmières Diplômées on the rue de la Culture[48] in what was at that time a suburb of Brussels. The nursing school consisted of four town houses. Marie Depage assisted Edith Cavell at the school, often defusing conflicts between her hardheaded husband and the equally stubborn Cavell.[49] When Marie Depage left Brussels in the spring of 1915, both she and her friend Cavell had become criminals in the eyes of the Germans because of their efforts to aid the enemy. As she left for America, Marie urged her friend,

"You will exercise every caution, will you not?"[50] Neither woman would survive the year.

After the Germans entered Brussels (August 20, 1914), the city filled with German wounded. Cavell and her nurses tended German soldiers because, as far as she was concerned, a wounded man was a patient who needed help, regardless of what language he spoke. An American businessman and his wife residing in Brussels knew Edith Cavell. A few days after the Germans arrived they advised her to leave and go to London. She declined.

> "I intend to devote my services to the relief of suffering humanity, and whether they are English, French or German, I will serve them just the same." Under her direction all empty houses were converted into hospitals for the wounded, and my wife and myself had a ward with 150 beds in it to look after.[51]

Cavell also aided the enemy, at least the enemy from a German point of view. Mons and other battles in Belgium stranded many British, French and Belgian soldiers behind German lines. To help these men escape, Belgians guided Allied soldiers from the countryside near the battlefields into the city of Brussels, and from there on to neutral Holland where ships transported the men to England where they usually rejoined their respective armies. The buildings on the rue de la Culture housed these men while they were in Brussels. It became the main Brussels safe house; by the summer of 1915, more than 200 men had been sheltered there and sent on. Understandably, the Germans went to great efforts to close down this underground railroad since the men who escaped returned to fight again.

> On August 5, 1915, Miss Edith Cavell, an Englishwoman, directress of a large nursing home at Brussels, was quietly arrested by the German authorities and confined in the prison of St. Gilles on the charge that she had aided stragglers from the Allied armies to escape across the frontier from Belgium to Holland, furnishing them with money, clothing, and information concerning the route to be followed. It was some time before news of Miss Cavell's arrest was received by the American Legation.[52]

After her arrest at the nursing school on the afternoon of August 5, a German guard escorted Cavell to the *Kommandantur* in the rue de la Loi for questioning. She spilled the beans about everything to her German interrogators, almost bragging about how many men she had helped escape; worse than that, she gave away the names of her confederates and the locations of other safe houses. The Germans asked and she talked. She had done the right thing and had no remorse; God and honor were on her side. She signed a confession that was devastating.[53] "This was a shattering statement, an astounding exposure of those with whom she had worked, and it just cannot be explained entirely in terms of her natural instinct always to speak the truth."[54]

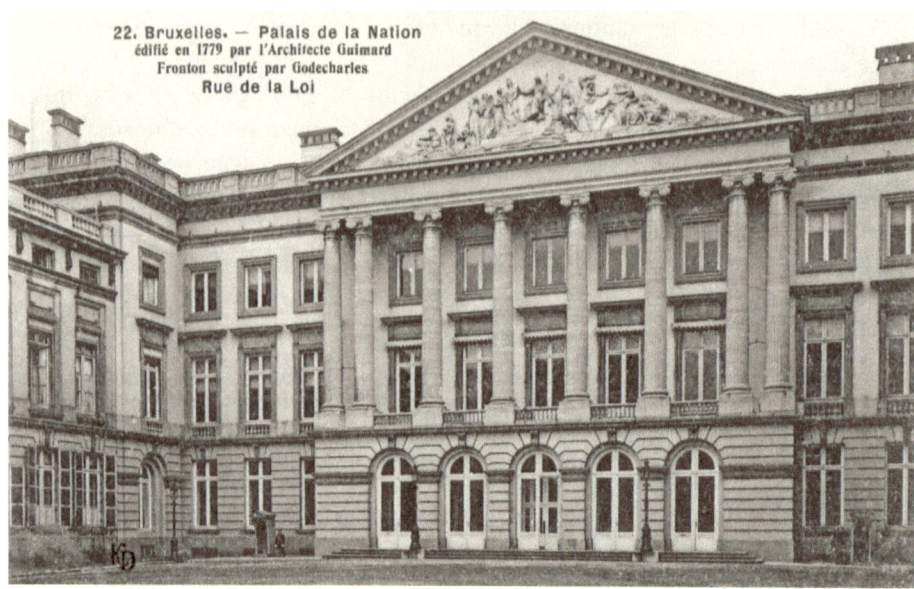

The Palais de la Nation, Brussels. It was in this building that the English nurse Edith Cavell was tried by a German military court, convicted and sentenced to death by firing squad. The Senate Chamber, where the trial took place, has a plaque with her name and others who suffered the same fate (Klekowski collection).

No one knew Cavell's motivation in confessing to all and implicating her friends. Whitlock described Cavell as "a woman of refinement and education; she knew French well; she was deeply religious, with a conscience almost puritan, and she was very stern with herself in what she conceived to be her duty."[55]

On August 10, the Germans transferred her to St. Gilles Prison, a castellated nineteenth century Gothic structure located in the suburbs of Brussels. Edith Cavell spent two months in her cell, mostly alone. She prayed and read. Whitlock tried to see her; he tried to get the American Legation lawyer, Gaston de Leval, to represent her. The German authorities refused to allow any contact or representation. "Lawyers defending prisoners before German military courts were not allowed to see their clients before the trial and were shown none of the documents of the prosecution. It was thus manifestly impossible to prepare any defense save in the presence of the court during the progress of the trial."[56]

On October 7, 1915, the authorities moved Cavell to the *Kommandantur* for trial in the Belgian senate chamber.[57] The charge was conducting soldiers to the enemy, for which the penalty was death. Cavell was her own worst witness; again, she admitted everything. Unfortunately, the German judge in charge had lost a son at the front fighting the English. The trial ended the following day and the prosecution asked for a sentence of death. On the afternoon of October 11, the court delivered a verdict, death by firing squad on the morning of October 12. The American Legation did not learn of the death sentence until nine o'clock that evening. Now came a frenetic evening as Hugh Gibson, the American Legation secretary, Gaston de Leval, the American Legation lawyer,[58] and the Marquis de Villalobar, Minister of the Spanish Legation, drove around Brussels trying to get some member of the German command to stay the execution to allow time for mounting a plea for clemency.

> When everything else had failed we asked Lancken [Baron von der Lancken, head of the Politische Abteilung, political department] to look at the case from the point of view solely of German interests, assuring him that the execution of Miss Cavell would do Germany infinite harm. We reminded him of the burning of Louvain and the sinking of the *Lusitania*, and told him that this murder would rank with those two affairs and would stir all civilized countries with horror and disgust.[59]

The nurses from Cavell's school were at the American Legation under the care of Mrs. Whitlock. Brand Whitlock was in bed, collapsed from stress. No one really believed that the verdict would be death. Who would shoot a nurse who had cared for German wounded? She would probably just get a prison sentence—why kill her? It was insane.

Early in the morning of October 12, the gates of St. Gilles Prison[60] opened and an automobile emerged, entering the square in front of the prison. Its passengers included Edith Cavell and one of her confederates, a Belgian named Philippe Baucq; their destination was the Tir National,[61] the national shooting range.

> Nurse Cavell was brought in a gray motor car with Baucq, the Belgian, who would probably not have been shot except that it would not be decent to shoot only one Englishman. There must be a Belgian as well. Both were marched near the place where there are platoon ranges. There was a chair. Nurse Cavell had to sit on it. They bound her eyes, and twelve soldiers shot her dead.[62]

With the stresses of dealing with the German occupation and then the Cavell affair, Whitlock was on the verge of a nervous breakdown. The experience of being a city mayor in Ohio, even with its cutthroat politics, never prepared him for fifteen months in Brussels under German occupation. The sensitive novelist in him cracked. Hearing of his condition, the U.S. State Department granted him a two-month leave of absence to recover his health. On November 6, 1915, Brand and Nell Whitlock left Belgium for Holland; in Rotterdam they boarded the Holland-America liner *Ryndam*, sailing on November 10 for New York. The crossing was a rough one, with northwesterly gales pummeling the ship and destroying two lifeboats. Two days late, the battered ship entered New York harbor. Whitlock said the sea journey benefited him greatly, foul weather being less stressful than dealing with German authorities. To friends he appeared almost cadaverous. Immediately, Washington insiders speculated about the real reason for his return. It had to be more than health. "No one in this old and disillusioned and cynical Europe ever believes anything a diplomatist says, but seeks in his utterances every meaning save that which they would seem to have been framed to convey."[63]

Cynical Americans were just as bad. Many speculated that Brand Whitlock really came home to become the Democratic candidate for Vice-President in the 1916 Woodrow Wilson reelection bid. Others believed that he would be the Democratic candidate for Governor of Ohio.[64] He really just came home to recuperate, make his report to Washington, and see his friends and family in Ohio. It was only a working vacation! Cynical Europeans questioned whether he would return to Brussels; few believed he would. He did. The Whitlocks arrived in Rotterdam on January 9, 1916, and proceeded by automobile to the American Legation in Brussels the following day.[65]

Chapter 7

Is Food a Weapon?

All measures which conduce to the attainment of the object of war are permissible and these may be summarized in the two ideas of violence and cunning. What is permissible includes every means of war without which the object of the war cannot be attained. All means which modern invention affords, including the fullest, most dangerous, and most massive means of destruction, may be utilized.[1]—*Kriegsbrauch im Landkriege*

Now although according to the modern conception of war, it is primarily concerned with the persons belonging to the opposing armies, yet no citizen or inhabitant of a State occupied by a hostile army can altogether escape the burdens, restrictions, sacrifices, and inconveniences which are the natural consequence of a State of War. A war conducted with energy cannot be directed merely against the combatants of the Enemy State.[2]—*Kriegsbrauch im Landkriege*

A critical question facing the Imperial German Army in the fall of 1914 dealt with noncombatants: was it to Germany's advantage to allow the citizens of occupied Belgium to starve or was it advantageous to make some arrangement to feed them? Fortunately, Germany chose the latter. The decision was self-serving and followed the spirit of the *Kriegsbrauch im Landkriege*—it averted food riots behind German lines.

Although nearly all arable land in Belgium was under cultivation, there was never enough food to sustain its seven million inhabitants. Even in times of peace, Belgium imported 75 percent of the food necessary to feed its population; it was an industrial economy dependent upon trade to earn cash to purchase food and was probably the most industrialized country in Europe. The war isolated the country and brought manufacturing and trade to an end. The war also greatly reduced the farm yields for 1914. Because the Germans invaded in August before the harvest was complete, the locally produced food quota was considerably less that year. Many crops rotted in the fields when both the Belgian and German armies commandeered farm horses to pull artillery or wagons. Farm workers disappeared as the young men who worked the land joined the Belgian Army. Finally, the Germans requisitioned what little was left to sustain their invasion drive. By the end of September 1914, the local population faced starvation.

> The complete commercial isolation of a land, its encircling by a steel ring that permits no import of foods or raw materials for industry or commodities for commerce, and no export of manufactures or money or exchange even, may or may not mean swift catastrophe to the country. It depends on the degree of the country's self-sustainingness.... It has not spelled speedy catastrophe to Germany. But to a highly industrialized land like Belgium, whose imports and exports are, in normal times, greater per capita than those of any other country, whose annual production of bread-grains equals but one-fourth of its annual bread-consumption, whose self-sustaining agricultural class is but one-sixth of its total population, such an isolation means swift catastrophe and horror. The steel ring means starvation to the people inside of it.[3]

The major obstacle for provisioning Belgium using international sources of food was Great Britain. The same reason that compelled Germany to support the import of food into Belgium made the British view food as a weapon. Food riots in Belgium could threaten German supply lines, forcing the commitment of troops and resources away from the front. The British also must have read the *Kriegsbrauch im Landkriege.*

> The shooting down of starving mobs in city streets by machine guns is no indication of a successful civil administration of a land.... Peace and quiet are indications of successful civil administration, but people do not starve peacefully and quietly, and a starving population of ten millions [in Occupied Belgium and France] would, even without guns or bombs, be a serious group to handle.[4]

In the fall of 1914, prominent members of the British Cabinet, including Lord Kitchener at the War Office, Lloyd George at the Exchequer, and Winston Churchill at the Admiralty, "vehemently opposed shipping any food whatever into Belgium."[5] Since the British Navy controlled the sea ways, Belgian aid depended upon British acquiescence.

Back in Brussels and unaware of possible British opposition, — after all the British had entered the war to help Belgium — business leaders founded a charitable organization to import and distribute food. Named the Comité Central de Secours et d'Alimentation, its mission was to feed Brussels' needy. Soon, however, recognizing that starvation was nationwide, the Comité Central metamorphosed into the Comité National with an expanded mission to feed the entire country. Both organizations listed the American and Spanish Ministers to Belgium, Brand Whitlock and the Marquis de Villalobar, respectively, as formal patrons. On September 20, the Comité Central sent Millard Shaler, an American mining engineer living in Brussels, to purchase food abroad. He carried with him a letter of credit for $100,000 (£20,000) and a written assurance from the German governor-general of occupied Belgium.

> The first agreement given by the German authorities in immediate control of Belgium granted permission for the import of food into Belgium by way of the Holland frontier and guaranteed that all such imported foodstuffs would be entirely free from requisition by the German Army. This guarantee was given in early September, 1914, by Baron von der Goltz, then Governor-General of Belgium, to the Americans.[6]

Arriving in London on September 26, 1914, Shaler readily purchased 1,500 tons of cereals. The purchase turned out to be the easy part; getting an export permit from the British government proved to be a bit more difficult. Red tape, conflicting diplomatic demands, obstructionist rules and unforeseen requirements conspired to keep the cereals in Britain. On October 6, a frustrated Millard Shaler, still without an export permit, met his old friend and fellow mining engineer Herbert Hoover.[7]

When the war began, Herbert Hoover had been living in London for ten years. A partner in a prestigious mining firm, Hoover directed a global network of mining and engineering projects ranging from gold mines in Australia and copper mines in Russia to oil companies in California. He was a graduate of Stanford University (class of 1895), nearly forty years old, very wealthy, and highly regarded in British financial and government circles. For the first month of the war, Hoover worked with Ambassador Walter Hines Page and the American Embassy assisting thousands of "busted Yankees" stranded in England, i.e., American tourists who found themselves without funds since traveler's checks were nearly impossible to cash and letters of credit not honored during the first days of the war. By the end of September 1914, most of these travelers were on their way home. On October 3, Hoover's wife Lou and their two sons boarded *Lusitania* for New York. Three days later, Hoover met Millard Shaler and learned of the plight of the Belgians and the intractability of the British regarding the shipment of food aid. He agreed to meet with the British government.

October became a month of meetings focused on getting food to Belgium, and Hoover chaired them all. The Comité Central sent Baron Léon Lambert and wealthy Belgian banker Emile Francqui to London. Whitlock fretted that Francqui might give the wrong impression because "He presented the appearance of one too well-fed to be exhibited in London as an example of a starving *Belgium*."[8] The Belgians met with Hoover, Millard Shaler, Hugh Gibson, the American Ambassador Walter Hines Page and the Spanish Ambassador to Great Britain Alfonso Merry del Val to work out ways to feed Belgium. Communicating via cable, Hoover included Brand Whitlock, the Marquis de Villalobar, James W. Gerard, American Ambassador to the German Imperial Court in Berlin, and Jongkeer de Weede, the Dutch Minister to the Belgian Government at Le Havre. Together with other business leaders in the United States and Belgium, the group became the nucleus of the Commission for Relief in Belgium (C.R.B.) with Herbert Hoover as chairman.[9] The C.R.B. eventually would become the most important volunteer relief organization of the war. For the present, there was still the "small" problem of British export permits. The British wanted assurances that the imported food would feed only the civilian population; under no circumstances could the German Army use these imports. To guarantee this control, the food should be under the supervision of an American staff in Belgium. The Germans countered with demands that the British would not stop the C.R.B. ships and that the C.R.B. could purchase foodstuffs in Britain and its colonies.

> As each government wished the other to give its assurances as a prerequisite to giving its own, some manœuvering was necessary to effect a practical simultaneousness of agreement. This was effected, however, before the end of November.[10]

In the meantime, the C.R.B. began to purchase cereals (wheat, rice, peas, and beans) with Belgian funds ($500,000) secured by Emile Francqui from the already existing Belgian Relief Fund. By the last week of October, the C.R.B. had purchased 10,000 tons of cereals and had chartered four steamships, one English and three Dutch, to transport the food to Rotterdam for canal transport into Belgium. All that was missing was the British export permit. With the last sack of food stowed aboard and the hatches bolted down, Hoover went into action; his *modus operandi* was, "If a thing was really necessary, we did it first and asked permission afterwards."[11] Rather than adhering to proper British procedure and following the maze of red-tape-clogged channels almost designed to delay rather than to expedite, Hoover went in person to the Cabinet Minister in charge and brazenly asked for the permit.

> "Out of the question," said the distinguished Minister. "There is no time, in the first place, and if there was there are no good wagons to be spared by the railways, no dock hands, and no steamers; moreover the Channel is closed for a week to merchant vessels while troops are being transported to the Continent."
>
> "I have managed to get all of these things," Hoover replied, quietly; "and am now through with them all except the steamers. The wire tells me that these are now loaded and ready to sail, and I have come to have you arrange for their clearance."
>
> The great man gasped. "There have been — there are even now — men in the Tower for less than you have done," he ejaculated. "If it was for anything but Belgian Relief — if it was anybody but you, young man — I should hate to think of what might happen. As it is — er — I suppose there is nothing to do but congratulate you on a jolly clever coup. I'll see about the clearance at once."[12]

You either loved the high-handed young man from Stanford or hated him. Hoover's forceful personality set the tone for the C.R.B.; he valued action over delay, achievements instead of excuses. On November 4, 1914, the first shipment of food from outside Belgium arrived in Brussels. While the British and German governments were debating the conditions under which the C.R.B. would operate, the C.R.B. was operating.

The next possible "deal-buster" dealt with native foodstuffs. Although Belgian farms produced little, the British stipulated that what the farms did produce should be for Belgians only. Of special concern was the up-coming harvest of 1915.

> The British insistence that we could not continue to take food into Belgium unless the Germans agreed not alone to refrain from requisition of such imported foodstuffs, but to refrain from taking for their army any of the native foodstuffs, made it necessary for us to use all effort to get such a guarantee and get it quickly.[13]

This was a much tougher negotiation since it was normal for a conquering army to live off the land. The German government steadfastly maintained that in accord with international practice in time of war it had the right to maintain its army of occupation on the products of the occupied country. In April 1915, the British threatened to shut down the C.R.B. unless Germany agreed on the native food question. Hoover and Ambassador Gerard pushed negotiations in Berlin, while Whitlock, the Marquis de Villalobar and Dutch Chargé d'Affaires Mynheer Vollenhoven vigorously pursued the matter with Governor-General von Bissing in Brussels. On July 4, 1915, when von Bissing formally gave his assurance not to requisition native foods, another crisis passed. The only exception allowed was the "occasional small personal purchases by individual soldiers not representing the army's commissary department."[14] A Belgian farmer could sell an apple to a German soldier but not a bushel of apples to an army cook.

The C.R.B. had its principal offices in New York, London, Rotterdam and Brussels. The port of entry for all C.R.B. ships was Rotterdam. As such, this port city became the most critical link in the supply chain, with all C.R.B. foodstuffs funneling through the Dutch port. Hoover appointed his friend and fellow mining engineer Captain J.F. Lucey in charge of the Rotterdam office. A fellow Californian and the same age as Hoover, both were 40 in 1914, Captain Lucey had previously served in the U.S. Army in the Philippines and worked in the goldfields of Alaska as well as mines in Mexico and the American West. He was in Romania when the war began. He left there on October 10, 1914, arriving in London on October 22. The following day Hoover called and convinced Lucey to help the C.R.B. Three days later, he was in Rotterdam with seven Rhodes scholars as staff.[15] However, they were all that was in Rotterdam; there were no relief ships.

As a matter of fact none arrived for two weeks, not because the commission could not obtain the food, but because of the red tape in the British War Office, certain officials of which considered the move to feed the Belgians a mistake from the military standpoint.[16]

In the meantime, across the border people were starving. In the city of Liège, 100 miles (161 km) away, 600,000 men, women and children had only 3 days of rations left. Liège was the first Belgian city to fall to the Germans and consequently was in the direst need. Captain Lucey tried to purchase foodstuffs in Holland, but the French and British Legations thwarted him. "We did not want red tape; we wanted food, and at once," he said.[17] Then the captain learned there were 10,000 tons of grain stowed aboard several ships docked in different ports on the Dutch coast. The ships were someone's war booty; however, their ownership was debatable. The ships were originally from Antwerp and their cargos belonged to German merchants. During the final days of the siege of Antwerp, the Belgians requisitioned the ships and sailed them to Holland. Under Dutch law, since the ships had entered in time of war, they were Dutch property. Lucey devised a plan to steal the grain, valued at $1,000,000, from the German/Belgian/Dutch ships. "I dictated a statement giving me absolute authority to get the grain on behalf of the Belgian Government, which claimed it, and I concluded it had as much right to the grain as the German or Dutch Governments. I got the members of the Belgian committee to sign this statement."[18]

With 50,000 francs to cover unforeseen costs, Captain Lucey set off to the port holding 3 of the ships. He immediately ran into bureaucratic problems; the captains of the ships, understandably, refused to honor his dubious papers. They required something signed by the Belgian Consul in Holland. A representative of the Consul arrived and convinced the captains to go along with the scheme. Lucey immediately hired 500 stevedores to transfer the sacks of grain to other ships, a feat they accomplished in record time; he rightly thought that if he sailed into Rotterdam harbor in the original vessels eyebrows might raise. Soon he was ready to sail. "Then the problem of clearance came up. There was no time to bother with red tape, and we issued clearance papers ourselves. They were not forgeries: we merely assumed the authority of issuing them."[19]

Bearing their ersatz clearance papers, the ships arrived in Rotterdam where stevedores quickly loaded the grain into a special train. The sacks of grain arrived in Liège just as the city's food rations ran out. Lucey managed to steal 5,000 tons of grain before the Dutch and Germans found out about the "Grain Caper." When they did, their diplomats howled. Captain Lucey took Hoover's *modus operandi*, "If a thing was really necessary, we did it first and asked permission afterwards," a step further. For Lucey, "If a thing was really necessary, we FORGED the permission and did it, and dealt with the consequences afterwards." Lucey remained in charge at Rotterdam for 4 months and organized the sea to land transfer port for C.R.B. foodstuffs.

> Once in Rotterdam, the great ships become the centres of extraordinary activity. Giant floating elevators come up to them, sometimes one or two on each side, and a group of empty canal boats cluster around. The hungry pipes of the elevators are thrust down into the mass of wheat in the hold, and other pipes are let down into the lighters; then the precious wheat streams run up and out of the ship and down and into the canal boats.[20]

If the cargo consisted of boxes, barrels or sacks of foodstuffs, stevedores took the place of elevators in loading the canal boats. From the ship, tugs towed long strings of boats into the canals of Holland and then Belgium. Some boats had their own gasoline engines and traveled independently.

In the first months of the war, Belgium's incredible network of canals, the principal basis of its internal transportation system, was in tatters. When the German Army requisitioned large numbers of canal boats for its own transport needs, many canal-boat captains took their boats out of Belgium to escape seizure. The canals themselves were not navigable, with sunken barges and blown-up locks blocking many stretches. Nor was the Belgian railroad system in better shape; most of its rolling stock was in France and the Belgian Army had destroyed many critical railroad bridges during its retreat. Thus, food ships could reach Rotterdam readily enough, but in the final months of 1914, getting their cargos into Belgium was another matter. Captain Lucey and his staff succeeded in opening the constipated Belgian canal system, converting the main transportation network for the food aid.

> Practically all the food comes in from Holland by the three canals *via* Maastricht and the Meuse, *via* Brussels, or that through East Flanders to Mons and Charleroi. When the Commission opened its work all three of these waterways were blocked, but in some places with the help of the Germans, and in some where they were allowed to approach the canals with the aid of the Belgians, the Americans have now succeeded in making all three navigable for their small lighters.[21]

Railroads did contribute to the distribution of foodstuffs. There were two types of railway systems operating in Belgium: standard-gauge main trunk lines and narrow-gauge lines that connected the villages with the large centers. The German Army relied upon standard-gauge railways to move men and supplies across Belgium, so these railroads were mostly unavailable to the C.R.B. Since narrow-gauge lines were less important militarily, these lines moved food from warehouses served by canals into small villages and hamlets.

> The Dutch Government generously gave the Commission free railroad transport on all the Dutch railroads, and an agreement was reached with the German

Government whereby only one half the regular tariff should be paid by us for freight inside of the occupied territory.[22]

The Comité National, headed by Emile Francqui, worked through communal, regional and provincial committees to distribute the food to the Belgian needy. Thirty-five thousand Belgians gave volunteer service to the Comité National.

Thirty-five to forty Americans, known as delegates or *délégués Américain*, supervised the transport of C.R.B. foodstuffs from Rotterdam to distribution centers in Belgium and from these to areas of the greatest need. The delegate's task was to satisfy the British that imported food went only to the Belgians and that the Germans were living up to their guarantees concerning C.R.B. aid and locally grown foods. These delegates in the field were essentially referees for a gentleman's agreement between two belligerents who never really trusted each other. Baron von Bissing, the Governor-General of Belgium, did his best to stand by the agreement. He ordered notices safeguarding the supplies from German requisition affixed to all C.R.B. warehouses, canal boats, railroad cars, motor trucks and wagons.

> Comité National de Secours et D'Alimentation
> Commission for Relief in Belgium
> Service of storage of foodstuffs, provisions and divers merchandise
> By order of his Excellency, the Governor General in Belgium,
> all stocks stored in this warehouse, belonging to the Comité National de Secours et d'Alimentation, or to the Commission for Relief in Belgium, and intended for the civil population of Belgium shall be neither seized nor requisitioned by German military or civil authorities.
> Brussels[23]

The German Government in Belgium lived up to its guarantees respecting the Commission's imported food in such measure that we may honestly say that the Germans got practically none of this food.[24]

American C.R.B. delegates had about twenty-five automobiles with Belgian chauffeurs assigned to them. German authorities issued passes permitting delegates to travel nearly anywhere, except near the front. Often in out-of-the-way places, *Monsieur le Délégué* became a voice of reason, smoothing German/Belgian frictions. After a day in the field, *Monsieur le Délégué* returned home. For one group of eight delegates based in Brussels, home was rather sumptuous. They lived in an elegant residence on one of the most prestigious avenues in the city.[25]

"The life of an American delegate is a hard life," Maverick [Robert V. Maverick, Princeton] one day said whimsically. "Here we are forced to live in a place quite as humble as the average house that you see on Fifth Avenue overlooking Central Park. I am reduced to the humiliation of riding about in an Overland car with a chauffeur only in half livery. To-night I shall probably be obliged to dine at the Taverne Royale."[26]

Another occupant of the "elegant residence" was Edward D. Curtis (Harvard). He served as a courier, carrying mail between Brussels, Antwerp and Rotterdam two or three times a week. He made the trip in a long, low, rakish automobile provided by Mr. Ernest Solvay, the president of the Comité National and probably the richest man in Belgium. Curtis and his chauffeur "turned up in every German *Kommandantur en route,* usually under arrest."[27] The Germans arrested him seventeen times! After the war, Belgium decorated him as a Chevalier of the Order of Couronne for his service.[28]

Because they traveled so widely and some frequently crossed back and forth between Belgium and Holland, C.R.B. delegates were always under suspicion of espionage. German road guards frequently stopped C.R.B. autos to search for letters, contraband newspapers, or written materials concerning the German military. The checks were not trivial and the delegates had strict instructions never to carry anything suspicious.

> Two soldiers inspected the car, prodding cushions, examining the hood, washing their hands in the gasoline tank, which, by the way, they were surprised to find (by means of a wire which they thrust into it) was divided into compartments. At first they thought they had made a great discovery — secret compartments for letters, and God knows what else; but after consultation with an under-officer in the garb of a motor-cyclist, they decided to accept our explanation of the phenomenon, finding that there were some German cars with tanks built that way, to keep the gasoline from swashing around too much.[29]

There were some delegates, while not carrying written materials, certainly made injudicious remarks about what they had seen in Belgium. In late 1915, these remarks reached the Rotterdam C.R.B. office where an American, later described, of course, as unbalanced mentally, reported what he had heard to the German intelligence staff at The Hague, who in turn passed it on to Brussels. The Germans, rightly, filed espionage charges against three delegates: the ones with the loose lips and the Rotterdam contact. Hoover came to their rescue, first arguing that the charges were untrue but eventually conceding the argument and removing the Rotterdam man and agreeing to replace any delegate who did not scrupulously observe the obligation of neutrality. Back in New York, the ex–Rotterdamer immediately became associated with a leading pro–German organization, confirming suspicions about his bias.[30] Fortunately, this case was an exception; most delegates observed the neutrality rule.

The majority of the difficulties between American delegates and German military were testosterone-based. Arrogant German officers and impudent (cheeky?) Americans proved to be a volatile mix. Mild infractions of military courtesy such as failing to salute or address officers as *Herr Leutnant* or *Herr*

Hauptmann (Captain) or *Herr Major* infuriated Prussian sensitivities. Sometimes Prussian sensitivities reacted to the strangest provocation, such as simply hearing English spoken. The Teutonic hatred of the English as an enemy translated into hatred of the language. The American author Julia Helen Twells resided in Brussels during the war; she recalled an instance of language intolerance that nearly led to a diplomatic incident.

> One day a number of Alimentation-Commission men, all Americans, were seated together in a café; and, as all mention of the war was, by their own decision, prohibited, were jovially recounting reminiscences of happier times. Not far from them sat five young officers stiffly upright in gilt-buttoned parade dress and high red collars. They constantly turned their sheared heads to cast severe glances at the merry group who, though noting the angry eyes flashing under pale, knitted brows, paid no attention.[31]

Finally, the Germans could no longer stand the presumed insulting behavior of the Americans; a well-fed officer swaggered over to their table.

> "You shall not speak English where officers of the German army are seated!" he ejaculated, through lips pale and quivering with rage.
> "Indeed? Why not?" inquired one of the party, an athletic creature who could have pounded the little fatty to a pulp.
> "Because *I* say it!" was the reply; "the English language is distasteful to us, and should be officially forbidden in Brussels."
> "But it isn't!" retorted the other in Americanized German.[32]

And so it went, each exchange increasing the likelihood of a fistfight. Fearing a scandal brought upon the Commission, especially after the American called the officer a "D--- little swine!," the saner Yanks at the table separated the two and hustled their hot-headed colleague out of the café.

Then there was the time a delegate named Ridgley Lytle (Princeton) smashed his automobile into an auto belonging to a German official. The American was not repentant.

> Lytle's letter to the Governor of the province of Luxemburg [a province of Belgium and where the accident occurred] was not calculated to smooth the feelings of the Governor, and the Governor wrote back stating that Mr. Lytle's letter and his bearing at the time of the examination and detention were such that he, the Governor, felt called upon to "proceed against him for insult"—unless Lytle personally apologize. Lytle preferred to leave the country and so the matter rested.[33]

Official histories of the C.R.B. published during or immediately after the war omitted anything that might reflect negatively on the behavior of delegates in occupied Belgium. The writers presented a sanitized, somewhat-mythical story where everyone acted properly, with restraint, prudence and tact being the rule. C.R.B. regulations censored what the delegates said in letters home, controlling the message even to family and friends.[34] Since such letters often appeared in local newspapers, the C.R.B. controlled the message at that level also.

> Altogether about two hundred Americans represented the C.R.B. at various times inside of Belgium. They were mostly young university men, representing forty different American colleges and universities in their allegiance. A group of twenty Rhodes Scholars whom Hoover hurriedly recruited from Oxford at the beginning of the work was the pioneer lot. All of these two hundred were selected for intelligence, honor, discretion, and idealism.[35]

Using Rhodes scholars made for good publicity back home, but on the ground in Belgium there were difficulties. Although never mentioned in their published works, both Brand Whitlock and Hugh Gibson, in their private letters, believed using Rhodes men was a blunder. They proved to be too young, too inexperienced, too impulsive and too headstrong to fulfill their mission — whatever that was. Both Whitlock and Gibson pleaded with Hoover to send the Rhodes boys back to Oxford; they were better suited to graduate school than gallivanting about Belgium. Gibson wrote, "Most of the Rhodes scholars are half-baked kids who ought not to be allowed to leave school." Whitlock described them as, "a lot of impulsive, ignorant young doctors of Philosophy." Both the German Army and the Belgian authorities were for once in agreement; the young Americans joy riding about the country in fast automobiles and intervening in things that they knew little about had to stop. The traits that made a tactful C.R.B. delegate were evidently not those the Rhodes selection committees looked for. But, of course, there were exceptions. Some Rhodes men gave extraordinary service.[36]

A few C.R.B. delegates came from the ranks of journalists. Edward Eyre Hunt (Harvard) survived the siege of Antwerp to become the C.R.B. delegate in charge of the province of Antwerp. Hunt originally traveled to Belgium as a war correspondent, free-lancing for American magazines such as *The New Republic, Collier's* and *The Outlook*. On August 25, 1914, he sailed on the Holland-America liner *Nieuw Amsterdam* from New York harbor, bound for Boulogne and Rotterdam. Also on board were 400 German-Americans and 250 Austrian-Americans volunteering to fight for their respective fatherlands; the German-speaking would-be soldiers spent their time singing "Die Wacht am Rhein" and other German airs, drilling, marching about and generally making pests of themselves. Thousands of reservists had arrived in New York in August 1914, where "Germans, Austrians, and Hungarians paraded the streets singing the songs of their fatherlands and shouting hochs to Emperors William and Franz Josef."[37] Boarding whichever liners would take them, they headed for Germany. Unfortunately for them, British and French war ships intercepted many of these trans–Atlantic liners and made their Teutonic voyagers prisoners of war.[38] *Nieuw*

Amsterdam suffered this fate off the coast of France.[39] The armored French liner *La Savoie* stopped her and determined there were German and Austrian reservists on board; *La Savoie* shepherded the neutral ship to the fortified harbor of Brest and internment for the reservists. This was Hunt's first war experience and probably his first war story.[40] He must have wondered what the reservists had been thinking about when they booked passage on a ship scheduled to stop at a French port (Boulogne) before going on to Rotterdam. The French Army never would have let them leave Boulogne.

Hunt left *Nieuw Amsterdam* at Rotterdam, crossed into Germany and traveled to Berlin where he spent about a month. He then entered Belgium, somehow made it through the German siege line fronting Antwerp and entered the city on October 6, 1914, one day before the Germans commenced the final bombardment of the city. In Antwerp, Hunt headed for the Hôtel Saint Antoine, the war correspondents' hang-out. There he met a brash American war photographer.

> "I'm Donald C. Thompson," he said, "photographer for the New York *World*. Guess I'm better known in America now than President Wilson is. I've been taking *the* pictures of this little war!"
> I showed interest. "Are you going to stay and take pictures when the Germans come in?"
> "You bet your sweet life!" exploded Thompson, recovering his animation.
> "I'm staying too. But is there really going to be a bombardment?"
> "Yes," he said, "you bet your hat there is! Come stay at my house, won't you? I've got a fine little shack with all you want to eat and a good bed. It belongs to some Belgian friends of mine, but they've gone to Holland."[41]

That was how Edward Eyre Hunt became a denizen of "Thompson's Fort" during the final days of the siege of Antwerp[42] (see Chapter 4). Hunt watched the German Army occupy the city and after a few days wandering streets deserted, "except for a few weeping women and children," he had seen enough.[43] He walked out with the refugees to Holland. Thompson opted to remain in Antwerp to photograph Germans, intent upon his quest of becoming more famous than Woodrow Wilson! Hunt visited refugee hostels and camps in Holland as well as in war-ravaged Belgium, where those who stayed now faced starvation. In Rotterdam, he met Captain Lucey on November 23, 1914, and learned of the newly formed C.R.B. There was an immediate need for Americans with business experience who spoke German and French to oversee the distribution of food in Belgium. The following day Hunt traveled to Brussels to see Brand Whitlock.

> On December eleventh I was again in Antwerp, this time holding Mr. Brand Whitlock's power-of-attorney as chief delegate of the Commission for Relief in Belgium in charge of the fortress and province — a territory as large as the State of Rhode Island, and with a population of more than a million.[44]

His first impressions were very pessimistic; it all seemed so overwhelmingly hopeless. Perhaps 30,000 refugees had returned to Antwerp to find no food, no heat and no work. Many were without homes, the bombardment having targeted some of the middle class residential areas rather than the city center. After a long meeting with the Provincial Relief Committee to discuss means of distributing the food when it arrived, Hunt went alone into the city. Walking down streets bordered with smashed and burned houses, he sought a familiar address, 74 rue du Péage,[45] the address of Thompson's Fort. He found Donald Thompson's name still penciled on the unlocked door.

> There were two candles in the hallway, and a box of matches, just as we had left them.... Down in the kitchen was the familiar clutter of bottles and pans; in the cyclone cellar where we had weathered the bombardment were the names of the four of us — Thompson, Weigle, de Meester, and me — just as they had been written for the eyes of our heirs on the night the shelling began.[46]

Shells had struck the top two floors, bringing down piles of plaster and wall debris; smashed and broken furniture, torn books and charred bed linen, all tumbled chaotically together by explosions, marked what once had been bedrooms. In addition to high explosive shells, shrapnel shells also must have struck the building because lead pellets littered the floors.

Hunt's next assignment after meeting with the Provincial Relief Committee was to make sure the canals linking his province with Rotterdam were still open — they were. Then came an unexpected visit by Herbert Hoover, who said almost nothing while sitting quietly in a chair in a dark corner of Hunt's cramped office at the American consulate. Hoover's only advice was to get a better office.

> One of the thrilling experiences of the first month's work was the coming of the "Christmas Ship," — the steamer full of Christmas gifts presented by the children of America to the children of war-ridden Belgium. I was amazed to find that before the ship docked in Rotterdam the Belgian children knew all about it.[47]

James Keeley, proprietor of *The Chicago Herald*, conceived the idea of the Christmas Ship. Newspapers from all over the United States picked up the project, including the *New York World*, the *Kansas City Star*, the *San Francisco Chronicle*, the *Cleveland Plain Dealer*, the *Pittsburg Leader* and about 200 others. The toy drive began in late August 1914. The Christmas Ship would take toys and clothing donated by Americans, many of them children, to the war orphans of Great Britain, France, Belgium, Germany, Austria, and Serbia.[48] The American response was astounding: public schools, colleges, factories, large department stores and small local stores, rich and poor, grown-ups and children all sent gifts or money for the Christmas Ship. Children collected pennies to buy toys or sent their own treasured playthings. A school in Iowa collected $231 in pennies; in Massachusetts, the Amherst Woman's Club contributed $39.50; convicts in Joliet prison raised money to purchase leather to make 500 pairs of children's shoes; elderly women in nursing homes knitted and sewed children's clothing; a mother sent $1.11 and the following note:

> Dear Children:
> I have two little boys. They have no father. They are poor like some of you, and last Christmas their cousins received some gold fish. All the year my little boys have been saving their money to buy some goldfish for themselves this Christmas. This is the goldfish money.[49]

All through the fall, trains of freight cars filled with gifts converged on a terminal in Brooklyn where soldiers from Fort Hamilton loaded the United States Naval Auxiliary steamship *Jason*—the Christmas Ship. On November 14, 1914, under the command of Lieutenant Commander C.E. Courteny, U.S.N., *Jason* sailed for Europe. She got a spectacular send off as whistles on dozens of ships saluted her while the Boy Band from St. John's Home in Brooklyn added musical accompaniment to the noisy departure.[50] Her first port of call was Falmouth, England, to unload presents for the English and Belgians, then Marseilles to deliver the French gifts, then Genoa where trains took presents to Germany[51] and Austria and, finally, to Saloniki for the Serbians. The Christmas Ship Hunt described entering Rotterdam was actually an English ship carrying the Belgian consignment of American gifts.

> There were scores of dolls, French bisques smiling pleasantly, pop-eyed rag dolls, old darky mammy dolls, and Santa Clauses; picture books, fairy books, and story books. One child had written in the cover of her book, "Father says I ought to send you my best picture book but I think that this one will do."
> I remember six linsey-woolsey dresses of a sort worn only in the Kentucky and Tennessee mountains, pitifully ugly and cheap, but symbolizing as fine charity as anything among the gifts. And there were bunched ears of corn tied with twine, given by Americans as poor as the Belgians for whom they were intended. These things made American sympathy more real to me than all the rest. My countrymen had "given what they could."[52]

In November 1914, the first relief ships reached Rotterdam: two ships from London arrived, then a flotilla of small ships (lighters) brought in wheat and flour "requisitioned" by Captain Lucey, followed by more ships from London. The first North American vessel was *Tremorvah* from Halifax, Nova Scotia, bringing 176 tons of flour, 49 tons of meat and bacon, and 2,338 tons of miscellaneous — "everything edible which could be got on short notice by the generous Nova Scotians and thrust into a ship."[53] *Massapequa* from New York followed with 3,500 tons of food, then a few more ships from London. A total of 26,000 tons of food worth about $1,000,000 reached Rotterdam the first month of C.R.B. operations. However, Belgium required approximately 100,000 tons of food per month to feed its population so fifteen ships had to reach Rotterdam every month. The price tag for this monthly aid was enormous, about $4,000,000! Here was a problem that required the genius and experience of someone like Herbert Hoover; under his leadership, the C.R.B. raised awareness worldwide of the plight of Belgium; money and in-kind donations of food and transport sufficient to feed 6,500,000 people per month — that was the C.R.B. mission. Although worldwide in scope, most of the resources came from America.

Hoover appointed Lindon W. Bates,[54] a civil engineer, as head of the critical New York office. Located at 71 Broadway, this office coordinated food relief and its transport from the entire United States. Bates developed an incredibly effective C.R.B. national organization with state committees and subcommittees reaching into counties and even into small communities. These committees gathered food and cash. Perhaps remembering the grass-roots response that resulted in the Christmas Ship, Bates and his volunteers tapped into the American desire to help Europe's starving — it was the least a rich neutral immigrant nation could do. The amount of giving was astounding.

In America, C.R.B. state committees and sub-committees collected and sent foodstuffs to state assembling depots, usually donated space in private warehouses in a city with good railroad connections. Of special importance were foods containing the maximum amount of calories: grains, legumes, pork fat backs, bacon and oleomargarine. The C.R.B. also accepted food donations from individuals, issuing specific instructions about what constituted an "Ideal Box." For example, the "Infant Ideal Box" should contain the following:

20 1-lb. tins of sweetened condensed milk
2 1-lb. tins patent barley flour
2 1-lb. cotton sacks rice
1 3-lb. sack rolled oats
1 3-lb. sack yellow corn meal
1 ½-lb. sack salt
1 can opener
All packed in a wooden box 18 × 12 × 6.5 inches, total weight 36.5 lbs. This will support one infant for four weeks.[55]

Of course, there were instructions defining "Ideal Boxes" for adults and for families. Individuals mailed their boxes free of charge (the C.R.B. reimbursed postage) to the 71 Broadway office. The C.R.B. also sought cash donations from individuals, private foundations and governments to purchase food on the international market and offset transportation costs. Donors were both the rich and the not so rich. During the first year of the war, the Rockefeller Foundation contributed $1,000,000, a sum sufficient for five relief ships; the

Belgian government in exile gave $500,000; the American Society of the Daughters of the American Revolution contributed $150,000; Allied bazaars held in various cities raised about $150,000; the Rocky Mountain Club contributed $246,000; private individuals totaled more than $500,000; little girls in a charity home in Cooperstown, New York, sent $1 each month.[56]

> A little country school near Montara lighthouse, on the Pacific Coast, gave its playtime to knitting wool caps and mittens and mufflers, and then the school children brought pennies from their little metal banks, and jars of preserved fruit, and home-made jam, and the girl school teacher put them all, pennies, jam, and mittens, into her one-horse buggy and drove forty miles through a storm to bring these more than royal gifts to the California Committee's office in San Francisco.[57]

From the state assembling depots, railroads carried the food to seaboard port terminals, usually at much reduced freight rates or even gratis. Seaboard ports included Montreal, Boston, Philadelphia, Baltimore, Norfolk, Charleston, New Orleans, Galveston, Seattle, Tacoma, San Francisco and, of course, New York. From the ports, C.R.B. ships carried the food to Rotterdam. The ships flew the C.R.B. flag and displayed conspicuous markings showing C.R.B. identification to prevent accidental torpedo attacks from German U-boat captains.

> Each ship carried a pair of great cloth banners, 9 x 100 feet, stretching along the hull on each side; also two 50-foot pennants flying from the mast heads, a house flag 12 x 15 feet, a pair of deck cloths, 12 x 50 feet, to be stretched across the deck face up, one forward and one aft, and two huge red- and white-striped signal balls, eight feet in diameter attached at the tops of two masts. The balls and flat deck cloths are for the benefit of airplane pilots; the side cloths, pennants, and house flag are for sea raiders and submarines. All the flags and cloths are white, with the Commission's name or initials (C.R.B.) in great red letters on them.[58]

Soon after the opening of the C.R.B. office in New York City in 1914, state committees went into action. They achieved almost immediate results. The state of Washington filled the steamer *Washington* and dispatched it to Rotterdam; Louisiana and Alabama sent *Wabana*; Georgia, North and South Carolina sent *St. Helena*; and Ohio sent the largest vessel, the steamer *Naneric*, loaded with 8,500 tons of food.

> Ex-Governor W.R. Stubbs of Kansas organized every county in Kansas and gathered the food that went over in the ship *Hannah*. The ninety-nine counties of Iowa each gave a carload [freight car] or more of food. California organized early, and she has stayed organized. Her people collected three hundred thousand dollars' worth of food within three weeks, and by December 8 [1914] had it aboard the steamer *Camino* and started on its way to Rotterdam, via the Panama Canal.[59]

In Rotterdam, Dutch stevedores quickly emptied C.R.B. ships and filled canal barges. The unloaded ships departed for more food, and tugboats towed strings of barges into the Belgian canal system and ultimately to distribution centers in the country.

C.R.B. delegates inspected at every step, insuring that the food supplied only the Belgians and none leaked to the German Army or the black market. In Belgium, through the Comité National de Secours et d'Alimentation, the food reached the hungry in the communes. A commune issued every individual in its domain a ration card, good for 2,000 calories of foodstuffs per day per adult. The menu was skimpy. It included a 250 gram loaf of bread (about three to four slices) and the following: "These were bacon (trifle over 1 oz.) lard (trifle over ⅔ oz.), rice (2⅓ oz.) dried beans and peas (1⅔ oz.) cerealine (1⅓ oz.) potatoes (10½ oz.), and brown sugar (trifle over ⅔ oz.)."[60]

FARMERS
Help the Belgians

500,000 Belgians driven out of their Country are needing food and clothing. For their benefit there will be a

GIVING PARTY
at Academy Hall,   OLD DEERFIELD
at seven o'clock

WEDNESDAY EV'NG, NOV. 25

Bring what you can, if it is only a few potatoes, onions, apples or beans. Warm clothing will also be received, and toys for the children.   Money also is wanted.

The urge to do something to help the plight of the Belgians resulted in efforts large and small to collect food, money and clothing for relief. This 1914 poster from a village in Massachusetts advertised an event that had 97 attend. It raised $50, collected three boxes of groceries, seven cases of clothing, 10 bags of potatoes and onions, and a barrel of apples, all which went to Boston for a ship to Rotterdam (Pocumtuck Valley Memorial Association Library, Deerfield, Massachusetts).

Obesity was not a health problem in occupied Belgium. The average Belgian got about 2,000 calories a day, with a low intake of proteins and fats. Belgians might have been hungry, but they lived longer. The death rate in Belgium during the war, eight per thousand per annum, was half that of New York City in 1914.

The Comité National distributed the same amount of food to rich and poor. Although the rich paid for their food, the poor did not. Depending upon the commune, the means of distribution varied. There were C.R.B. stores

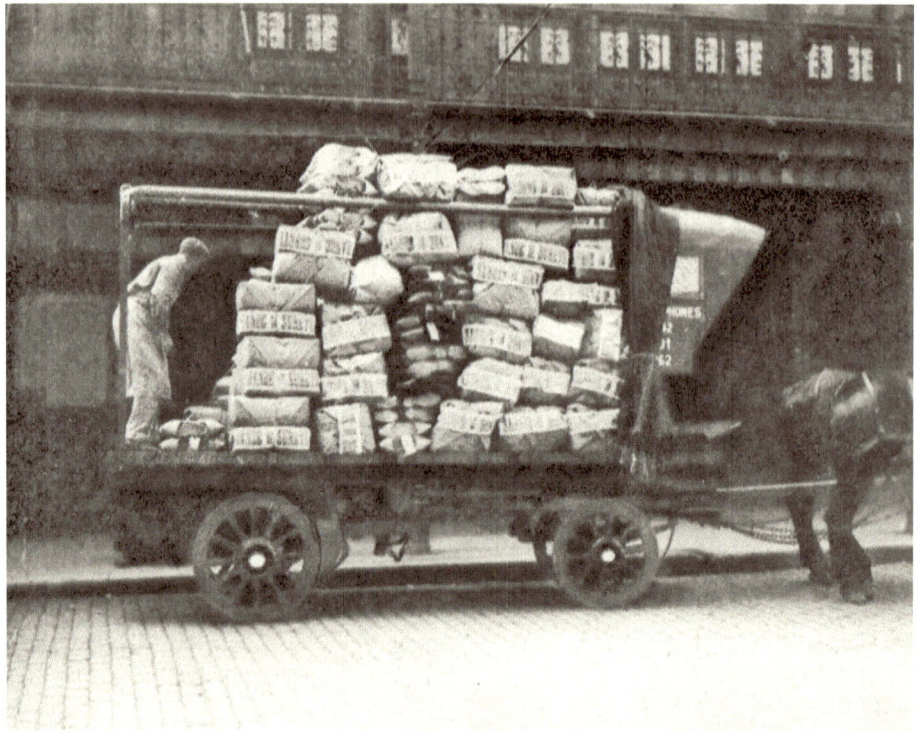

The C.R.B. distribution network began in Rotterdam and ended in depots in Belgian cities, towns and villages. Here a wagon delivers boxes of used clothing to a depot in Brussels (*Illustré*, 1914).

where rich and poor could obtain food, but most Belgians probably obtained their daily individual or family ration at the *soupes,* the bread and soup kitchens.

> Each person standing in line at the distributing station brings a pitcher, a saucepan, an old coffee pot — any receptacle that can be used to carry the soup away.[61]

> And, once the applicants had their pitchers filled and bread in hand, they did not waste any time. When I asked, I learned some of them had to go several blocks to get home and the family was sitting around with waiting soup bowls hoping to get their meal while it was still hot.[62]

A Brussels aid organization, The Little Bees, paid special attention to babies, children and the elderly. In other parts of Belgium, similar organizations filled the Little Bees function. The Little Bees established canteens near schools to feed the young a more nourishing meal than that available at the *soupes.* The cantines were dining areas or eating halls established in vacant garages, cellars, convents, stores, or private homes. Volunteers spruced up the places, making

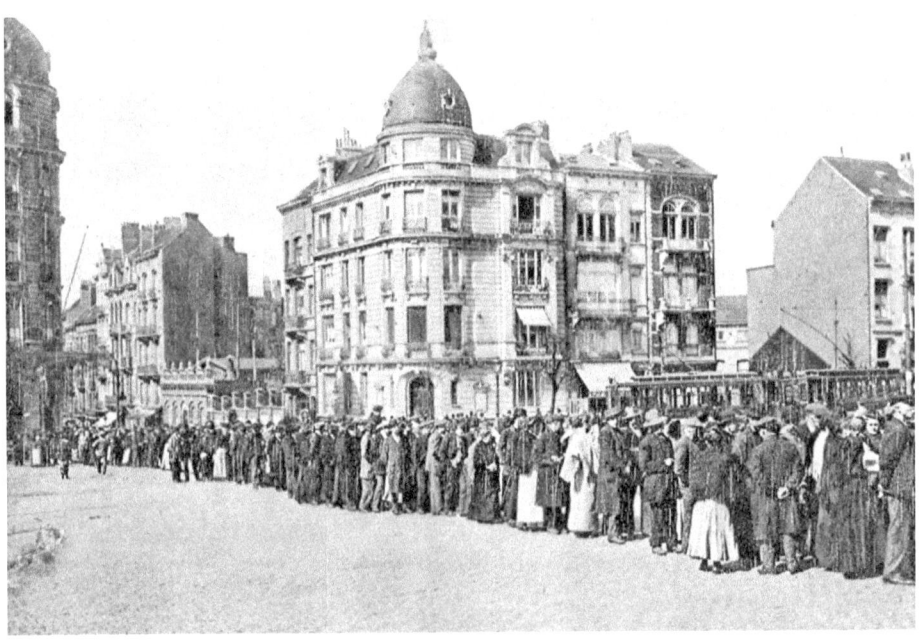

A food line in Saint Gilles, a district of Brussels. Such lines were common sights in Belgium during the war (*Illustré*, 1914).

them bright and cheery. Invariably American flags, pictures of President Wilson and embroidered C.R.B. flour sacks with messages of gratitude were part of the decorative motif. The young (ages three to fourteen) came from school at 11:00, had their ration cards checked, and took their places on benches in front of long tables. At each place setting was a cup (for milk), a large bowl and a spoon. Volunteers served bread and a thick stew of potatoes (or rice or macaroni), carrots and green vegetables and small pieces of meat (three days a week were meat days). The favorite course came last; it was phosphatine dessert.

> The phosphatine dessert (of which the children can not get enough) was already served at a side table. The "Little Bees" originated this phosphatine dessert, which is a mixture of rice, wheat, and maize-flour, phosphate of lime and cocoa.[63]

Mothers with their new babies attended a special canteen late in the afternoon after the children returned to school. Physician and nurse volunteers examined the children at the canteens. The infirm elderly had rations brought to their homes.

In addition to soup-lines and canteens, some cities opened special restaurants to supplement diets and add a bit of variety to Belgian life. Going by names such as the *Diner Economique* or *Diner Bourgeois* and with subsidies from local relief committees and a staff of unpaid volunteers, these diners provided a meal at very little cost. However, one still had to pay; consequently, the customers felt they were not accepting charity. The restaurants were very popular. Antwerp had 10 such restaurants and served 10,000 dinners a day. Liège converted a large indoor skating-rink into a mighty restaurant that served 4,000 dinners each day.

> The dining-rooms are always attractive, often bright with flags and flowers, the women are cheery in their service. Priests, children, artists, men and women of every class sit at the tables.[64]

As well as foodstuffs and cash, the C.R.B. also collected clothing as part of Belgian relief. Stevedores loaded bales of clothing freighted to New York from throughout the country into C.R.B. ships bound for Rotterdam. From Rotterdam, the clothing traveled by canal barges to Brussels or Antwerp for processing. In Brussels, 500 men and women worked in the Hippodrome to fumigate the clothes and then to cut them apart for reuse by seamstresses and tailors. In the Antwerp music hall, 1,200 worked to make new clothes from old. They saved every scrap, for even flour sacks supplied cloth for men's shirts and babies' clothes. Making new garments from old clothes gave thousands a paying job. Although paying only about 60 cents per week, it was paying work — a rarity in occupied Belgium. Since so many people sought employment in the garment processing works, an individual could work only 2 weeks per month in an effort to spread out the jobs to the greatest number of individuals.

> A young woman was putting together an attractive baby quilt. She had four pieces of an old coat, large enough to make the top and lining, and inside she was stitching literally dozens of little scraps of light woolen materials. Another was making children's shoes out of bits of carpet and wool.[65]

Initially, the Germans restricted C.R.B. activities to only part of Belgium. Areas near the front, in both Belgium and Northern France, were off limits despite the fact millions of civilians were starving in these areas. Hoover's next mission would be to bring C.R.B. aid to these millions.

Chapter 8

Feeding the Etappen Zone and Social Darwinism

> We were not haters of Germany when we went to Belgium. We have simply, by inescapable sights and sounds and knowledge forced on us, been made into what we have become. If we hate Prussians and Prussianism now, it is because Prussia and Prussianism have taught us to hate them. Whom have they ever taught to love them?[1]— Vernon Kellogg, C.R.B. officer

> Individuals with a strong homicidal mania, who just manage to suppress their paranoiac tendencies, will welcome war since it removes for them the burden of constant inhibition, and unfortunately such poorly balanced individuals have rather too frequently been the leaders of governments.[2]— Jacques Loeb, Columbia University, 1917

In the immediate post-invasion period, German authorities divided Belgium into three functional zones and governed each differently (see Chapter 6). From west to east, the first zone was the *Operationsgebiet,* which included the front lines and areas immediately behind the trenches and defensive positions. The *Operationsgebiet* began at the North Sea near Nieuport, followed the Yser Front, then skirted the Ypres Salient and continued south toward Armentières in France. East of the *Operationsgebiet* came the zone of communications and supply, the *Etappengebiet,* which included the Flemish cities of Ghent and Bruges as well as the ports of Ostend and Zeebrugge. The military commander in charge of the army operating in the area governed his sector of the *Operationsgebiet* and the *Etappengebiet.* The rest of Belgium, the largest and most populous zone, was the *Okkupationsgebiet, General-Gouvernement.* It included Brussels and Antwerp and was under a governor-general who answered directly to the Kaiser. C.R.B. activities described in Chapter 7 occurred only in the *Okkupationsgebiet, General-Gouvernement* of Belgium. However, by the end of 1914, food shortages and the possibility of food riots in the *Etappengebiet* threatened to destabilize the zone. The threat of starvation was especially immediate in the cities. It was imperative for the German military to find a way to extend C.R.B. aid into the *Etappen* zone and those Belgian villages still inhabited in the *Operationsgebiet,* i.e., East and West Flanders. Again, as in the *Okkupationsgebiet,* England was at first a roadblock. Her troops were fighting and dying in the Belgian *Operationsgebiet,* so it seemed insane to allow the importation of food behind the lines and possibly help provision the enemy.

> It must absolutely be avoided having any of the breadstuffs thus supplied to the communes taken by the troops, because England has declared her willingness to permit the importation of grain only under the condition that none of these shall be used for the provisioning of German troops.[3]

In December 1914, the army commanders gave their assurances that C.R.B. foodstuffs would be safe from requisition by the German Army. Jules A. Van Hee, former American Vice Consul at Ghent, represented the C.R.B. in East and West Flanders and was responsible for bringing food to approximately 200,000 Belgian civilians. In October 1914, as the German Army closed in on Ghent, Van Hee used his automobile to evacuate Belgian wounded from the city to a military train bound for Ostend.[4] Such an action certainly did not fall into his job description as a diplomatic representative of a neutral country. However, his action earned him not only respect from the Belgians but, remarkably, the confidence of the Germans that he would do the correct thing. In the case of feeding the *Etappen,* the correct behavior was the scrupulous observance of neutrality. Therefore, C.R.B. delegates in the *Etappen* could make their inspections only when accompanied by a German officer. Freedom of movement as experienced by delegates in the *Okkupationgebiet* was *verboten*. The German military was understandably very weary of foreigners traveling willy-nilly in the *Operationsgebiet* and *Etappengebiet*. Chance

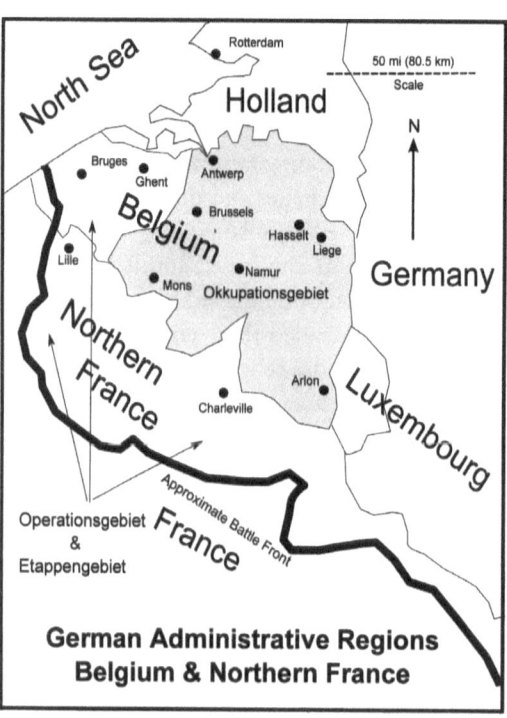

German Administrative Regions
Belgium & Northern France

observations of depots, staging areas or secret camps by C.R.B. delegates made the Germans nervous about the possibility of espionage. "In general it was the American delegate's duty to keep an eye upon the situation, to keep his ears open and his mouth shut."[5]

That November and December, Hoover shuttled between the continent and Britain, arguing his position and the importance of the C.R.B. with almost any important personage who would listen — in Belgium, he cajoled the Belgians and Germans; in London, he did the same with the British. Prime Minister Asquith, after suffering through a lengthy Hoover session, thought Hoover a most undiplomatic, yet very effective, diplomat.[6] Hoover seemed to thrive on convincing others to do what he wanted and making organizational schemes to implement his wishes. He often left ruffled feathers in his wake. Whitlock, who could not be more different in temperament, marveled at the man. Emile Francqui, Hoover's counterpart in the Comité National de Secours et d'Alimentation, was another organization man who also did not shy from confrontation. Then there were the German conquerors, a group not noted for flexibility in negotiations. It was the lot of Whitlock, who hated committee work and strongly disliked confrontations, to pacify the C.R.B. belligerents.

> The minor task of keeping peace in the family seemed, by some unkind fatality, to fall to the lot of the person who happened to be American Minister at Brussels, and seemed to offer a convenient human substance to absorb all the numerous shocks.... It seemed to be my rôle for a long time to induce men of various nationalities and widely separated points of view and different habits of thought to meet at the Legation and, over a cup of tea, notoriously an innocuous and soothing beverage, to compose or forget their differences and to allow those poor Belgians, who had had no quarrel with anybody, to go on eating.[7]

Besides Hoover, Francqui and German bureaucrats, the American Minister often had to deal with fools.

> I shall always recall with something like horror the long hours of discussion with a certain fellow-citizen who wished everything to be done by everybody in his way and in no other; he was not quite sure just how it should be done himself, and when in despair I told him to proceed at once and carry out his plan of organization with a free hand, it seemed that he had no plan. He would sit for hours at the Legation trying to convince me, and I never could be sure of what he was trying to convince me. The worst of him was that he used long sentences, without verbs, which was maddening.[8]

Whitlock yearned for the old days — a bit of novelizing and then an afternoon round of golf with Hugh Gibson. How life had changed.

Herbert Hoover, along with his wife Lou, arrived in Brussels on December 20, 1914. Although Frederick Palmer, an American journalist, was in the Hoover party, he traveled separately from Rotterdam to Brussels with the C.R.B. currier

Edward D. Curtis in his long, low, rakish and chauffeured automobile. Palmer identified him with the pseudonym "Harvard 1914" and commented that he was the quietest of traveling companions, hardly speaking for the entire journey; Palmer described him as sphinx-like.[9] Hugh Gibson described Curtis as one who "exudes silence and discretion."[10] Mr. Curtis evidently was not given to small talk. Curtis dropped Palmer at the Palace Hotel. Herbert and Lou Hoover probably stayed there as well. Gibson dined with them.

> Mr. and Mrs. Hoover arrived last night.... We dined together at the Palace. They were full of news, both war and shop, and I sat and talked with them until after eleven, greatly to the prejudice of my work. Had to stay up and grind until nearly two.[11]

Then came, as usual, rounds of meetings at the American Legation dealing with everything from immature Rhodes men, the sensitivities of Belgians and Germans, new rules from the British and the hurt feelings of a Spaniard. Hoover and the Marquis de Villalobar locked horns over C.R.B. stationery during the visit. In a Spanish rage, Villalobar confronted Hoover; evidently, the Spaniard felt affronted at the placement of his name on C.R.B. letterhead and thought Hoover was hogging all the glory for himself and the Americans (He probably was.). Did not Villalobar and Whitlock push for a food aid program soon after the Germans arrived? Were they not equal patrons of the C.R.B.? Hoover finally agreed to the revised letterhead after two days of wrangling. For Hoover and Villalobar confrontation was a sport, for Whitlock it was not.

Christmas 1914 approached; in Brussels, only the Germans were celebrating. The Teutonic good cheer was almost more than Whitlock could stand.

> In the Parc Royal there was an enormous tree, blazing with thousands of electric lights in coloured bulbs, like the one in Madison Square at that season, and German soldiers gathered around it and sang their choruses. There were little Christmas-trees in all the blazing windows of the *ministères* in the Rue de la Loi; at the King's palace at Laeken a great dinner for the officers. For weeks they had been cutting down fir-trees in the Belgian woods for their Christmas-trees; there were celebrations for the soldiers everywhere.[12]

The Whitlocks hosted a Christmas Eve dinner at the Legation for the Hoovers, Hugh Gibson, three officers of the Rockefeller Foundation on a "fact-finding" junket and Frederick Palmer. On this first Christmas of the war, there was little to be merry about for either side. As the Western Front celebrated its first Noël, a spontaneous Christmas truce along some stretches of the trenches stopped the killing for a day — but only for a day. The Christmas Ship loaded with gifts for war orphans had come and gone — unfortunately, there were more orphans than gifts. The dinner had one significant high note; Whitlock learned that the Rockefeller Foundation "was prepared to aid the *ravitaillement* to the full extent of its resources."[13] So at least until September 1915, the Belgians would not go hungry. After that, it was up to Hoover to raise more cash.

The following day, Christmas, was cold and brisk. A hoar frost gave even war-time Brussels a festive appearance. In the afternoon, the Americans motored to the palatial home of Lewis Richards. A native of Michigan, Richards had attended the Royal Conservatory of Music in Brussels, graduating with distinction in piano. He married a Belgian, had two children, and was a well-known concert pianist, touring in both Europe and America. Unknown to most, Lewis and his wife Berthe had been supplying food to the children in their neighborhood. For Christmas, the couple planned something special.

> He has a big house at the edge of town, with grounds which were fairy-like in the heavy white frost. He had undertaken to look after 660 children, and he did it to the Queen's taste. They were brought in by their mothers in bunches of one hundred, and marched around the house, collecting things as they went. In one room each youngster was given a complete outfit of warm clothes. In another, some sort of toy which he was allowed to choose. In another, a big bag of cakes and candies, and, finally, they were herded into the big dining-room, where they were filled with all sorts of Xmas food. There was a big tree in the hall, so that the children, in their triumphal progress, merely walked around the tree.... The children were speechless with happiness, and many of the mothers were crying as they came by.[14]

In occupied France, Christmas 1914 was very bleak with conditions being much worse than almost anywhere in the Belgian *Okkupationsgebiet*. Occupied France, also referred to as Northern France, consisted of a band of territory between the Belgian frontier and the trench lines. This area began just north of the city of Lille and continued south to the vicinity of Verdun. Paralleling the Western Front and nearly always proximal to the active combat zone, it fell directly under the German military, being *Operationsgebiet* or *Etappengebiet*.

> Living behind the German lines in Northern France were some 2,150,000 French whose situation was even more desperate and precarious than that of the Belgian population. Unlike the people of the greater part of Belgium, this population were living under an absolute military regime. They enjoyed no liberty of movement and were practically prisoners within their own communes.[15]

The industrial population of this area was very dense and always dependent upon food imports for its sustenance. The war essentially stripped Northern France of food. Initially, the French Army lived off the countryside as it retreated through the land, and then came the German Army in pursuit, consuming what the French Army had missed. The local councils succeeded in negotiating that a fraction of the harvest of 1914 be set aside for the citizenry; nonetheless, by Christmas 1914 there were major food shortages in many places. Hoover wrote to the President of France about the situation (February 17, 1915); remarkably, the French government was reluctant to pay for food aid. One is reminded of another callous French personage who, when faced with bread riots, is supposed to have said, "Let them eat cake." Well in late 1914, there was neither bread nor cake, but fortunately, there was Hoover!

> If your Excellency could see the mobs of French women and children which surround every German camp from daylight to dark to gather refuse from the German soldiers, your Excellency would then believe that these French people will pay the last penalty unless someone comes to their rescue.[16]

The Allies, whether British or French, hated assisting Germany in feeding civilians in the occupied lands. They viewed food riots in the *Etappen* zone positively — food was a weapon. Hoover literally had to shame them into putting aside war aims and doing the right thing. Hoover's letter to the President of France ended with a political appeal to the French people; after all, France was a republic with an elected president. "In conclusion, before taking the heavy responsibility of saying to these people 'you shall not have bread,' I make a last appeal to the French people themselves in the name of their own countrymen and countrywomen."[17]

The President of France then argued against setting a precedent. If France paid for the importation of foodstuffs to feed its citizens, should not Germany have the right to pay for the importation of food to feed German citizens? By the last week in March, French officials and Hoover's men devised a face-saving tactic to resolve the impasse. The French government would stick to its position about not paying for food aid in Northern France; instead it would borrow the funds from the Belgians.

> The Belgian Government, in conformity with the views of the French Government, advances to the C.R.B. a sum of twenty-five million francs for which the French Government will repay them later. This sum is destined to the immediate purchase of a stock of provisions for feeding the invaded parts of France.[18]

While negotiating with the French, Hoover was in contact with James W. Gerard, the American ambassador to the Imperial German Court in Berlin. Gerard negotiated the German guarantees necessary to satisfy the British that the foodstuffs would provision only French citizens in Northern France. The negotiations were straight forward as the German Army was anxious to get food aid into the French *Etappen*. German authorities signed an agreement on April 13, 1915.

> It was stated that the supreme command of the German army gave its consent to the Commission undertaking the provisionment of the population of the occupied French territory; that all goods imported for this purpose would be reserved exclusively to the French population; and that strict orders would be

sent out by the supreme command to the effect that these goods must never be seized and that all goods not distributed should remain at the exclusive disposal of the C.R.B.[19]

The C.R.B. appointed American delegates to confirm the German military lived up to the guarantees negotiated in Berlin. Since they were in an active war zone, a German officer (Begleit-Offizier, accompanying officer) always accompanied the American delegate on inspections. The officer spoke English and French and the two men shared accommodations, ate together, drank together and traveled together. The delegate's correspondences, whether official or personal, both incoming and outgoing, were first read by the Begleit-Offizier; thus censorship was total. A delegate in the *Etappen* "would be required to take on himself the obligation to carry out his duties in such a manner as may be expected from an honorable citizen of a neutral state."[20]

> In the course of time these begleits-offiziers came practically to take into their own hands most of the details involved in the work of provisionment. For the most part these officers showed a great interest and took an immense pride in the work of the Commission. They came even to consider themselves as part of the Commission. Most of them adhered faithfully to the obligations of their position and took a sincere interest in the welfare of the population of their district. They came to regard any violation of the German guarantees in France as a personal reflection upon themselves, because it was their duty to see that such violations did not occur.[21]

The C.R.B. and German authorities divided Northern France into six districts for the purpose of foodstuff distribution, each district roughly coinciding with one of the five German field army's positions on the Western Front in France in 1915. Each district had a delegate and a Begleit-Offizier. Foodstuffs for Northern France entered through the port of Rotterdam, then traveled via canals across Belgium, and finally by rail or canal to the districts for distribution. Delays in food distribution occurred if a battle was ongoing in a sector of the front that included a particular district because then, understandably, the German Army monopolized all transport.

Each German field army was a law unto itself, answerable only to the Kaiser and the General Staff of the Army. Therefore, the C.R.B. officer in overall charge of the food relief in Northern France needed to be near the headquarters of the supreme command. In mid–September 1914, the location of the Großes Hauptquartier (G.H.Q.) was in the French town of Charleville, about 10 miles (16 km) from the Belgian frontier. Consequently, Charleville became the headquarters for C.R.B. activity in occupied France. It was here that Herbert Hoover, Vernon Kellogg (Director of the C.R.B. office in Charleville, June 1915–November 1915) and C.R.B. delegates dealt with matters pertaining to the sustenance of the civilian population in occupied France. However,

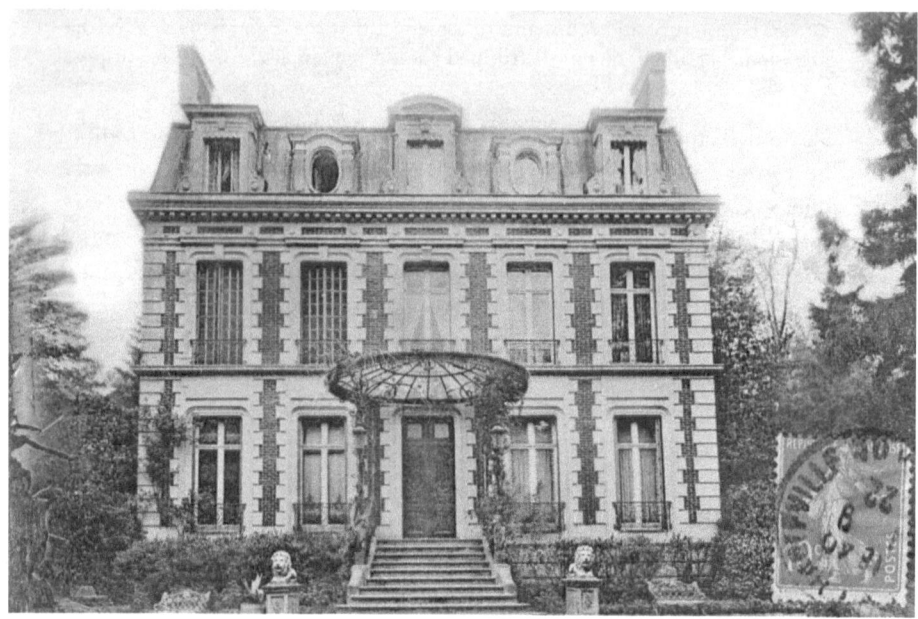

Château Corneau in Charleville, Kaiser Wilhelm's residence, was located opposite a park fronting the railway station. The Château Corneau no longer exists, having been razed to make way for a modern building (Rainer Hiltermann collection).

because life at the G.H.Q. was at best a bit bizarre, it is worth a diversion to show the kind of world the Americans witnessed.

Charleville is located inside a broad bend of the Meuse (Maas) River, a river with many war time connections. It flows past Verdun, Charleville, Namur, Liège and into the North Sea at Rotterdam. With a pre-war population of 21,000, Charleville's chief industry was the manufacture of small hardware goods. It had (and has) an attractive town square, the Place Ducale. *Baedeker for Northern France* (1909) advised the traveler that "the rest of the town is uninteresting." The movers and shakers of Imperial Germany established themselves in this provincial backwater in the fall of 1914. Kaiser Wilhelm's residence was in the Villa Corneau near the railway station, facing the Square de la Gare where military bands gave concerts. Proximal to the station was the military house of prostitution (*maison close* or pouf) for troop trains stopping on their way to the front. The owner of this profitable Temple of Venus was the Kaiser's friend, staff-surgeon Dr. Wezel.

> Situated as it was near the station, all the troops passing through Charleville devoted to it a part of their short visit, where they met their comrades of the garrison. It was always crowded, and the entrance was blocked in the morning by an impatient band of clients.[22]

8. Feeding the Etappen Zone and Social Darwinism   159

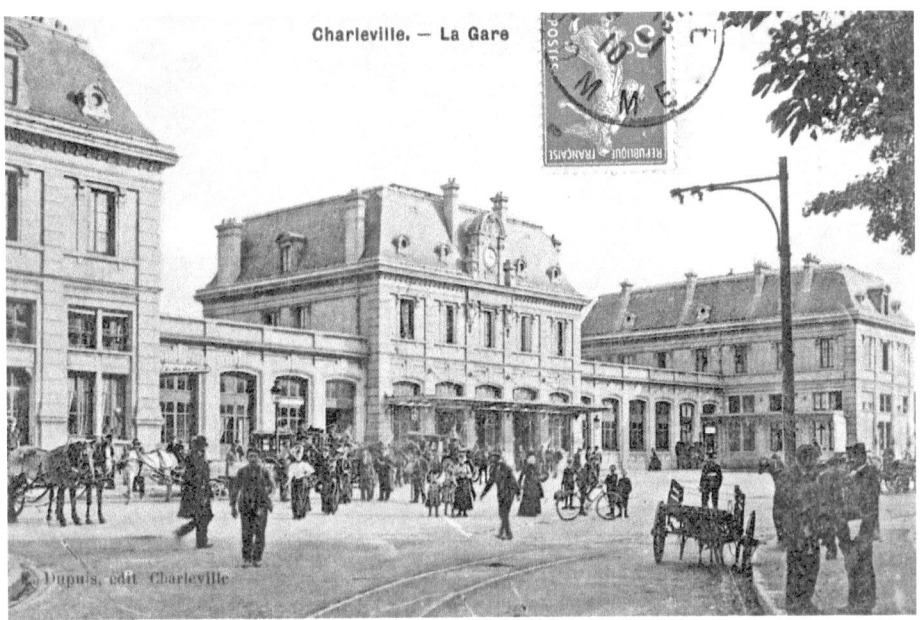

Charleville railway station (La Gare). All the major German personalities involved in the strategic planning of the war passed through its doors. Located on the main north-south railway line (Metz-Lille) that supplied the Western Front, the station often swarmed with soldiers waiting for troop trains. Having survived both world wars, the station looks much the same today (Klekowski collection).

Near the "Imperial Pouf," authorities requisitioned mansions for the Ministry of War and the offices of the Imperial Chancellery. The Chancellor of the German Empire, "scrap of paper" Bethmann-Hollweg[23] (see Introduction), resided regally on the Avenue de la Gare in the former home of a banker.

> Charleville became the capital of the Central Powers. The modest Ardennes city had the misfortune to contain the most eminent officials of the Empire. The Wilhelmstrasse had been transferred to the Avenue de la Gare, and the Villa Corneau took the place of the Potsdam palace.[24]
>
> Just around the corner from the Kaiser, within stone's throw of his back door, is another red brick house with terra cotta trimmings — rather larger and more imposing. The names of its new residents, "Hahnke," "Caprivi," and "Graf von Moltke," are scrawled in white chalk on the stone post of the gateway. Further up the same street another chalk scrawl on a quite imposing mansion informed me that "The Imperial Chancellor" and "The Foreign Office" had set up shop there. Near by were Grand Admiral Tirpitz's field quarters.[25]

Germany's allies sent emissaries to the new capital of the Central Powers on the Western Front. They all had grandiose titles; the streets and byways of

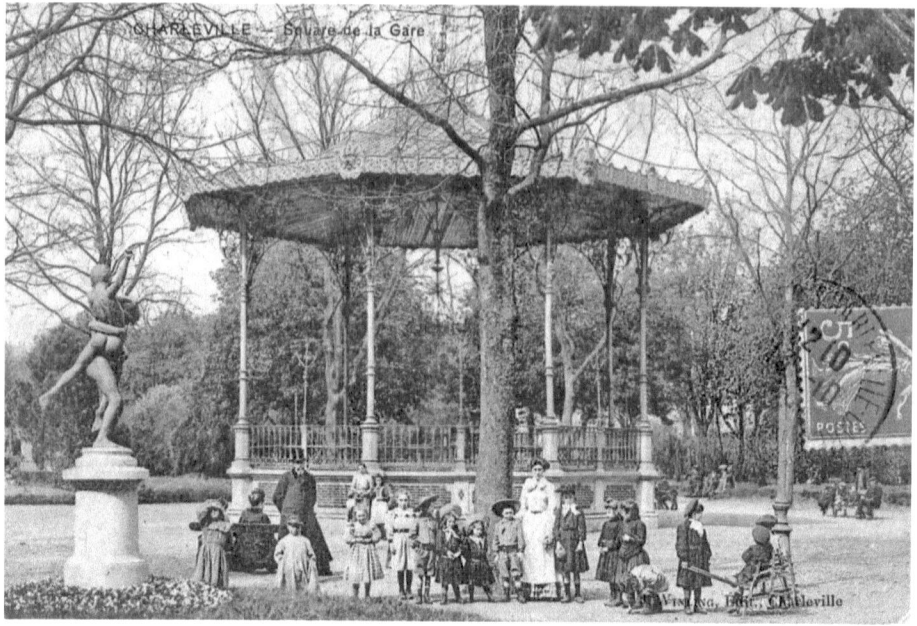

A pre-war photograph of the bandstand in the park between the railway station and the Château Corneau. Concerts given there serenaded the Kaiser and welcomed dignitaries arriving in Charleville (Klekowski collection).

Charleville teemed with petty kings, grand dukes, crown princes, princes, counts and lowly generals. Franz Joseph, the Emperor of Austria and the Kaiser's partner in the crime known as the First World War, sent Field-Marshal von Sturgh. The Field-Marshal left the largest impression on the folks of Charleville.

> Field-Marshal von Sturgh was a huge giant, repulsively fat, with the bearing of a hippopotamus. Too obese to mount a horse, he always went about in a royal car. Now and again he risked a short walk, and this mass of flesh moving with difficulty sweated and groaned piteously. He spent his time feasting. He was always to be found eating. He took no exercise, and all his movements had to be assisted by his faithful orderlies.[26]

Another significant partner in the war was Turkey; its emissary spent much of his time visiting the houses of prostitution in Charleville, presumably exercising a hobby dating from his harem days. The Kaiser's married son had the same hobby. The Crown Prince led the life of a royal rake. He settled down with a French mistress from Charleville, whom the locals referred to as the second crown princess. When not dallying with the ladies, the Crown Prince enjoyed scattering free cigarettes among a gang of young ragamuffins who prowled Charleville's streets.

How many times did the members of the municipal council witness the spectacle of a band of fifty to sixty young urchins pulling the Prince by the sleeve or by the edge of his tunic and shouting at the top of their voices: "Cigarettes, Kronprinz, cigarettes!"

One would have thought it was a masked figure at Carnival time followed by the jeering crowd of cheeky children.[27]

Kaiser Wilhelm could not have been more different from his son. The Kaiser was monogamous, very proper and straight-laced, and very religious. He truly believed the motto embossed on German soldiers' belt buckles, *Gott mit uns* (God is with us). He was also strangely fastidious about his clothing, changing uniforms, under linen and silk stockings several times a day. His greatest fear while at Charleville was from French air raids targeting the Großes Hauptquartier district, located near the train station. French bombing aircraft needed only to follow the railroad tracks to their targets: the G.H.Q. and the Kaiser's residence. A *New York Times* correspondent, who managed surreptitiously to enter Charleville in October 1914, thought the town a great target to which the French had not paid enough attention.

I could not help wondering why the Allies' aviators weren't "on the job." A dozen, backed by an intelligent intelligence department, could so obviously settle the fortunes of war by blowing out the brains of their enemy.[28]

The first air raid finally occurred in April 1915, damaging houses near the Villa Corneau. A frantic Kaiser ordered the strengthening of the Corneau residence cellar for use as an imperial bomb shelter. A subsequent raid the following year caused more damage and some casualties. That raid prompted the Kaiser to move his residence to the suburbs, to the Villa Renaudin at Bélair. Still feeling insecure, he issued orders to bomb proof the entire villa.

He could never be sufficiently protected from bombs. The children's bedrooms were on the floor above immediately over the royal bedroom. Enormous iron beams were brought and placed to support a layer of solid concrete, a yard thick. Henceforward his Majesty thought he could sleep in peace.[29]

Charleville reflected the personalities, needs and foibles of Kaiser Wilhelm II, his feckless son and heir Crown Prince Wilhelm, their associates and sycophants. In addition, there were more than 600 officers at G.H.Q., each having orderlies, drivers and gofers. The General Staff, based in the Hotel de Ville on the Place Ducale, supervised military hospitals, medical services, telegraphs, railroads, munitions and ordinance, etc. As many as 1,500 German officers and enlisted men lived in the town. Troop trains stopping at the station on their way to the front brought thousands of day-trippers looking for entertainment. Charleville was, at times, literally awash with foot-loose German soldiers. The men's urgency to experience life before it was too late brought a moral deca-

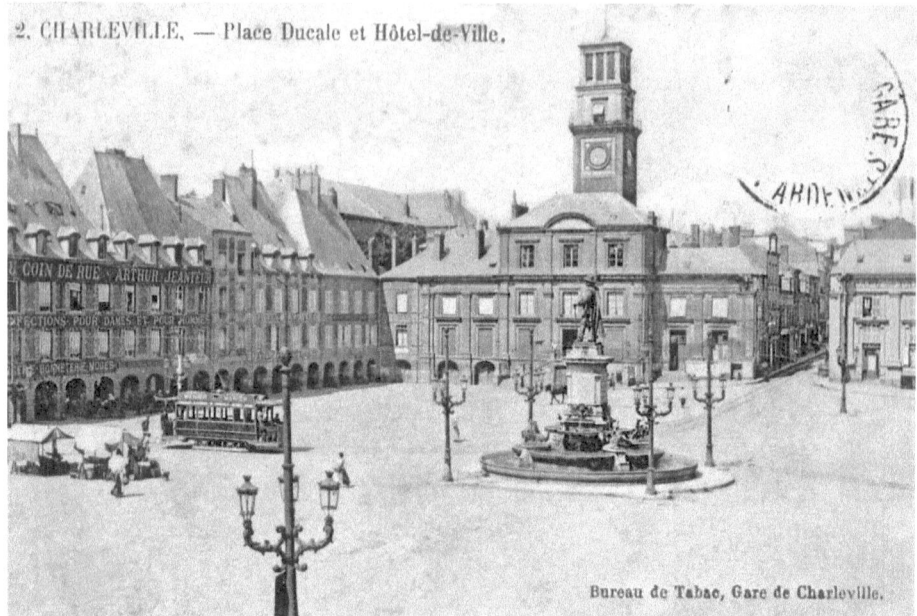

Place Ducale, Charleville. The town hall, the building with a tower, housed the German General Staff. A German pre-war traveler's guide described the Place Ducale as the only thing of interest for a visitor, the rest of the town being not worth a diversion. The town's visitor attractions greatly increased with the coming of the Kaiser and his entourage (Klekowski collection).

dence to once-sleepy Charleville. For French observers, however, it was more depravity than simple decadence.

> The theatricality of the Kaiser, the orgies of the Crown Prince, the obscene conduct of the officers, their men's indulgence in every kind of infamy, the requisitioning of French women, and the consequent association of respectable women and girls with prostitutes of the lowest type, theft, nameless bestiality — all this turns one sick.[30]

Vernon Kellogg arrived in Charleville in June 1915 to organize the C.R.B. aid effort in occupied France. On leave from Stanford University where he was a professor of entomology (the study of insects), Kellogg was 48 years old. He shared a room with his Begleit-Offizier in a large town house with other officers. In such a small town, Kellogg could observe the major players at the G.H.Q.

> Here also were Von Falkenhayn, the Kaiser's Chief of Staff, and sometimes even the All-Highest [Kaiser Wilhelm] himself, who never missed the Sunday morning service in the long low corrugated-iron shed which looked all too little like a royal chapel ever to interest a flitting French bomber.[31]

Kellogg's postgraduate studies included a couple of stays at the University of Leipzig in 1893 and 1897; thus he spoke German and had German colleagues, most of whom where now in uniform. Surprisingly, a Leipzig colleague, now an infantry captain, lived in the same house as Kellogg and his Begleit-Offizier. Although Kellogg referred to him with the pseudonym Captain-Professor von Flussen, he was the noted German zoologist Otto zur Strassen.[32]

> I lived as the Commission's chief representative for North France among these gray-uniformed officers, who busied themselves assiduously all day in their plain offices with maps and dispatches, with telephones and telegraphs tying them to every part of the various fronts, east as well as west, and playing on little tables the great game of war and destruction and death. At night they would dine and drink their requisitioned French wines, and then they would talk and debate anything from music and poetry to German militarism and American munitions-sending. [American factories manufactured and shipped munitions to the Allies.][33]

Kellogg participated in these wine-lubricated dinner discussions, and when Captain zur Strassen was at the table, the discussion revolved around genetics and social Darwinism. The key question was whether waging war was genetically beneficial or deleterious for a nation and its population. Captain zur Strassen and the other German officers viewed the war as a positive factor in human genetic evolution. They earnestly believed that the German nation, by waging war and winning resources from its neighbors, improved itself not only economically but also genetically. The latter was the key point, did waging war result in genetic improvement? Was war eugenic? Did it result in an increased frequency of "good" genes in the race or nation that waged it? The German thesis was a mixture of social Darwinism and group selection.

> That human group which is in the most advanced evolutionary stage as regards internal organization and form of social relationship is best, and should, for the sake of the species, be preserved at the expense of the less advanced, the less effective. It should win in the struggle for existence, and this struggle should occur precisely that the various types may be tested, and the best not only preserved, but put in position to impose its kind of social organization — its *Kultur*—on the others, or, alternatively, to destroy and replace them.[34]

The above description by Kellogg of the German thesis is clearer than the pseudoscientific writings of German theorists of the time:

> War is a biological necessity of the first importance, a regulative element in the life of mankind which cannot be dispensed with, since without it an unhealthy development will follow, which excludes every advancement of the race, and therefore all real civilization.[35]

> Without war, inferior or decaying races would easily choke the growth of healthy budding elements, and a universal decadence would follow.[36]

War is elevating, because the individual disappears before the great conception of the State.[37]

The German view that the group or state was of more importance than its citizens, i.e., "that the individual is nothing, the State all,"[38] appalled Kellogg. He conceded that group selection was possible in social insects: ants, bees, wasps, termites. A colony of such insects could be viewed as a group or state in the German sense, and group selection as colonies competed for survival could result in positive evolutionary change, especially since the members of the colony were closely related genetically, being essentially members of a very large family. Kellogg believed that to apply such ideas to genetically variable states such as Germany or France or England was nonsense. He went further, arguing that waging war was dysgenic rather than eugenic, i.e., it resulted in genetic degradation rather than promoting "good" genes. War selectively killed off the best and left the least healthy home to breed.

> Of the men gathered by conscription, as in France and Germany, or by voluntary enlistment, as in Great Britain, from 40 to 50 per cent are rejected by the examining boards as unfit for service because of undersize, infirmities, or disease.[39]

In Kellogg's view, an army creamed a population of its healthiest young males. Since in war more soldiers perished than the infirm males who remained at home, the latter contributed more of their genes to the next generation. Ergo, war was dysgenic.

Kellogg's dinner discussions with his German colleagues converted him philosophically; he was no longer a pacifist. Although outwardly neutral as his position demanded, he came to despise the German super-race attitude.

> The Germans do indeed recognize the value of social evolution inside the race or nation, but its advantage is all for the sake of building up a powerful organism to fight effectively and viciously with all other races and nations. The different peoples are to be looked on as the analogues of different brute species, all terribly and everlastingly at war with each other, each using everything possible to it to gain the upper hand. Everything that can be construed to be of military advantage in this struggle is justified as biological advantage.[40]

If one had to single out one place in the French *Etappen* that felt the heaviest hand of German social Darwinism, that place would be the city of Lille. An industrial city with a wartime population of about 623,000, Lille was less than 10 miles (16 km) from the active front. Every day Lille heard the echoes of artillery fire and drew the attentions of English fliers. The Bavarians under Crown Prince Rupprecht[41] occupied the city; Kellogg had little good to say about the Bavarians.

8. Feeding the Etappen Zone and Social Darwinism   165

> Lille has been occupied by a particularly large and particularly brutal army, the Bavarians under Prince Rupprecht. There has long been a popular belief that the Bavarians are gentler Germans.... Well, whether the royal Bavarian commander is a particularly brutal man, ... or Bavarians as soldiers are particularly brutal,...—it is notorious that the French in the Lille district, ... have suffered a constantly and mercilessly cruel treatment at the hands of their masters. Perhaps these masters have all along been a little afraid of their slaves.[42]

Five months after Kellogg left Charleville, James W. Gerard, the American Ambassador to the Imperial German Court, visited G.H.Q. Charleville. There he learned the sad story of the Lille deportations.

On the evening of April 28, 1916, Gerard and his staff boarded a special saloon car in Berlin and arrived in Charleville the following morning. "We were received at the railway station by several officers and escorted in one of the Kaiser's automobiles, which had been set apart for my use, to a villa in the town of Charleville."[43]

Gerard was in town to confer with the Germans about their resumption of unrestricted submarine warfare and to meet with C.R.B. delegates working in occupied France. As part of the agenda, he toured some villages, visiting food distribution facilities. In the countryside, he saw something that the Germans wished he had not.

> During this trip about the country, I saw a number of women and girls working, or attempting to work, in the fields. Their appearance was so different from that of the usual peasant that I spoke to the accompanying officers about it. I was told, however, that these were the peasants of the locality who dressed unusually well in that part of France.[44]

Dismissing Gerard's observation, the party returned to Charleville. As part of the agenda, the G.H.Q. arranged for Gerard to meet C.R.B. delegates working in occupied France. Since these men were at a meeting at their own headquarters in Brussels, G.H.Q. ordered up a special train to bring them to Charleville. There, Count Wengersky (probably Count W- in Kellogg's writings), who was the G.H.Q. liaison with the C.R.B., hosted a tea party at his residence so everyone could chat informally. Everything was warm and fuzzy and goodwill gushed until a bombshell exploded at the tea party.[45]

> We had tea and cakes in these lodgings, and then some of the Americans drew me aside and told me the secret of the peculiar looking peasants whom I had seen at work in the fields surrounding Charleville.[46]

It turned out the Germans were using what was essentially slave labor in the fields around Charleville. Moreover, the slaves were women, girls and men from the French city of Lille. These were the well-dressed peasants Gerard had seen during his tour! The Germans intended to enslave 50,000 to work in agriculture — Gerard had seen the first cohorts. The following proclamations (abridged) described the new "work program."

> Proclamation of the German Military Commandant of Lille
>
> The attitude of England makes the provisioning of the population more and more difficult.
>
> In order to relieve the distress, the German Government has recently asked for volunteers to go to work in the country. This offer has not had the success anticipated.
>
> Consequently, the inhabitants will be evacuated by order and removed to the country. The evacuated persons will be sent to the interior of the occupied French territory, far behind the front, where they will be employed in agriculture, and in no way on military works.
>
> Lille, April, 1916   The Commandant
>
> Annex 2.
>
> All the inhabitants of the house, with the exception of children under fourteen and their mothers, and of the aged, must prepare themselves to be transported within an hour and a-half.
>
> An officer will decide definitively what persons are to be taken to the concentration camps. For this purpose, all the inhabitants of the house must assemble in front of the house; in case of bad weather they may remain in the passage. The door of the house must remain open. No protest will be listened to.
>
> Each person will be entitled to 30 kilogrammes of luggage; if the weight is excessive, the whole of the luggage of the person concerned will be peremptorily refused.
>
> Any person endeavouring to avoid transportation will be punished without mercy.
>
> Etappen-Kommandantur[47]

The Lille C.R.B. delegate, Lawrence Wellington of Amherst, Massachusetts, a graduate of Williams College (1912), provided detailed information about the deportations.

> The deportations commenced on 22d April, the day before Easter, and the order, coming through the German ranks as a military command, was naturally carried out in a blunt, brutal, military way. A whole regiment was placed in a given quarter of the city and machine guns were placed in the streets, and six, eight, or ten fully armed soldiers entered each house to remove all inhabitants capable of doing field labor.[48]

He reported that in addition to homes being entered, industrial schools with several hundred young women students suffered the same treatment. Soldiers rounded up the pupils as if they were cattle, packed them in tramcars and sent them to the railway station for deportation. The parents never knew what happened to their daughters — they just vanished.

> Young girls of irreproachable life — who have never committed any worse offence than that of trying to pick up some bread or a few potatoes to feed a numerous family ... have been carried off. Their mothers, who have watched so closely over them, and had no other joy than that of keeping their daughters beside them, in the absence of father and sons fighting or killed at the front — these mothers are now alone.[49]

Lawrence Wellington's information served as the detonator for the diplomatic explosion that rocked the Charleville tea party. Ambassador Gerard confronted Quartermaster von Zoellner, a Bavarian general attending the tea. Of course, the Bavarian feigned great surprise, promised to investigate and to summon the general commanding Lille to Charleville for an explanation, etc. Gerard's protests eventually stopped the deportations, although by then 22,000 were already in work camps.

> The young girls and women were kept together in camps which in many cases were located within the district of actual operations. These districts were necessarily overflowing with the passing thousands of German soldiers on their way to and from service in the trenches. Girls of the best families and character were herded with women with no character at all. The moral consequence of such contact, under the conditions that prevailed, can easily be imagined. By showing complacence to the lusts of the soldiery these women could gain for themselves protectors in the army of their enemies; they could be exempted from labour, could receive better food and better treatment. The inevitable result was the moral degradation of a considerable proportion of these girls in camps near the front.[50]

When the young women finally returned to their homes, nearly one in three was pregnant. For the theorist, their plight was an example of wartime social Darwinism in action. For everyone else, it was legalized rape.

Because the deportations surfaced when a C.R.B. delegate broke his pledge of "see no evil, report no evil" neutrality, relations between Germans and Americans in occupied France soured. After the spring of 1916, more and more restrictions limited the travel of delegates and very much curtailed their ability to carry out inspections. German officers took over many of the tasks of the delegates. With their new tasks came a new name; they were no longer *Begleitoffiziers* (accompanying officers) but now *Verplegungsoffizers* (aid and provisioning officers). Most took their missions seriously.

Because food was going into areas just behind the active front, the British and French constantly opposed C.R.B. activities, which in their view aided the enemy. On the other hand, the Germans considered C.R.B. delegates as spies for the Allies. Caught between the warring belligerents, Hoover and his administrators in Brussels somehow always managed to negotiate an accommodation; the C.R.B. continued to function in Northern France until America broke off diplomatic relations with Germany (February 1917) prior to entering the war.

The United States finally entered the war on April 6, 1917. Because the United States was now a belligerent, American leadership (i.e., Herbert Hoover's leadership) of the C.R.B. ended. The Dutch and Spanish Legations, the remaining neutral legations in Brussels, took charge of the C.R.B. operations, although most of the aid still came from the United States. By any reckoning, the C.R.B. achievement under Hoover had been incredible. The C.R.B. had handled more than $200,000,000 in charitable gifts and government subsidies, with no hint of scandal and with administrative costs under 1 percent. It had acquired and transported across submarine infested seas more than 2,500,000 tons of foodstuffs to Rotterdam. From that port it moved the food via canals and rail to 4,700 communes in Belgium and Northern France, covering an area of nearly 20,000 square miles. The C.R.B. rescued 9,000,000 from hunger for more than two and a half years. Around the world, it had 130,000 volunteers participating in one aspect or another of this humanitarian effort. In charge of this effort were, on the average, 55 C.R.B. members including approximately 36 in the field in Belgium and 6 in Northern France.[51] At the top of this chain of command was one man, Herbert Hoover. The C.R.B. was essentially a twentieth century piratical nation; it negotiated treaties, had a navy of transport ships, an army of volunteers, its own flag and a pirate chief (Hoover). In 1915, a British parliamentarian recognized his qualities. "If England could have availed herself of such talent for organization as H.C. Hoover has displayed in feeding the Belgians, we would be a good year nearer the end of the war than we are to-day."[52]

Herbert Hoover was always very humble about his achievements in Belgium and Northern France.

> I always feel an infinite embarrassment at the reception and overestimation of the part that I may have played in what is really an institutional engine, and the credit for which belongs, not to myself, but to some fifty thousand volunteers who have worked for a period now of nearly three years.[53]

Chapter 9

Battles Around Ypres

> We saw them gay, and we saw them gassed; we found them idling or writing letters on the running boards of our cars, and we found the dark stains of their fading lives upon our stretchers; we passed them stealing up like stalwart ghosts to action, and we left them lying in long brown rows beside the old roads of Flanders.[1] — Henry Sydnor Harrison, American ambulance driver

> As one report modestly observes, "The difficulties of this part of the country are worthy of note. The trenches are very wet, and water is up to the men's knees in most places." Such phrases as "men knee-deep in water," "trenches full of liquid mud 2 to 3 feet deep," ... "trenches untenable owing to flooding," "ground so wet only able to dig down 2 feet," occur in endless repetition.[2]
> — Douglas W. Johnson, professor of physiography, Columbia University

The West Flanders town of Ypres (Ieper) became the focal point of the most horrific battles fought in Belgium. The fighting, although essentially unceasing for four years, attained peaks of butchery in the fall/early winter of 1914 (First Battle of Ypres), in the spring/summer of 1915 (Second Battle of Ypres) and in the summer/fall of 1917 (Third Battle of Ypres). All told, either defending or attacking this Belgian backwater cost nearly one million casualties, making it one of the most expensive pieces of real estate on the Western Front.

The town of Ypres was within range of German artillery fire for four years, "never more than seven miles from the front line, and sometimes less than three."[3] The first shell fell on the town on October 7, 1914, the last, on October 14, 1918. In the interim, countless high explosive shells and bombs from aircraft pummeled the town, leaving nothing at the war's end but piles of rubble marking where churches, public buildings and houses once stood. Conveniently for German artillerists, a prewar travel guide by the Leipzig publisher Karl Baedeker gave a clear description (including a detailed street map) of the Ypres target.

An old town on the *Yperlée* [a tributary of the Yser River] (now vaulted over), with 17,400 inhab., who are chiefly occupied in the manufacture of Valenciennes lace, possesses broad and clean streets and imposing old buildings of the 13–14th centuries. It was formerly the capital of West Flanders. The cloth-making industry here dates back to 1037, and about 1217 Ypres is said to have been the wealthiest and most powerful commercial town in Flanders.[4]

The most notable medieval edifice was the *Halle des Drapiers* (Lakenhal) or Cloth Hall (1304) on the Grand Place, a gigantic building of three stories with a frontage of 433 feet. In the center of the Cloth Hall, a belfry rose to a height of 230 feet, providing an easy target. Just north and across a narrow lane from the Cloth Hall was the Cathedral Church of St. Martin, dating from the thirteenth century and considered the most imposing example of ecclesiastical architecture in Belgium. Its 190-foot bell tower also made a useful targeting point. Both the Cloth Hall and cathedral towers were clearly visible from the German lines.

> The woodwork of the Cloth Hall and the cathedral-roof blazed and was burned in spark-shot veils of smoke, and the great Church of St. Nicholas lay partly in ruins.... The dull clash of falling masonry, the shrill whine of shell-splinters ricocheting from roofs, echoed and re-echoed in the deserted cloisters of the church. Inside the cathedral all lay piled in disorder — crosses, marble statues from tombs, old oak choir-stalls, rags of burned canvases that once were priceless pictures — all smashed beneath masses of fallen masonry and plaster from the roof. Here was a carved angel's head, here a fretted pinnacle. Over all glittered with the sheen of many jewels broken lozenges of stained glass that once had made the cathedral-windows glow with sumptuous coloring.[5]

> When the last shell had fallen on the town of other days, and the last fire had been extinguished, there remained of the noble Halles [Cloth Hall] but a fragment of the Belfry and portions of the neighboring walls. The Cathedral was represented by a shattered tower and ruined walls.[6]

However, until the last week of October 1914, Ypres was still relatively unscathed. In the north, the Belgians and French held the Yser Front from the North Sea to Dixmude (see Chapter 5). After much maneuvering by all armies, including a temporary incursion by the German Cavalry into the town of Ypres, a relatively stable front materialized south of Dixmude. By October 21, the French held the line from Dixmude along the east bank of the Yser Canal[7] to the village of Bixschotte (Bixschoote), five miles north of Ypres. From Bixschotte, the British held a front that swung east in an arc around Ypres forming a salient into the German lines. The front crossed the Ypres Canal about four miles south of Ypres and then continued to Armentières and beyond, deeper into France.

Even before King Albert of the Belgians ordered the inundation of the Yser Front (October 25), and the resulting flood stopped the German attacks (October 29), German assaults began on the Ypres Salient. On October 23, units of poorly trained but very patriotic student-volunteers and cadets from German universities recklessly attacked British trenches near the village of Langemarck (Langemark). The result was a catastrophe for the former students.

> The new German levies, many of whom had had scarcely two months' training, hurled themselves on our trenches with incredible courage and resolution. They were mown down by our fire, but they came on again and yet again, till human endurance reached breaking-point. The corps that attacked that day lost 75 per cent of its effectives.[8]

The German military cemetery at Langemarck contains the remains of more than 3,000 student-volunteers and cadets who fell that day. Immortalized as *Kindermord bei Ypern*, the Massacre of the Innocents at Ypres and Langemarck entered Nazi mythology.

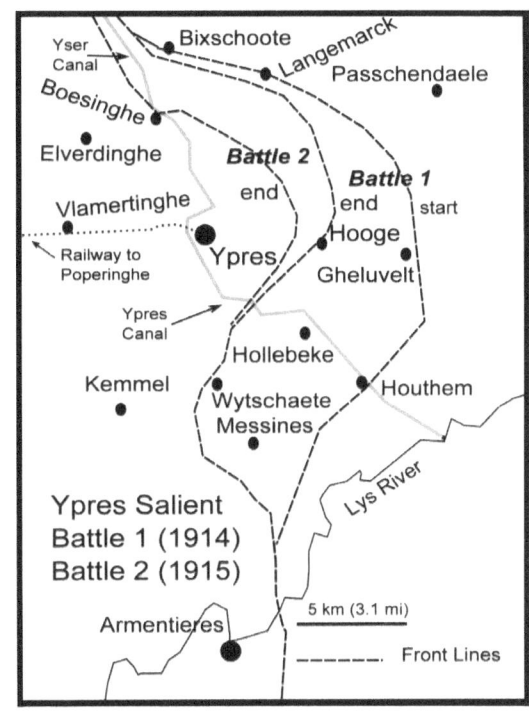

The same day (October 23) the Germans attacked the midpoint of the salient at the village of Becelaere (Beselare), about six miles due east of Ypres. By October 27, the Germans managed to push the British back about a mile but at great cost. However, Langemarck and Becelaere were only prologues to what the Germans planned next. On October 29, they launched a massive attack against the southern portion of the salient. The Germans vigorously pressed the offensive from October 29 until November 15, 1914, the First Battle of Ypres.

> The German plan of attack was to concentrate as many guns as could be massed in the locality chosen for the attack, and prepare the way for infantry to advance after resistance had been weakened by overwhelming artillery-fire. Infantry were sent forward in battalions, regiments, and even brigades, massed together after the fashion of the Macedonian phalanx, which were often seven or eight deep, the men standing shoulder to shoulder.... In thus trusting to mass-formations the Kaiser omitted to take account of the increased power conferred on the defense by the destructive effects of modern weapons, with which a few men entrenched could check a column ten times their strength in numbers.[9]

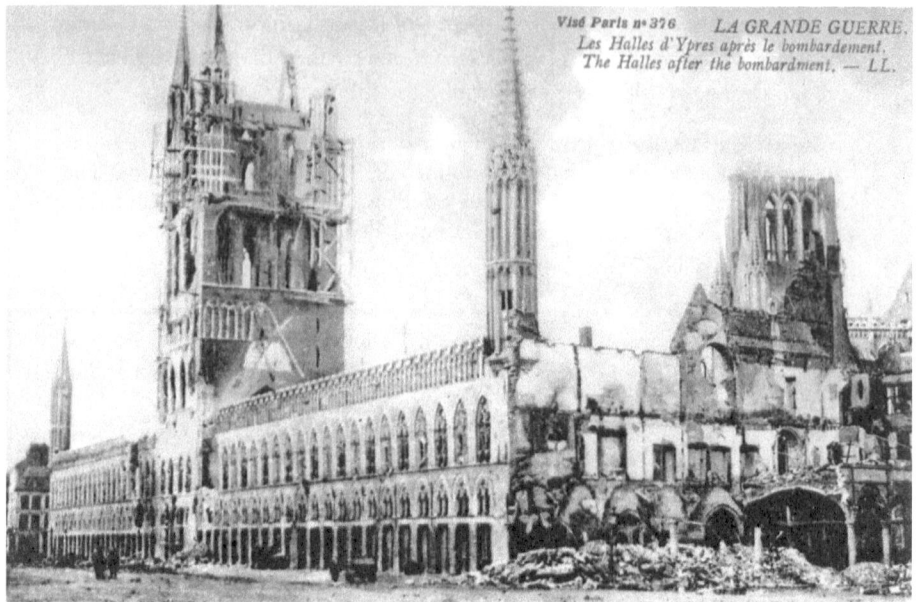

The famous Cloth Hall at Ypres at the beginning of the city's bombardment (1914-1915). The square tower on the right is the Cathedral Church of St. Martin. By the end of the war only the skeleton of the tower of the Cloth Hall remained; the rest of the building had been reduced to a few jagged standing walls and mounds of rubble. The Cathedral Church suffered the same fate (Klekowski collection).

The Allies manned hastily-constructed shallow trenches lacking barbed wire defenses. The battle was truly an Allied affair, with a French Cavalry Corps of four divisions and two divisions of French Territorials fighting alongside the British. The suicidal massed assaults eventually overwhelmed Allied positions, essentially smothering them with German bodies.

> The attacks had been growing stronger; across the lines the British heard the Germans singing as though working themselves up, German fashion, to a Berserk courage; captured orders showed that the Kaiser had commanded a great assault which should clear the way to Calais and to Paris.[10]

However, before the British retired from any position, they exacted a heavy price. Fierce volleys of rifle fire scythed down attackers. Armed with the Lee-Enfield rifle with its overly large ten-round magazine, a rifleman could fire fifteen aimed shots a minute.[11] Wounded men loaded for their comrades. The rapid volleys of bullets convinced the Germans they faced machine guns rather than rifles.[12]

> The odds in favor of the Germans were at times nearly ten to one, but owing to the nature of the ground they could only attack in mass formation along

roads and open spaces.... Nothing but masses of men and reckless disregard of carnage could have inspired the German with any hope of subduing the terrible superiority of British fire.[13]

Outnumbered and outgunned in terms of artillery, the British fell back. Their commander, Sir John French, replied to a request for reinforcements, "I can send you my two sentries."[14] There was no one left; everyone, including cooks, was fighting. The French Corps was equally desperate. Cooks, hewers of wood and drawers of water and even a French general's cavalry escort joined the fight. Napoleonic cuirassiers, resplendent in silver helmets with flowing manes, steel breastplates, cavalry boots and sabers, took part in a bayonet charge using sabers rather than bayonets.[15] Adding to the chaos, a lucky German shell hit General Douglas Haig's headquarters from which he commanded First Corps, about 36,000 men. "A shell had burst in the house. Haig was outside at the time, but nearly every staff officer of the 1st Corps was killed or wounded. The army up there was almost headless — was fighting as individuals on primitive fighting instinct."[16]

On October 31, near the village of Gheluvelt (Geluveld), the Germans nearly broke through. Upon learning this key part of the British line was collapsing, Sir John French violated World War I military tradition; the commanding general went to the front line during a battle. He was the last reinforcement.

> He jumped into his automobile and rushed to the line of the 1st Division. He had not so far to go as he thought. The line had retired four miles. Through his glasses he could see the close-locked quadruple ranks of German infantrymen attacking everywhere.[17]
>
> In the thickest of that day's fighting he left his motor-car and ran on foot to a wood where a brigade was giving ground. As he rushed in, a wounded private staggered back into his arms, French laid him gently down and went on talking to his men, encouraging them, rallying them, until they held.[18]
>
> He rallied a part of the broken 1st Division and threw it at the flank of a German attack which was proceeding on the reckless theory that the English were totally beaten. The Germans broke; the British retook Gheluvelt on the original line.[19]

On November 11, in despair that the battle was not going as planned, the Kaiser mustered his best troops in an attempt to crack the salient, and open the way to the Channel ports. Again, as on October 31, the Germans attacked near the apex of the salient. Two brigades of the famous Prussian Guards hit the line at Gheluvelt, a small village on the Menin Road, situated on the principal road leading to Ypres. They attacked at parade march in the early hours of the morning, a devastating volley of rifle fire greeted them. But still they came "and at three points they pierced our front, and won the woods to the west."[20]

Again the dense masses poured in; again the very officers fired until their rifles grew too hot to hold. When, that night, the strength of the German attack was spent the better part of the Prussian Guard lay dead in a wood — lay at some places in ranks eight deep.[21]

The enterprise of an American journalist, Will Irwin, brought the events of the First Battle of Ypres before the British and American public. Since he published his story in defiance of British military censorship, his story is worth telling. Irwin arrived in Belgium during the first weeks of the war in 1914 and was in both Brussels and Louvain. After the German Army occupied Brussels, filing news stories out of the city became nearly impossible. Irwin decided to leave Brussels for England, where he could use the trans–Atlantic cable. He took a train from Brussels to Aachen with a connection to Holland, where he boarded a ship to England. His fellow train travelers were the American journalists Richard Harding Davis, Arno Dosch, Gerald Morgan and Mary Boyle O'Reilly. This was the train with the famous layover in Louvain and from the windows of their coach, the Americans watched the city burn (see Chapter 2). Arriving in England, Irwin traveled to London where he met his old friend and Stanford classmate Herbert Hoover. Hoover convinced Irwin to volunteer as publicist for the Commission for Relief of Belgium — without pay, of course. Irwin traveled to New York in December 1914, to organize publicity for the C.R.B. and returned to England on *Lusitania* at the end of January 1915, as a correspondent for the *Saturday Evening Post* and the *New York Tribune.*

Now a mystery man entered the story, one George Gordon Moore, a wealthy and socially well-connected American living in London.[22] Moore was at British headquarters in Ypres when the Prussian Guard attacked. Why he was there was a source of controversy.

The remarkable George Gordon Moore merits a digression. An international financier and multimillionaire, Moore began his career in business when he took over the Michigan United Traction Company, an 18-mile railway that he expanded to rank among the largest in America. In 1910 aboard ship to England, he met Sir John French. The two men soon became very close; in 1911, they leased a house in a fashionable part of London, which they later purchased, mostly with Moore's funds. The two lived together and shared common interests: "good food, high society, and beautiful women."[23]

> They [London swingers] especially enjoyed parties given by George Gordon Moore, an American millionaire, because they lasted from dinner to breakfast and were bursting with red and white camellias and "rocketing with champagne and the new sound of Negro Jazz and Hawaiian bands."[24]

Although married, Sir John pursued beautiful women with the passion of Casanova. Moore noted in his unpublished memoirs, "The Field Marshal was famous for his love affairs. For several months we spent all our evenings together with feminine friends."[25] When Sir John became commander of the British Expeditionary Force (B.E.F.) and established his headquarters near Ypres, he invited Moore to live with him. Moore told a *Washington Post* reporter, "Yes, Sir John French and I lived together. I see nothing strange in that. I think a great deal of him and I hope the feeling is mutual. When the war began Sir John asked me to dine with him in France, and I was very glad to accept."[26] The British press thought it strange, in fact, very strange, that an American civilian was living with, and perhaps influencing, the man in charge of the B.E.F.[27] On a visit to London, Moore encouraged Irwin to write the battle's story and in this way to promote the career of his friend Sir John. Moore introduced Irwin to the men who directed the battle and those who fought it. He also guided him in finding confidential documents about the battle. Irwin based his story upon these sources. Hoover, when learning Irwin was writing the story, advised him against defying the censor. "You're new over here," Hoover said. "You'll get your fingers burned."[28]

Irwin brought the Ypres story to Lord Northcliffe, publisher of the London *Times* and the *Daily Mail*. Northcliffe felt that censorship of the military, which only permitted brief official communiqués to appear in newspapers, was a disservice to the public. Irwin's story was very different; it had color and human interest, just what the public wanted. Northcliffe decided to publish and damn the censor. It would appear simultaneously in the *Times* and the *Daily Mail* in London and the *New York Tribune*. To avoid interference from the censor if sent via the trans–Atlantic cable, the story traveled by special courier on a fast ship to New York.

When the story appeared, it caused a sensation. The British public loved it. Irwin became a celebrity; invitations poured in from London society, and he attended a luncheon at 10 Downing Street with Prime Minister Asquith; Northcliffe republished the story as a penny pamphlet, selling out the first edition of a half-million copies. *The British Weekly* (London) described the story as being "in every sense of the word an amazing performance." The commentary continued, "Few of us at home had the faintest idea of the peril in which our Army, our nation, and our Empire were placed in this battle."[29] Meanwhile, the censor seethed, it would get even.[30]

A letter published in *The Globe* newspaper of New York presented a more tragic picture of the consequences of the First Battle of Ypres.

> Through the glasses the ground seemed carpeted with the dead. The Greenish-gray of the German uniform, the khaki of the English, and the brilliant red and blues of the French were mingled in a frightful fellowship. There were rods [a measure of length —1 rod = 16½ feet] where the dead were piled and heaped upon each other.

> Neither Germans nor British could rescue their injured. During the day a movement might here and there be seen in that litter of misery. But no sound came. If they cried, the thunder of the guns, the staccato rattle of the mitrailleuses, drowned their voices.... There had been no attempt on either side to bury the bodies.... The corpses have burst their clothes.
> It was at a distance of five miles — five miles — that the witness first became aware of this bivouac of the unburied dead. He became faint and ill. No one knows the numbers of thousands of dead men there. All that is known is that over a segment of a circle, perhaps five miles long and a mile wide, they lie elbow to elbow and head to head. On either side their living mates glare lividly across that field toward the entrenched enemy.... The world should know what war of to-day is. "Shells fall upon that field continually," said the eye-witness. "Then the sickening odor that arises becomes a physical torture."[31]

If Irwin's patriotic prose upset the British censor, then *The Globe* letter probably caused it apoplexy. This image of the war was not for public consumption, especially for the families of the men who perished.

There was at least one American citizen in the German Army at Ypres. Karl Llewellyn was in Paris at the outbreak of the war. When a youth, he had lived in Germany for three years. As almost all young men of 1914, he responded to the war mania; in his case, the experiences of his youth pushed him to volunteer for the German Army. He traveled by train to Germany and joined the infantry. Soon his division was near Ypres attacking the English trenches.

> That advance! It was the first disillusionment, and a pretty bitter one. None of that music-playing, colors-flying, quick-time work you read about; none of the enthusiasm that sets danger sweetly at naught. Instead a terrible nervous strain, with your comrade shot beside you, whom you may not help; and a pounding undercurrent of thought you try to force back: "Are they going to get me now?"[32]

Firing his Mauser rifle wildly at imaginary targets as bullets whistled by his head, Karl continued forward. His five-round magazine was empty, but there was no time to reload, he must keep up with his line and advance. Finally, what was left of the line reached the English trenches and he reloaded. The enemy soldiers were retreating.

> Now there they are, the men that were shooting at you, running, running wildly! It isn't nice; it isn't civilized; but there is a fiendish joy in watching them drop or turn somersaults as you shoot, a joy the greater from your sense of new-gained safety after peril.
> There is dormant, I believe, in most of us a savage love of shooting at a live mark — the hunting instinct. When it comes upon us for the first time we cannot answer for ourselves. But it fades as quickly as does the glamour of war.[33]

While the Prussian Guard exhausted its vitality[34] against the British on the Menin Road near Gheluvelt, a different German formation attacked the French lines at the northern end of the salient at Bixschotte.

The fight raged round Bixschoote, which speedily became a charnel house full of unburied dead. The capture of the place would have given the Germans a position astride the Ypres-Dixmude canal and railway, and enabled them to turn the defence of Ypres from the north.... To achieve this end, battalion after battalion was hurled against the village.[35]

The French held; the German assault ebbed after four days of butchery. By November 17, following four weeks of fierce fighting, warfare fizzled to spasmodic assaults. "The weather had changed to high winds and snow blizzards, and in a tempest the Battle of Ypres died away."[36] Most of the combatants, whether French, British or German, were either dead, or wounded, or missing, or just too worn out to continue. All had literally exhausted their vitality! To what end? The salient, albeit a bit more compressed, still held, blocking the Germans from the Channel ports. For the contested ground, based upon rough accounting, the British suffered 60,000 casualties (including 24,000 dead); the Germans had 165,000 casualties (including 50,000 dead).[37] The French losses are not given. Perhaps the lesson, if there was one, was that given the weapons of 1914, especially magazine rifles and machine guns, soldiers attacking defended trenches suffered more than those defending them did.

December 1914 to mid–April 1915 was a period of relative calm. Trench fighting and raids were continuous and men died; however, there were no major assaults. In Ypres, people accommodated to whatever insanity war threw at them.

> By degrees Ypres became a show place; every soldier required picture postcards of the famous ruins; souvenirs were eagerly acquired, and a small kerbstone industry in shell fuses, stained-glass fragments, and relics of all kinds sprang up. Small boys acquired wealth, and the Cathedral guide must have accumulated a substantial balance. The shelling which sometimes occurred did not seem to disturb the townsfolk; they had grown accustomed to it.[38]

The American novelist Mary Roberts Rinehart arrived in Ypres in February 1915. The previous month she had toured the Yser Front, researching a series of articles for *The Saturday Evening Post* (see Chapter 5). A Belgian general, General M---, agreed to take her to Ypres where perhaps she might see something of interest. Near the town, the general's auto pulled over to allow troops to pass; a column of soldiers filed by just out of the trenches. From the comfort of his car and swathed in rugs for warmth, the general saw only heroes. Rinehart, who by then had a jaundiced view of the war, saw these men not as heroes but as the pawns of kings and emperors. The soldiers appeared tired, dirty and depressed. She learned later that the men described themselves as "cannon food" and that they had fought the night before from trenches that were in places waist-deep in water. "Scarcely a man lifted his head to glance at us. They went on drearily through the mud under the pelting sleet, drooping from fatigue."[39]

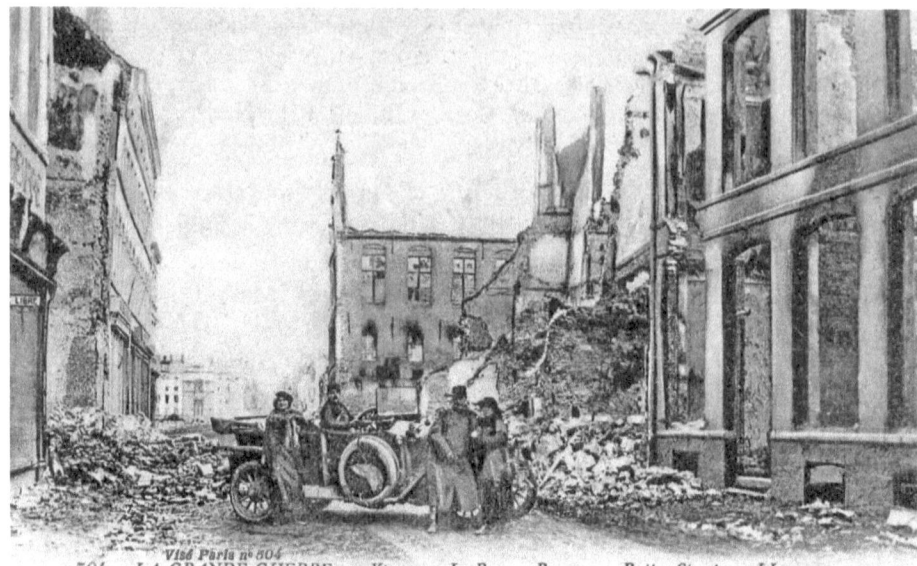

504 LA GRANDE GUERRE. — Ypres. — La Rue au Beurre. — Butter Street. — LL.

A couple of adventurous women and their companions making an automobile tour of the ruins of Ypres. They have stopped on the main street leading into the Grand Place and the Cloth Hall; the street is partially blocked by piles of masonry from shelled buildings. Mary Roberts Rinehart probably had a similar tour (Klekowski collection).

In Ypres, she toured the ruins of the Cloth Hall and cathedral, even finding an artillery shell nose cone and a bit of a fallen gargoyle. As she collected souvenirs, new reserves marched through the Grand Place on their way to the trenches. "Almost every man had an additional loaf of bread strapped to his knapsack at his back. They were laughing and talking among themselves, for they had had a sleep and hot food; for the time at least they were dry and fed and warm."[40]

After her tour, Mrs. Rinehart visited French headquarters in Poperinghe (Poperinge), a small village 6 miles (9.6 km) west of Ypres. While sipping coffee to warm up, the commandant showed her a postcard found on the body of a dead German soldier the previous night. With the card was a photograph of a woman, the soldier's wife. They were Otto and Hedwig. Rinehart found it all so tragic and sad. The wife said she was busy making clothes for their children, asked if he had received the packages she had sent, hoped he would have a chance to write, and said she thought of him often.

> So she was making clothing for the children and sending him little packages. And Otto lay dead under the stars that night — dead of an ideal, which is that a

man must leave his family and all that he loves and follow the beckoning finger of empire.

"For king and country!"[41]

That evening Rinehart and her Belgian general left Ypres. Packed in the car and wrapped in newspaper were her mementoes, the nose cone and the gargoyle. Probably her most lasting memory of Ypres was the postcard from Hedwig to Otto — not the city that lay in ruins.

About the time Rinehart was touring Ypres, an American journalist crouched in a German front line trench about three miles south of the town, firing a Mauser rifle at the nearby French defenses. Robert Dunn of the *New York Evening Post* was on special assignment with the Bavarian Army. Part of the junket included dining with Crown Prince Rupprecht of Bavaria at his villa near Lille. Dunn described the Prince as a greyish, tall, sinewy man with a strong oblong face and a long mouth that in smiling turned down at the corners. Because of a connection between the owners of the *Evening Post* and a member of the Prince's staff, Dunn received, in addition to the dinner invitation with the Prince, permission to visit the Bavarian firing line. He traveled north from Lille in a royal Bavarian motor car flying the Prince's flag on the radiator. A soldier-chauffeur, tooting a bugle-call reserved for sovereignty, warned traffic to give way. Their destination was the village of Houthem on the Ypres Canal, the divisional headquarters for the sector of trenches Dunn would visit. From Houthem, he and his guides walked toward the front line near the village of Hollebeke.[42] As Dunn said, "And then began the night of nights." The communication trenches (*Laufgraben*) were only safe at night, a safety that was relative since every night saw men killed or wounded.

> It was seven o'clock, drizzling hard. Ahead, over the swelling battlefield, the boom of artillery was dying fitfully, only to be replaced by glimmering rocket-lights shot from the trenches, which, like flashes of greenish lightning, reticulated the torn timber and tottering walls of houses. The soupy mud was ankle deep.[43]

Rifle bullets kicked up mud around him; his guide instructed that the party should walk ten meters apart and stop all conversation. More rifle bullets struck like pops of "venomous firecrackers." They pushed into a ruined village, "It was as if walls had enclosed us in a shooting-gallery."[44] Dunn had second thoughts, but in order not to lose face, he kept following his guide, closer and closer to the first line trench. The communication trench they traveled in was a water-filled ditch. The group literally floundered along in the darkness with lunged fists into the mud walls on either side to stay balanced. "And never two feet from us, through the ruff of earth, did those crackling reports cease, or the taut singing overhead." Finally, they reached the firing trench, only 140 meters from the enemy. Every couple of yards riflemen crouched behind steel shields, taking occasional pot shots at the enemy. One soldier handed his Mauser to Dunn and motioned him to try his luck at the French *Schützengraben* (front line firing trench). "The next moment it was in my hands, with the muzzle pointing through the eyehole atop the bank, across that short and hellish space. Be it on my head, I did it, fired twice."[45]

In less than a minute, Dunn had violated his code of neutrality as an American journalist. He realized his actions, performed in the heat of the moment, were a mistake and later attempted to rationalize them by saying that although he fired he did not aim.[46] "I cannot consider, either, that my neutrality, except perhaps technically, was in any way violated."[47] Later, trench rockets illuminated No Man's Land, that short hellish space he had fired over.

> The horror and climax of the night lay in the space between. Bodies, bodies unburied, unrecognizable, unless we had been told. Lumps of matter, like swollen sacks, in hundreds, scattered haphazard upon one another, heaped like sacks. Without visible flesh or clothing; all mud-coloured, drenched, gleaming terribly with the slimy pallor, like verdigris, of that awful field.[48]

The geology and weather of Flanders proved to be nearly as great an enemy as the Germans. The subsoil of the Ypres Salient is clay. In places, the thin topsoil is sandy loam. The clay acts as an impervious barrier, preventing rainwater from naturally percolating through the soil horizon and draining away. Canals and ditches crisscross the landscape to promote drainage. In the fall and winter, the weather, for lack of a better description, is nasty. Bitter winds from the North Sea lash seemingly endless rain squalls across the landscape. Water pools in any depression and ditches fill with water. The Ypres Salient was probably the most unforgiving environment on the Western Front in which to wage trench warfare for a prolonged period, let alone for four years! Water filled the trenches, which consequently could not be very deep; water filled the dugouts; water filled the shell craters, of which there were hundreds of thousands. Men waded up to their knees, or even waists, through communication trenches to reach the front line. Shelling and the transport of artillery, munitions and supplies destroyed the drainage ditches and plowed up the landscape so water had no place to go. Every hoof mark remained a puddle full of water for weeks. Trenches continually collapsed as their sodden walls gave way.

> On so flat a surface the rainfall finds it difficult to flow away. Nor can it escape readily underground, for the clay is one of the most impervious formations imaginable. Unable to sink downward or to flow laterally, the water remains stagnant over large areas, forming ponds and marshes, or rises until it slowly creeps, halting and hesitating as to what course to take, toward one of the sluggish rivers which wander with apparent aimlessness over the level land. The ground is saturated with moisture, whether it be the clay itself outcropping at

9. Battles Around Ypres 181

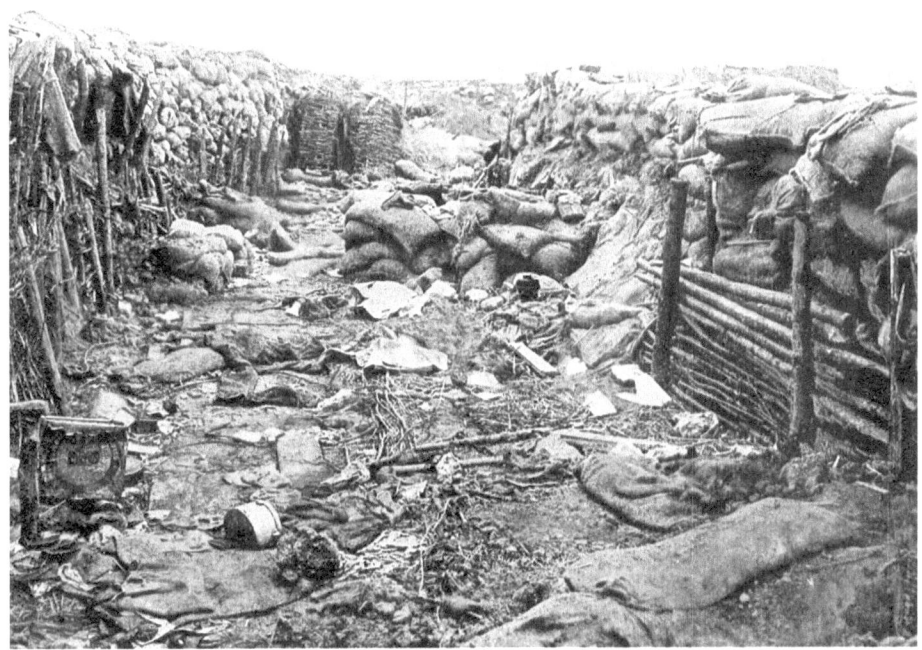

German photograph of a captured English trench in the Ypres Salient. The corpses and wounded have been removed. The trench's construction reflects the high water table; it is little more than a broad shallow ditch with sides raised by sand bagging. It offered essentially no protection from artillery fire (*Kriegs-Album des Marinekorps Flandern 1914–1917, 1918*).

the surface or the thin deposit of clayey loam resting as a mantle upon it. Either one gives a sticky, slippery mud which is the abomination of Flanders.[49]

The notorious Flanders mud, a mixture of organic matter and clay, was greasy, brown and glutinous. The mud stuck to everything and everybody. It stuck to boot soles so that walking involved lifting nearly a pound of mud with each step. Even the simple task of digging became arduous because one had to scrape away the mud stuck to the shovel before each stroke. Mud-smeared corpses were everywhere, whether dead a day, a week or a month. As if resurrecting, they sometimes "emerged from the quaking slime beneath men's feet in the trenches."[50]

> The damage done by artillery fire was greatly reduced when the shells exploded in a sticky clay. Shell holes filled with water which could not drain away, turning the battlefield into an almost impassable morass which blocked the advance for which the bombardment was supposed to be a preparation.... Assaulting columns found it difficult to scramble out of the slippery trenches and were mowed down by enemy fire as they advanced slowly through a tenacious clay

into which they sank more than ankle deep. Rifles became so clogged that they could not be fired; and, when they were wrapped in cloth to keep the mechanism clean, were not ready for instant use. The wounded lay half buried in the mud, and many were suffocated.[51]

As winter approached, the temperature dropped to near freezing. Fires near the front drew enemy attention and were generally forbidden; consequently, the men manning the lines were cold, wet and miserable. Even pin-ups clipped from *La Vie Parisienne* and displayed on earthen walls of dugouts did little to raise spirits. However, as Christmas 1914 approached, the men hoped for something better — perhaps a miracle? The first portent occurred in Ypres a few days before Christmas. All roads into the salient passed through the great square near the ruins of the Cathedral Church of St. Martin. One early morning, as men marched across the square and German shells exploded nearby, the sounds of an organ playing "O, Come All Ye Faithful" came from the "gaunt carcass of the cathedral."[52] The music began softly and then swelled to fill the square. Traffic stopped, men whispered of a miracle and all heads turned toward the cathedral. As the last echoes of the organ died away, a Red Cross orderly emerged. In exploring the ruins, he found the organ undamaged and seating himself at the instrument, he played the Christmas hymn.

On Christmas Eve, the Royal Flying Corps dropped a carefully wrapped plum pudding on a German flying field at Lille; not to be outdone, German airmen reciprocated the next day with the gift of an airborne bottle of rum. The Christmas Eve festive spirit even manifested itself in sectors of the front, although not everywhere.

> On the night before Christmas the Germans made a fierce attack on French and Belgian positions recently won to the north of Nieuport, and the Allies made a successful counter-attack, which resulted in the winning of a little more ground in the dunes.[53]

At Ypres, candle-lit Christmas trees appeared on the parapets of German trenches making a "chain of light all the way along the endless German line of communications."[54] Special trains from Berlin brought presents from home to the men. At G.H.Q. Charleville, the Kaiser presided over the distribution of gifts to all ranks. "There were long rows of tables bearing Christmas-trees shimmering with lights. Every officer and man received spiced cakes, apples, and nuts as at home. Men also received tobacco pouches and cigars."[55]

At the end of the gift-giving ceremony, the Kaiser delivered a short invocation that ended with these honeyed words. "We stand on hostile soil, the points of our swords turned to the enemy, our hearts turned to God. We say as once the Great Prince said, 'To the dust with all the enemies of Germany.' Amen."[56]

Presumably, the All Highest was not referring to the Prince of Peace.

To lift the spirits of his soldiers in the trenches, the Supreme Warlord sent regimental bands to reserve areas behind the trenches. After dark, when the shooting stopped, the sounds of "Stille Nacht, heilige Nacht" ("Silent Night") and other carols drifted across No Man's Land and into British and French trenches. Soon both friend and foe joined in chorus.

Christmas morning on the Ypres front was bright and clear with a fine powdering of snow. There was no sound, no artillery firing, no random rifle shots, just a clear cold dawn. Even the twittering of birds could be heard as they searched for crumbs. Then the miracle happened, a few gray-clad soldiers appeared in No Man's Land, waving and calling in broken English, "Merry Christmas, Tommy!" or "Merry Christmas, Jock!"[57] Spontaneously, men began climbing out of their trenches on either side and scrambling into No Man's Land. They shook hands, cheered and sang. Farther along the line, more men in khaki (British) and field-gray (German) appeared. The nationalities were sometimes difficult to distinguish as both wore mud-smeared uniforms supplemented against the Flanders winter with gifts from home: stocking hats, woolen balaclavas, woolen gloves and scarves, sheepskin vests, leather coats and cardigan vests. The men put their rifles aside and, finding someone bilingual, wished each other well. Often they resorted to soldier–French as their common tongue. They exchanged cigarettes, cigars, pipe tobacco and souvenirs, the latter usually military badges cut from their uniforms. And they sang: "Die Wacht am Rhein," "It's a Long Way to Tipperary," and "Auld Lang Syne" were the most popular. Mid-day they returned to their trenches for Christmas dinner.

> I went over in the afternoon and was photographed in a group of English and Germans mixed. We exchanged souvenirs; I got a German ribbon and photograph of the Crown Prince of Bavaria. The Germans opposite us were awfully decent fellows — Saxons, intelligent, respectable-looking men. I had quite a decent talk with three or four and have two names and addresses in my notebook.[58]

The truce continued that afternoon; working parties began to bury the dead in No Man's Land, German and British soldiers digging graves side-by-side. The Christmas Truce of 1914 ended that evening.[59] The next day there was still no shooting, but no one ventured into No Man's Land. "The morning after, the work of death was resumed."[60]

Back in London, Will Irwin agitated to get back to the front. No longer a celebrity as the memory of his Ypres story faded, Irwin found it difficult to get permission to enter the war zone. He was American, thus an alien, and regarded by the military censor as untrustworthy. However, with the help of George Gordon Moore, he finally received permission. On April 22, 1915, Irwin arrived in Boulogne, a major port of entry for British troops destined for Ypres and the exit port for the wounded.[61]

> Not only are the French hospitals in the regions named being emptied of those able to travel, but the British themselves are preparing new hospitals the whole way along the coast from Boulogne to Havre—120 miles or so. Summer hotels are being turned into hospitals, as well as commandeered villas of wealthy people. Among the commandeered villas is that of the millionaire Count Constanovitch, who married an American, and villas of a number of rich Americans.[62]

The British permission restricted Irwin's movements to the port area. While in Boulogne, he learned that the Germans had violated The Hague Convention of 1907 and launched a gas attack somewhere in the Ypres salient. He telegraphed this story to his papers, the London *Daily Mail* and the *New York Tribune*.[63] Irwin then caught an empty hospital train to a *post de secours* near Ypres at a railway station where the Royal Army Medical Corps dealt with the flood of wounded. Irwin manned a stretcher and noted that the air stank and seemed to burn in his lungs. Mildly gassed, he persisted and got his scoop, the near-first-hand report of the Second Battle of Ypres. He recovered from the effects of gas exposure in a London hospital.[64]

> The work of sending out the vapor was done from the advanced German trenches. Men garbed in a dress resembling the harness of a diver and armed with retorts or generators about 3 feet high and connected with ordinary hose-pipe turned the vapor loose toward the French lines.
>
> The effect of the noxious trench gas seems to be slow in wearing away. The men come out of their violent nausea in a state of utter collapse. Some of the rescued have already died from the after effects.[65]

The roads upon which Allied supplies and troops reached into the salient all passed through the town of Ypres, which was "like the hub of a wheel from which all the communications eastwards radiated like spokes."[66] The town of Ypres was the logistical bottleneck for the Ypres Salient. Although the Germans shelled the town intermittently, heavy shelling was usually a prelude to a German attack somewhere in the salient. On April 20, such a bombardment began and continued through the subsequent few days.

> The enemy opened fire upon the town with the giant 42-centimetre siege mortars [big Berthas]—the guns that had crushed Namur and Liége.
>
> Suddenly and without warning the bombardment began. With a dull drone that filled the air the giant shell could be heard coming for some eight seconds. The noise of its approach increased till it sounded like the roar of the passing of an express train; then fell the shell, and the giant burst of detonation seemed to shake the solid earth.
>
> The Grand Place was filled with people passing about their ordinary avocations when the first of these monsters fell.... The Place was a shambles, for

bodies lay in all directions, some mercifully dead, others mere heaps of agony....
A child lay motionless, pinned down by a giant pile of wreckage.[67]

Every twenty minutes a 42-centimeter shell exploded in the town. The shots were not random. A German observation airplane whose mission was to target and destroy critical roads "wirelessed" corrections back to the battery; a hit could leave a road impassable, blocked by a crater thirty feet across and more than seventeen feet deep. Trucks loaded with stone and rubble from wrecked houses raced to fill these giant potholes. The most critical road-junction of all was just west of Ypres, where the main road from the village of Vlamertinghe (Vlamertinge) and the railroad crossed the Ypres Canal at the very entrance to the town.

> The shell fell with mathematical exactitude upon the level crossing and the centre of the old road, creating a thirty-foot crater and leaving the rails and sleepers of the level crossing projecting in the air like some giant comb.[68]

The Germans' intent, of course, was to disrupt Allied supply lines supporting the salient. However, where would they attack? On April 22, the shelling of the town reached a new intensity. That evening, out on the lines, the weather was pleasant, with a steady wind blowing from the northeast. At 6:30 p.m., as darkness closed in, a strange green cloud drifted with the breeze across No Man's Land, hugging the land as it moved west toward the French trenches. French troops held about six and a half miles of front from the Ypres Canal to just east of Langemarck. This was the northern most sector of the salient. The cloud was chlorine gas and it came from the forward German trenches. Upon reaching the French lines, it caused total chaos: blinded, gasping for breath, coughing in agony, everyone ran wild with terror. It was a rout.

> The gas was pumped from cylinders, and, rising in a cloud, which at its maximum was seven feet high, it traveled in two minutes the distance between the lines. It was thickest close to the ground, and filled every cranny of the trenches.... It was fatal to run backwards, for in that case he followed the gas zone, and the exertion of rapid movement compelled deep breathing, and so drew the poison into the lungs. Its effect was to fill the lungs with fluid and produce bronchitis. Those smitten by it suffered horribly, gasping and struggling for breath, with blue, swollen faces, and eyes bursting from the head. It affected sight, too, and produced temporary blindness. Even a thousand yards from the place of emission men were afflicted with violent sickness and giddiness. After that it dissipated itself, and only blanched herbage marked its track.[69]

Adding to this horror, the Germans sent artillery shells containing gas into the retreating troops. As the gas abated, German infantry, wearing gas masks resembling pig snouts, crossed No Man's Land. Between the gas, exploding shells, pig snouts and spiked helmets, it was a scene to conjure visions of hell.

How many of the men left unconscious in the trenches when the French broke died from fumes it is impossible to say, since those trenches were at once occupied by Germans.[70] No discredit attaches to those who broke. The pressure was more than flesh and blood could bear.[71]

In Ypres that night, panic reigned: giant artillery shells pummeled the town, lighting the sky in the east with the incessant flash of gunfire and bursting shells. Flare lights streaked into the heavens like meteors while flocks of shrapnel shells burst overhead. Crazed troops retreated through the streets, and everywhere the air was sickly with the strange metallic smell of gas. No one knew what had happened or what kind of horrible weapon the Germans had unleashed.

> The road to Vlamertinghe was choked with halted supply-wagons coming up, and a medley of Zouaves, civilian refugees, French soldiers, limberless gun-teams, pouring madly in a wide stream to the south.[72]

> Behind the flight rose the pyre of Ypres; ahead lay the little village and station of Vlamertinghe, bathed in the green moon glow and constantly red-lit by falling shell.[73]

All converged upon the railway station-yard in Vlamertinghe. An empty train stood in the station, its engine, a grey armored locomotive, "stood, menacing, like some antediluvian monster come to life."[74] The crowd surged toward the train and escape. Chaos followed with pushing and shoving and everyone for himself. The strong trampled the weak in their panic to board the train. This mob behavior ended when a young French officer appeared and took charge. By force of will and personality, he restored order and discipline. When the train finally left the station, it carried only women, children and badly wounded or gassed soldiers.

The retreat of the French in the evening of April 22 left a four-mile-long undefended gap in the northern sector of the salient. The Germans poured in, realizing this was a chance to breach the salient and make the run for the Channel ports.

> Ypres seemed within German grasp. Storms of high-explosive shell, shrapnel, and bombs filled with asphyxiating gases burst over, or on, all tactical points north of the city, which was itself once more heavily bombarded. Onward came the Germans, leaving the wall of gas, which was now beginning to break up into patches, behind them. At a distance they looked like a huge mob bearing down on the town. Never had the position in Flanders been more critical.[75]

Next to and east of the French, troops from Canada held the line. Canadian action on the night of April 22 and the following day essentially saved Ypres. These soldiers were products of their country: prospectors in the Yukon gold rush, fur trappers from the boreal wilds, farmers from the Manitoba prairie, and businessmen from Toronto. They were self-reliant, with a need to succeed or die in the attempt. Sadly, many would die. The American reporter

Frederick Palmer observed, "The Canadians enlivened life at the front; for they have a little more zip to them than the thoroughgoing British."[76]

> I could never quite accommodate myself to the wonder of a man from Winnipeg, and perhaps a "neutral" from Wyoming in his company, fighting Germans in Flanders.[77]

They might seem undisciplined to a drill sergeant, but in their view, they came to fight and not be toy soldiers for a martinet to play with. What they lacked in military etiquette, they made up in self-reliance and a "go to it" mentality when a crisis came. "'Their discipline is different from ours,' said a British general, 'but it works out. They are splendid. I ask for no better troops.'"[78]

The Canadian trenches were not directly in the path of the April 22 gas cloud. As the Germans pushed forward into the undefended trenches of the French, advancing three miles in five hours,[79] the Canadians attacked and greatly slowed the German advance, providing enough time for British reinforcements to fill the gap. The German drive slowed but still carried, pushing the Canadians and British back toward Ypres. On April 24, at 3:30 in the morning, the Germans unleashed the second great gas attack. Now the Canadian trenches were the target; however, this time the gas was less effective. It was not the surprise it had been to the French. A wet cloth (water or urine) over the mouth and nose gave some protection. When the gas dispersed most of the Canadians continued to fight. Still the Allies lost ground and the salient shrank. More British reinforcements arrived; they suffered more losses; and the salient experienced more shrinkage.

There was one American volunteer group present in Ypres during the battle. Members of the American Ambulance Field Service (A.A.F.S.),[80] 20 men and 10 ambulances, arrived in Belgium in January 1915. Assigned to Dunkirk, they moved wounded from hospital trains to hospitals. The American Hospital of Paris at Neuilly-sur-Seine was the A.A.F.S. sponsor. Support of the ambulance section came from American donors.

> June 11th, 1915.
> Miss Catherine K. Turnbull,
> Princeton, N.J.
> My dear Miss Turnbull,
> We have just received word from Mr. Hereford of your generous contribution of an additional $1100 for the support for 6 months longer of the ambulance which you contributed last December.... Your car has been working in the North around about Dunkirk and Poperinghe since early January.[81]

Miss Turnbull donated a Model T Ford ambulance, one of nine in the section. Another donor gave a Pierce-Arrow ambulance, the donor's son volunteered as a driver.

July 25th, 1915.

Mr. Augustus Hemenway,
Boston, Mass.

Dear Mr. Hemenway,

You will doubtless be interested to know that the Pierce-Arrow ambulance which you presented to us has been rendering valiant service during recent weeks. We brought it back from Dunkirk, where, as you know from the accounts of your boy [Lawrence Hemenway, Harvard] and Mr. Hussey, it rendered very important service, especially at the time of the second battle at Ypres.[82]

On April 23, 1915, as the Second Battle of Ypres began, the Americans moved from Dunkirk. Their new headquarters was in a small château in Elvertinghe (Elvertinge), a village about two miles from the front and along the Yser canal, northwest of Ypres. The château, serving as a first-aid hospital, was often under fire and eventually destroyed. Since the château was nearly always overcrowded with wounded, the Americans slept in their ambulances.

> Our labor consisted in going down to the *postes de secours*, situated in the Flemish farmhouses, perhaps four hundred or five hundred yards from the trenches, where the wounded get their first-aid attention, and then in carrying the men back to the dressing stations where their wounds were more carefully attended to, and finally in taking them farther to the rear to the hospitals outside of shell range.[83]

To lessen the danger from shellfire, the ambulances reached *postes de secours* after darkness; even so, most cars suffered damage from shell splinters and shrapnel. Traveling without lights, the ambulances dodged in and out of truck convoys and horse drawn artillery batteries to bring out their charges quickly. The ultimate destination for the wounded was Poperinghe, a railhead 6 miles (9.6 km) west of Ypres. At the railroad station, the Royal Army Medical Corps moved the wounded into hospital trains bound for Boulogne.

Another American was also present during the opening days of the battle. On the night of either April 22 or 23, the journalist Will Irwin reported from a railway station near Ypres, probably Poperinghe. When he arrived on an empty hospital train from Boulogne, he noted that stretchers filled the platform.

Officially, the Second Battle of Ypres ended on May 24. After thirty-four days of fighting, the Allies suffered 71,500 casualties, mostly British, and the Germans lost about 35,000. Of the 18,000 Canadians engaged, 2,000 perished.[84] The front line trenches of the salient were now only two to three miles from the center of Ypres. The Germans controlled the high ground surrounding the town. They occupied a semicircle of heights about thirty meters above the town, affording them a view beyond the Allied defenses.[85] By most measures, it was a German victory; however, it failed in one critical way. There was still a salient, albeit smaller, and it still blocked the way to the Channel ports.

As the fighting died down on the Ypres battlefield, things heated up in Sir John French's backyard. The British press wondered why Sir John's American friend George Gordon Moore enjoyed such extraordinary privileges at Ypres. Moore could come and go as he pleased at B.E.F. headquarters, even during the worst of the fighting, and Moore often brought his women friends with him on these Ypres junkets. Moore's close friendship with French had become a liability. In June 1915, responding to pressure from the British press, Sir John French's American friend returned home.[86]

> At the Hotel Manhattan Friday Mr. Moore denied that his leaving the continent was concerned with recent articles in London papers intimating that Sir John French was showing his American friend too great consideration.[87]
>
> George Gordon Moore of the Michigan United Railways Company, who has been the subject of comment in England because he was for some time a guest of Sir John French at the front, stopped in Detroit today on the way to his home in St. Clair.[88]

The Moore-Ypres-French saga was still not over. On January 25, 1916, a British newspaper, *Manchester Evening Chronicle,* published an article in which it alleged Moore passed military secrets to the Germans, secrets he learned while living with Sir John French in Ypres. Specifically, Moore supposedly passed information to Count von Bernstorff, the German Ambassador to the United States. The article stated the meeting between the two men occurred in Long Island.

> "But," the article continued, "It is interesting to note that, within a few days after his arrival in America, he is said to have been a guest at a Long Island house where Count von Bernstorff, the German Ambassador, also was staying."[89]

Moore responded by bringing a suit of libel against the paper's publisher. During the trial Moore testified that he was in Long Island soon after his return to America; however, he only visited the home of Colonel and Mrs. Roosevelt and Count von Bernstorff was most certainly not a guest of the Roosevelts. This aside drew laughs from the court.[90] Sir John French testified on behalf of his friend. With fighting still ongoing in the salient, the integrity and judgment of Viscount French of Ypres was unquestionable. The *Manchester Evening Chronicle* conceded, apologized, paid all court costs, and agreed to terms not disclosed.[91]

Chapter 10

Medieval U-Boat Nest

> The enormous significance of the Bruges and Zeebrugge harbours during the First World War are obvious when one considers that the German submarines based at Bruges alone sunk more than half of the allied and neutral ships that were lost during the four-year conflict.[1]—*Bruges and the Sea*, 1982

> Of all the cities of Belgium Bruges has best preserved its mediæval characteristics, in spite of the erection of many tasteless new buildings.[2]—*Baedeker's Belgium and Holland*, 1910

With the end of the Second Battle of Ypres, the major battles on the Western Front shifted from Belgium to France for the next couple of years. Of course, fierce fighting still occurred along the trenches of the diminished Ypres Salient as each contestant sought tactical advantage over the other. However, in Belgium, the more important action now moved to the coast, to an artificial harbor and canal constructed in the late nineteenth and early twentieth centuries (1895–1907) to link the medieval city of Bruges to the North Sea at Zeebrugge.

A nineteenth century traveler's guide described Bruges (Brugge) as "the Liverpool of the middle ages."[3] In the thirteenth century, Bruges was one of the great commercial centers of Europe, with a population estimated at 200,000. The silting up of its connection to the North Sea in the fifteenth century led to its ruin; by the eighteen-seventies it had a population of 48,000, including 15,000 paupers. According to an 1876 guidebook, "At present it wears an air of desolation; the people in its streets are few, and it has lost the indications of commercial activity." It warned visitors to "beware of touting street guides."[4]

A German travel guide published in 1910 by Karl Baedeker described Belgium's new North Sea port.

> Zee-Brugge is the new seaport of Bruges. Its large outer harbour communicates with a smaller inner basin at the beginning of the new Canal Maritime. This canal, which is 230 ft. wide and 26 ft. deep, allows sea-going vessels to reach (6 Mi) Bruges, where another harbour has been made.[5]

Baedeker, as if anticipating the needs of the German Navy, continues the description of the facilities at Zeebrugge: "The crescent-shaped Mole, protecting the outer harbor from the N.W. wind, is 1½ M. long. It is mainly constructed of blocks of concrete and is provided with elevators, warehouses, and railway tracks."[6]

With Zeebrugge, the Germans potentially would have a port close to English waters — and, of course, English targets since Dover was only three to four hours from Zeebrugge. However, prior to the arrival of the Germans in 1914, Bruges/Zeebrugge was a Flemish backwater. The ambition of an artificial port in West Flanders to rival Antwerp was stillborn. Antwerp flourished and Zeebrugge languished.

> Time after time sand filled the harbor, and almost continuous dredging was necessary. Only one steamship line established itself at Zeebrugge, running a boat to Hull (England) twice a week, and that only in Summer, the vacation season. Now and again a small boat would run in, looking as if it was by mistake. Finally the Belgians became accustomed to the idea that Zeebrugge was a failure, and a very expensive failure. And when Germans took possession of Zeebrugge the Belgians said, "After all, it is a good thing, as Zeebrugge is no good."[7]

The Germans captured Zeebrugge and the neighboring port of Ostend on October 15, 1914. Since both facilities were intact, work began immediately to turn them into military bases. Approximately 5,000 Belgian worker conscripts constructed port fortifications, facilities to repair naval vessels, and storage warehouses for munitions and supplies. The canal from Ostend to Bruges needed to be deepened and widened. The canal from Zeebrugge to Bruges was already wide enough and deep enough for light cruisers, torpedo boats and U-boats. Dredges began clearing the harbors of sand.[8] The first U-boat to enter Zeebrugge was probably the *U-19*, which arrived on October 25, 1914, for repairs after a British destroyer accidentally ran over it.[9]

Both Ostend and Zeebrugge were literally under the guns of the British Navy. The Germans forced Belgian workers to dig permanent gun emplacements in the North Sea dunes flanking the ports. By March 1915, 13 batteries (55 artillery pieces) guarded the coast, forcing British ships to keep their distance; the batteries had ranges from 10 km (6.2 miles) to 16.2 km (10 miles).[10]

What became known as the Flanders U-Boat Flotilla arrived at the end of March 1915. One of the first boats to arrive was the *UB-2*, under the command of Werner Fürbringer, then 25 years old. In his memoir,[11] Fürbringer described the *UB-2* as "admittedly not impressive." It was 27 m (ca. 88 ft) in length with a crew of 13. It had diesel and electric motors, developed 60 hp and sputtered along at a maximum surface speed of 5 knots per hour (ca. 6 mph) in a calm sea. The *UB-2* sailed from Germany (Wilhelmshaven), intending to

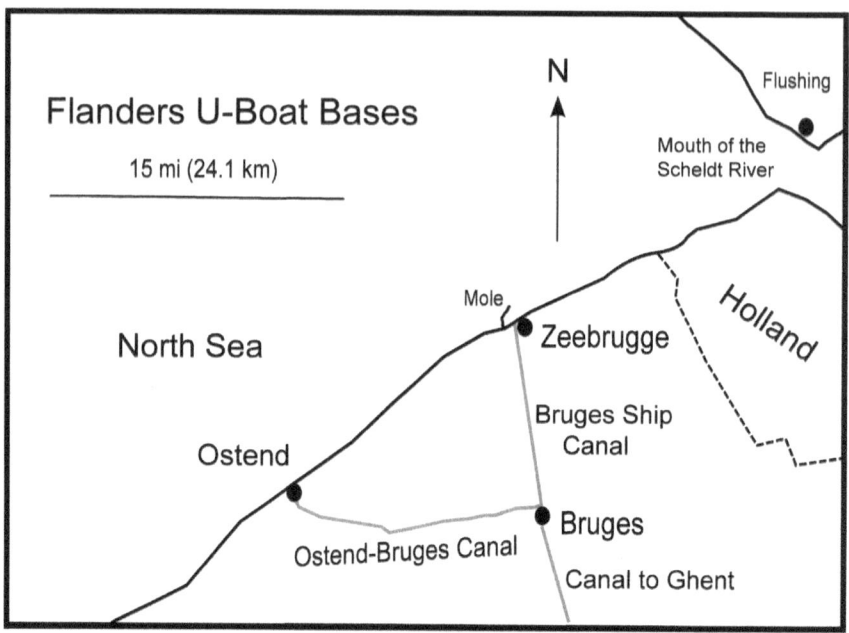

go around Holland before turning for Zeebrugge. What should have been an easy voyage was not. A heavy storm struck, nearly foundering the boat. Decidedly the worse for the experience, the *UB-2* limped into Zeebrugge harbor and berthed an hour or so later at Bruges.

UB class submarines formed the backbone of the Flanders U-Boat Flotilla early in the war. With a radius of action of 800 nautical miles on the surface, the small coastal U-boats soon proved their worth; the *UB-4* sank four steamships in April and the *UB-6* sank a British destroyer in May. Sentry patrols, on the alert for British landings that never came, occupied the UB-boats for the next couple of months. Finally, in July, Fürbringer's *UB-2* made her first war patrol; her assignment, along with three other UB boats, was to torpedo British troop transports in the English Channel. Operating 120 miles (193.2 km) from its home base at Zeebrugge, the *UB-2* had only two torpedoes with which to attack enemy shipping. She fired on two transports and missed. Unable to take any further offensive action, the *UB-2* started the long journey home having accomplished nothing. Fifteen minutes into the return trip, Fürbringer learned that the coupling between the diesel and electric motors had sheared. The U-boat could now move only on battery power, but the sheared coupling made it impossible to recharge the batteries. There was only enough juice in the batteries to travel at half speed (3 mph) for four hours. Fürbringer decided to try to drift with the tide east toward Zeebrugge. In the English Channel with every twelve-hour tidal cycle, for six hours the water flows east and for six hours it flows west. "We would drift on the surface when the flood was eastwards, and sit out on the bottom when it ebbed westwards.... Our calculations showed we should be able to advance eight to ten sea miles eastwards twice daily."[12]

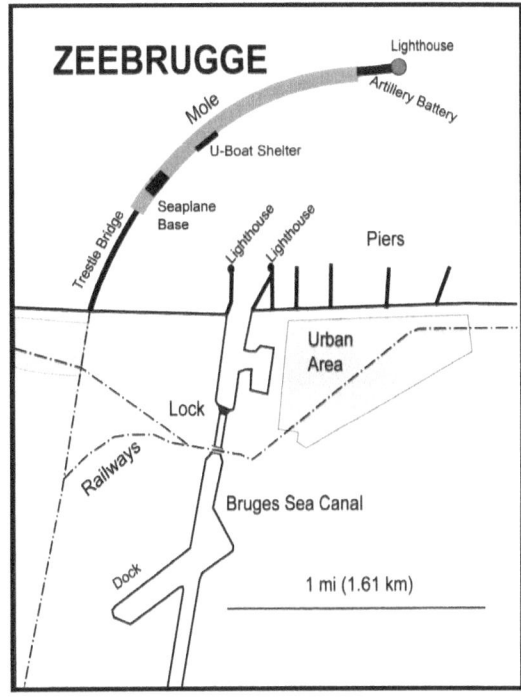

In addition to having insufficient food and water for the now extended voyage home, there was another problem. To save battery power, the U-boat rested on the bottom six hours without its electric fans circulating the often re-breathed air through carbon dioxide absorbers (potash cartridges). After six long hours, carbon dioxide levels reached near-lethal concentrations. The men suffered in total darkness, in order to save power. They were in a completely dark steel coffin, slowly suffocating. Then after six hours, the boat would rise to the surface and everyone would stumble on deck, prostrate with exhaustion. Necessity being the mother of invention, the men devised new means of surface propulsion to lessen the duration of the voyage. A sail made of canvas hammocks hoisted from a jury-rigged mast helped some; the men fashioned paddles from wooden bunk slats; the *UB-2* began to resemble a South Seas war canoe as it made its way through the Channel. Prior to diving, they would stow the sail and take deep breaths before closing up for six hours. Finally, after many tedious days she reached the coast of Flanders where a German U-boat spotted the *UB-2* and towed her to Ostend. A shipping canal linked Ostend to Bruges, so soon the *UB-2* was finally home. There the crew learned that the other three Channel U-boats also failed to sink anything. Not all forays against the enemy proved successful.

In addition to torpedo attacks, U-boats of the Flanders U-Boat Flotilla laid mine fields in areas frequented by British and neutral shipping. UC class boats were the minelayers.

> We loaded up the ten mines we carry in an hour and five minutes. They were lifted from a railway truck by a big crane and delicately lowered into the mine tubes, of which we have five in the bows. The tubes extend from the upper deck of the ship to her keel, and slope aft to facilitate release.[13]

The UC boat released mines from the bottom of the tube; they could be released either when the boat was cruising on the surface or underwater.

> About 20 miles from land, we dived to what we calculated would be the level of the mine-field, and laid our course to the south-west in continuation of the existing chain, the termination of which we had succeeded in discovering after three-quarters of an hour's search. The crew were all at their posts; look-out men were listening intently and the mine-layers were awaiting orders....
>
> The first mine sped from the shaft, plunged gurgling downwards and anchored itself automatically to the bottom. One after the other, at regular intervals, the whole number followed in rapid succession.[14]

A water-soluble plug attached the mine to its heavy sinker, which pulled the buoyant mine to the seabed. Later, after the U-boat had moved away, the plug dissolved, releasing the mine, which now floated to just beneath the surface, tethered by a cable to the sinker on the seabed. Sometimes the plug dissolved too quickly, allowing the mine to rise so that it struck the mine-laying U-boat's bottom — the resulting explosion was catastrophic, the boat having sunk itself![15]

There were sometimes interesting diversions from the business of war, especially when cruising underwater near the enemy coast.

> "Herr Grassl," [Navigating Officer Grassel of the Bruges-based *UC-70*] said the Commander, standing at the periscope, feeling cheerful now that the boat was safely on its way again, "just look through the periscope a minute.... Do you see the English bathing beauties?"[16]

Like the UB class boats, UCs were small coastal submarines. Sometimes small size could be an advantage. *UC-6* was mining the mouth of the Thames when its diesel engine stopped working. The situation was dire as the boat was only 17 miles (27 km) from the English coast in an area of high British traffic. Noting a northwest breeze, the crew fashioned a sail of canvas hammocks, and recalling the voyage of another sailing submarine, the *UB-2*, the *UC-6* set sail for Zeebrugge.

> At a speed of two to three knots they went on their way. Now and then British patrols appeared on the horizon, but fortunately not so close that they felt called upon to make a closer investigation of the "shabby little fishing smack."[17]

After 52 miles (83.7 km) of sailing, another U-boat found *UC-6* and towed her the remaining distance to Zeebrugge.

The UBs and UCs had a radius of action of 800 nautical miles on the surface (a range to and from the target zone of 1,600 nautical miles). Thus, the English Channel and east coast of England were the main fields of action for the Flanders boats. Karl Wiegand, an American journalist for the *New York World* and representative of United Press in Berlin, interviewed Grand Admiral von

Tirpitz at German headquarters in Charleville on the subject of submarines. The then sixty-six-year-old admiral expressed great concern about getting enough sleep.

> It is unquestionable that submarines are a new and powerful weapon of naval warfare. At the same time one must not forget that submarines do their best work along the coasts and in shallow waters, and for this reason the Channel is particularly suitable for these craft.[18]

Long voyages were possible said the admiral, as long as the crew had a place to rest.

> All that is necessary is that the crew gets an opportunity of resting and recuperating, and this opportunity can be afforded the men by taking the boat into shallow and still waters, where it can rest on the bottom and remain still in order that the crew can have a good sleep. This is only possible where the water is comparatively shallow.[19]

By the end of September 1915, U-boats of the Flanders Flotilla, when not sleeping on the seabed, accounted for 142 enemy vessels with a loss of only 1 UB and 1 UC.[20]

U-boats reached Bruges either one of two ways: either by sea from Germany, as the *UB-2* did, or inland via canals. Most vessels arrived via the safer inland route. Disassembled U-boats traveled by train from Germany to Antwerp shipyards for final construction. The prefabricated sections of a single U-boat required eight railway cars for transport to Antwerp. Assembly of the U-boat took two to three weeks, followed by a five-day journey through inland canals towed by two tugboats.[21] An April 1915 report in the *New York Times* documented the movement of three U-boats to Bruges.

> An eyewitness gives an account of the passage by river and canal from Antwerp through Belgium of three German submarines to one of the bases on the Belgian coast. They came up the River Scheldt as far as Ghent, and then by canal, running direct from there to Bruges through Rupelmonde....
>
> They had been constructed at Hoboken [a suburb south of Antwerp]. The canals have been deepened and widened at several points to allow their passage.[22]

Barges moving Commission for Relief in Belgium (C.R.B.) foodstuffs from Rotterdam into Belgium yielded right of way to U-boats. "Sometimes I've had to stop to make way for a submarine going to Bruges — had to wait till the monster had passed. Who would ever have thought it?— submarines in the Belgian canals!"[23]

The unrestricted U-boat campaign began in February 1915 and lasted until September 1915. U-boat commanders could now sink British ships without warning. Immune from attack were ships flying neutral colors; however, since British ships at times flew neutral colors as a deception, commanders were to use their own judgment based upon structure, place of registration and behavior of the ship. For example, even *Lusitania* had resorted to such deception, but not on her final voyage — perhaps she should have.

> The reference to the misuse of neutral flags was assumed to refer to an incident that had occurred on February 6 when the *Lusitania* arrived in Liverpool flying the American flag. Her captain had hauled down her Union Jack and put up the Stars and Stripes while in the Irish Sea, on receiving by wireless a warning of danger to his ship from German submarines.[24]

Consequently, mistakes occurred; the American flag was no protection. Hospital ships, unless they were transporting troops from England to France, and C.R.B. ships were both immune from attack. In April, the Flanders Flotilla entered the offensive, ultimately sending nine UBs and eight UCs into the fray.[25]

One of the notable achievements of the campaign was the sinking of the British liner *Lusitania* off the Irish coast on May 7, 1915, by *U-20* (not a Flanders boat). Among the 1,201 passengers who perished were 128 Americans, some of whom had enormous wealth and influence (see Chapter 6). Strongly worded protests from Washington to Berlin nearly brought the United States into the war. President Wilson first demanded a complete cessation of the U-boat campaign but finally settled for an assurance from the Germans that they would not sink passenger liners without warning. It was a dilemma for the Germans since cargo ships as well as passenger liners often carried American-made munitions in their holds. The war was big business for American factories; all their products went to the Allies.

> One metallic cartridge company [Remington Arms] obtained a contract to supply 3,500,000 rounds of ammunition weekly, and the understanding was that this would be increased to 7,000,000. A steel company [Bethlehem Steel] received an order for 8,000 field-guns and was turning out 12,000 shrapnel-shells every day. For one-pounders and smaller shells the rate was 50,000 a day. An electric company [Westinghouse Electric] was said to have an order for $100,000,000 worth of war materials. Reports of other large contracts became common items in American daily newspapers. Stocks in these companies traded in on the New York Stock Exchange advanced sensationally.[26]

Three months later, on August 19, a German U-boat (not from Flanders) sank the White Star Line passenger liner *Arabic*. Although she sank in eleven minutes, two factors contributed to minimizing losses. Since the ship was off the southern coast of Ireland in a war zone 50 miles (80.5 km) from where *Lusitania* went down, the captain ordered the life boats swung out. The passengers, having just witnessed the torpedoing of a British steamer, were prepared for the worst — it soon came. "In their fright the passengers had rushed

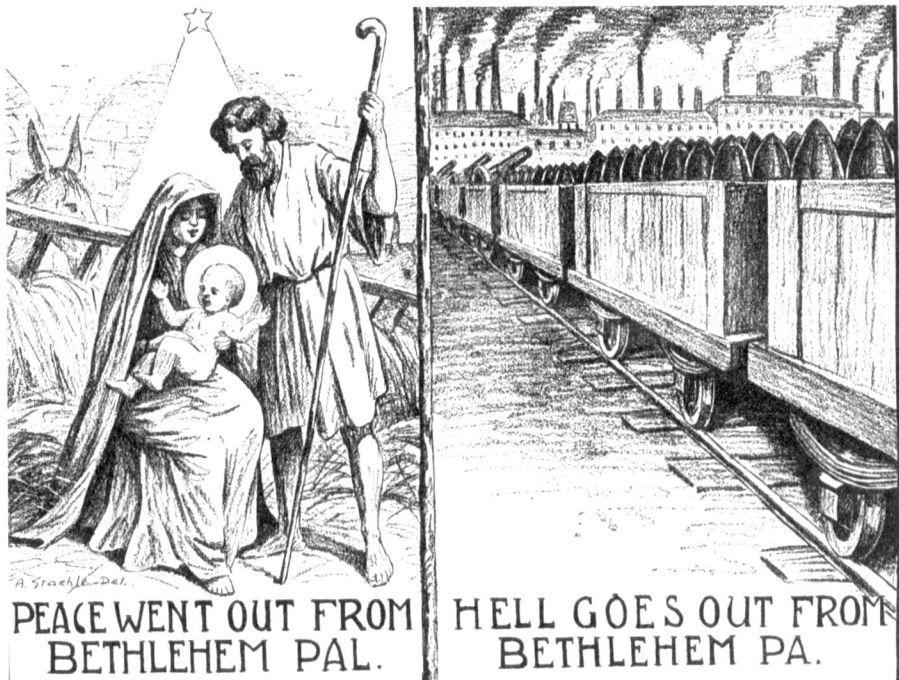

PEACE WENT OUT FROM BETHLEHEM PAL.   HELL GOES OUT FROM BETHLEHEM PA.

American-made arms and munitions greatly supported the Allied war effort, despite the country's "neutrality." *The Fatherland*, a German-American magazine published in New York City, agitated about American pro–Allies bias with a cartoon contrasting Bethlehem, Palestine (PAL), and the steel-making city in Pennsylvania (PA) with the same name (*The Fatherland*, 1915).

for life preservers, and had barely adjusted them when the German submarine turned its torpedo against the Arabic's side."[27]

These factors resulted in a minimal loss of life; of the 423 persons on board, 44, including two Americans, lost their lives. One survivor, a British comedian and actor, Kenneth S. Douglas, had the dubious distinction of being both a *Lusitania* survivor and an *Arabic* survivor.[28] He was on his way to Broadway.

The sinking of *Arabic* without warning nearly ruptured American relations with Germany — perhaps the powerful neutral might soon become a powerful belligerent. "The White House was silent, but President Wilson's concern was indicated by the fact that he canceled an engagement to play golf."[29]

Responding to American pressure, the Germans halted their unrestricted U-boat campaign on September 18, 1915. U-boat attacks would follow Prize Regulations: for military vessels nothing changed; however, non-military vessels now required a warning to allow passengers and crew to escape. Consequently,

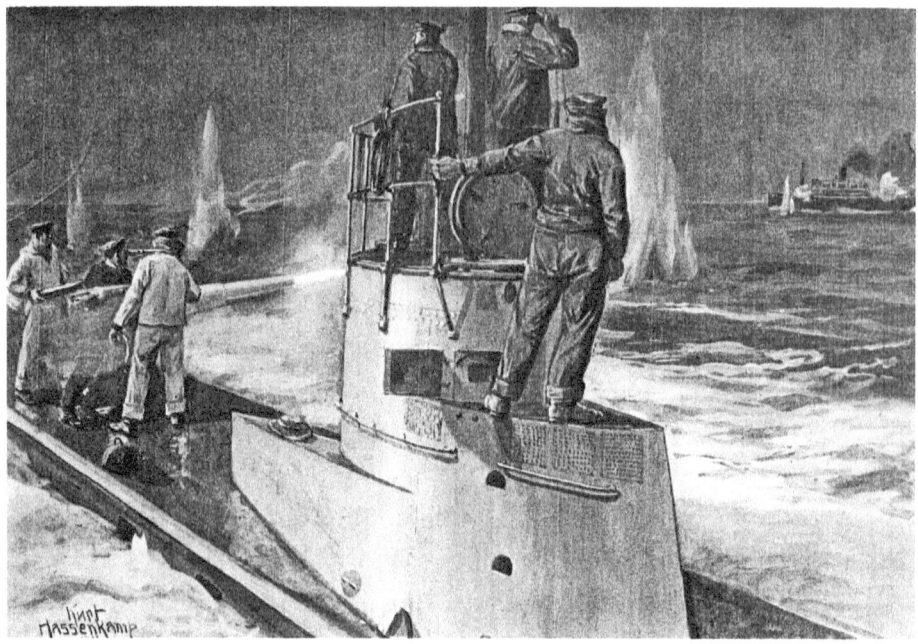

Under "Prize Regulations," a U-boat had to surface and warn neutral or British merchant ships, allowing crew and passengers a chance to escape before sinking the ship. On the surface, the U-boat was very vulnerable; to turn the predator into a prey, the British secretly armed merchant ships with concealed deck guns. Such ships, called Q-ships, attempted to lure the attacking U-boat closer and closer before firing, often tasking the more histrionic of the crew to lower life boats and feign panic and fright. The drawing depicts a running fight between a Q-ship and a surfaced U-boat, where the only advantage for the U-boat is that it is a smaller target (*Die Wochenschau*, 1916).

submerged U-boats could attack only military vessels. To warn a merchant vessel, the U-boat, of course, had to surface — somewhat defeating the point of being a submarine. Trans-Atlantic passenger liners, regardless of nationality, could not be attacked.

With the Flanders Flotilla raising such havoc along the east coast of Britain and in the English Channel, the British responded by aerial and naval attacks on Zeebrugge and Ostend and aerial bombardment of the Bruges base. Mostly these attacks were ineffectual.[30] The Germans response was a massive building program using reinforced concrete.

> We are alongside the mole [at Zeebrugge] in one of the new submarine shelters that has been built.
> The boat is under a concrete roof over three feet thick, which would defy the heaviest bomb.[31]

10. Medieval U-Boat Nest

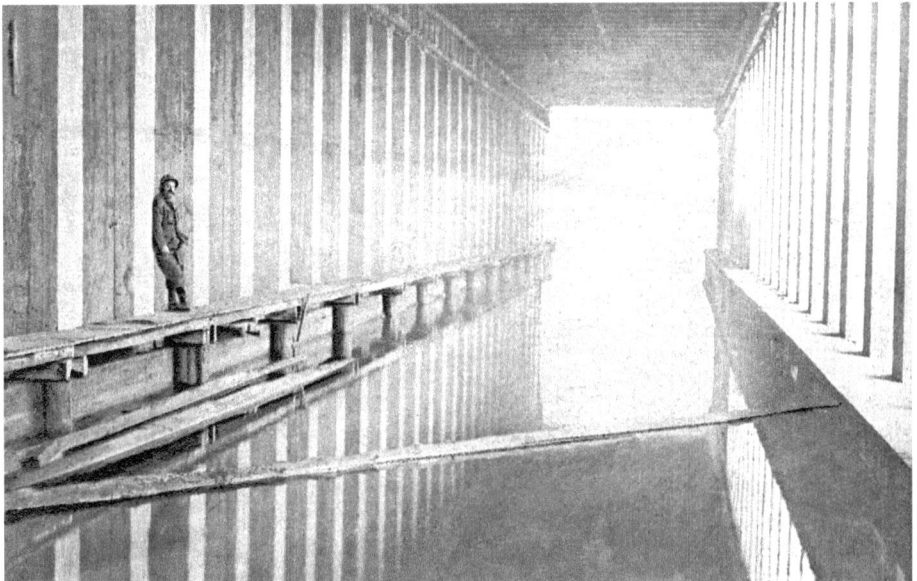

A rare photograph inside a U-boat shelter in Bruges. Capped with two meters of steel-reinforced concrete, the shelter could protect three U-boats from aerial bombardment (*Le Miroir*, 1919).

In Bruges, the defenses against aerial bombardment began at the city center where a concrete tunnel led to the military docks outside the city, allowing submariners and dock personnel safe access.

> The German submarine docks of Bruges were secured from attack from the air by a roof of reinforced concrete 7 feet in thickness, that concrete being in turn protected by a quantity of vertical steel rods, across the tops of which was stretched a curtain of steel netting. Some fifteen shelters of reinforced concrete in the neighbourhood of the docks afforded additional security for the workmen who might be prevented in emergency from reaching the main structure.... In this unassailable security the German submarines were fitted together in eight long galleries, each of which could contain three submarines.[32]

In contrast to the strict discipline at the High Seas Fleet base in Wilhelmshaven, life in Bruges was freer. The submariners stayed at the *Hôtel de Flandre*, rated by Baedeker as the best hotel in town. It boasted a lift, central heating and baths.

> Here, in Bruges, at any rate as far as the submarine officers are concerned, the matter is far different. When the boats are in, one seems to do as one likes, with a perfunctory visit to the ship in the course of the day....
> In the evenings there are parties, for which there are always ladies, and I find it is necessary to have a "smoking" [a dinner jacket].[33]

The Flanders U-Boat Flotilla bases at Bruges, Zeebrugge and Ostend were, understandably, off limits to foreign visitors, even neutral journalists. However, an American artist resided in Bruges throughout the occupation. A naturalized American citizen, S. Arlent Edwards was born in England (1862) where he studied art; he established himself as a book illustrator in New York in 1890. There he revived the art of printing in color from a mezzotint plate. He and his wife Annette came to Bruges in January 1914.[34] When the German Army arrived, Edwards obtained a document from the American Consul at Ghent stating that his house/studio was the property of an American citizen and promptly affixed the document to his door. Edwards was generally unmolested the first three years of the war and continued his color printing art business. He functioned as the ersatz American Consul in Bruges, helping redress grievances between Belgians and the occupiers. Edwards was also a member of the local C.R.B. committee. He recalled that among men returning from a voyage, license and debauchery were the norm.

> They might stagger, yelling in drunken ribaldry in the streets, with the lowest women on either arm, break windows, or molest citizens; they might even insult officers of the army — they were never punished.
> The Colonel of the Germans' Police Bureau was reported to have said when an army Captain complained of a gross outrage offered him:
> "What do you want me to do? A fortnight's arrest to them means a fortnight's respite. These men are 'tode geweiht' [consecrated to death]. An allied depth bomb will soon wipe out the memory of the insult you were forced to swallow."[35]
> The finest houses in Bruges were at their disposal as quarters, and the cream of famous Belgian wine cellars was "requisitioned" by the invaders. The favorite amusement of U-boat officers ashore was an orgy of champagne terminated by the demolition of every piece of crockery and furniture in the house. Several fine old mansions were set on fire as a result of such bouts, but instead of being punished the officers had a fresh dwelling immediately offered them.[36]

Each voyage out was a voyage of the damned. Of the 460 U-boats in action, 178 were lost by the war's end. Torpedoes from enemy submarines, mines, depth charges, net barrages, aircraft bombing, ramming, accidents and malfunctions took their toll. When a U-boat sank, there were usually no survivors; 5,132 men died on U-boats. The probability of surviving the war on a U-boat was less than one chance in two, less than 50 percent.[37] With just cause, they referred to themselves as members of the Suicide Club. Morphine and ether were common addictions, alcoholism was a given.

Walter Duranty of the *New York Times* arrived in Bruges soon after its liberation by the Belgian Army on October 25, 1918. In a rathskeller (drinking club) favored by U-boat men, he found the walls decorated with vulgar drawings and fatalistic graffiti.

> "Enjoy wine and women while you can. You live but once, and will be a long time dead...."
>
> "Have a good time while you can, because you don't know what awaits you tomorrow...."
>
> "Drink deep of wine, ye heroes. It will compensate and make you forget the dark days of hardship."[38]

The British used minefields to deter or, hopefully, to destroy U-boats. The British Navy laid minefields parallel to the Flanders shore, hoping to intercept U-boats entering or leaving Ostend or Zeebrugge. A mine barrage across the Dover Straights, consisting of over 7,000 mines, proved an inconvenient but surmountable obstacle to U-boat traffic.[39]

> As the level of the sea is constantly changing owing to the ebb and flow of the tides along the coast, the mines have to be fixed at such a point below the surface that a ship cannot pass over them at high tide without exploding them; nor must they float on the surface at low tide, in which they could be destroyed by gun-fire.[40]

Because of the great tidal range in the Channel and North Sea (ca. 3–4 m [10–13 ft] along the coasts), the latter condition was nearly impossible. Mines were usually floating on the surface at low tide.

> The enemy believed that he had blocked the channel to hostile U. boats, by means of an extensive minefield laid in several lines. I say "believed" because the mines, as already mentioned, float on the surface of the water round about the time of low water, and then we simply slip through the gaps.[41]

Slaloming with a submarine through a minefield at low tide was easier said than done, especially in rough seas. Minefields accounted for only 20 U-boats through the course of the war.[42] There probably would have been greater losses had British mines been more effective.

Fighting under Prize Regulations added a new peril to U-boats. Stealth underwater torpedo attacks on merchant vessels were forbidden, even if they were of belligerent nations. U-boats could only sink merchant vessels after examining papers and allowing the crews to lower life boats and escape. While all this was transpiring, the U-boat floated on the surface near its intended victim. To exploit this vulnerability, the British soon concealed deck guns on merchant vessels — the victim became the predator. The British called them Q-ships; to the Germans they were decoys. Regardless of nomenclature, Q-ships, a.k.a. decoys, sank 14 U-boats by the war's end.[43]

In early 1916, the German Navy, tired of fighting in half measures bound by the rules of the Prize Regulations, pressured the Kaiser to unleash the full force of the U-boats. Unrestricted warfare at sea resumed that February. Once again, the navy could sink neutral and Allied ships without warning. The

Germans were still insecure about the American response. These new orders violated the agreement reached with President Wilson after the *Arabic* sinking. Would he notice? He did after a Flanders boat, the *UB-20*, torpedoed *Sussex* on March 24, 1916. The English Channel steamer, on her way from Folkestone to Dieppe, exploded with a ferocity that blew her bow off. On board were 50 crew and 386 passengers, including 25 Americans. Although 50 people perished, all the Americans survived. Contributing to the loss of life was the fact that many of the lifebelts were rotten and useless.[44]

Some American newspaper editors called for President Wilson to break off relations with Germany over the incident. Wilson demurred; was *Sussex* sunk by a mine or torpedo? If a mine, then there was no problem as mines could come from anywhere. If a torpedo, then there was a diplomatic problem as the Germans had broken their *Arabic* agreement. The Germans first maintained there was no U-boat near the sinking. In the meantime, the French towed the wreck to Dieppe for forensic investigation. To answer the key issue of what sank *Sussex*, mine or torpedo, the Germans acknowledged that although there was a U-boat nearby, it had sunk another ship.[45] Then the French discovered a metal fragment in the wreck that could have come only from a German torpedo — or so they said.

Accepting that a German U-boat was the culprit, President Wilson dispatched an ultimatum to the German government.

> Our Government declared that "unless the Imperial Government should now immediately declare and effect an abandonment of its present methods of submarine warfare against passenger- and freight-carrying vessels, the Government of the United States can have no choice but to sever diplomatic relations with the German Empire altogether."[46]

The Germans capitulated; Wilson had won a diplomatic victory. The following order to German naval forces ended the unrestricted U-boat campaign — for the present at least.

> In accordance with the general principles of visit and search and the destruction of merchant-vessels, recognized by international law, such vessels, both within and without the area declared a naval war-zone, shall not be sunk without warning and without saving human lives unless the ship attempt to escape or offer resistance.[47]

Thus by April 1916, it was back to Prize Regulations for the U-boat war. During the first six months (May–October), Germans sank through mines and U-boat attacks 600 Allied or neutral vessels, not counting smaller ships such as trawlers.[48] Many of these ships were neutrals trading with Britain, e.g., Norway, Sweden, Denmark and Holland. The United States lost only 6 vessels of the seagoing class. Most of the losses were in the North Sea and English Channel; consequently, the Flanders U-boats played a significant role. For example, in September 1916, the Flanders Flotilla sank 53 ships, mostly British and Dutch.[49] The British laid a barrage of moored steel nets along the Belgian coast in an attempt to stop U-boats as they left or returned from missions. The idea was that U-boats entangled in the nets would surface, allowing British vessels to sink them. The British also attempted to block the English Channel with moored mine nets, but the strong tides made this difficult to achieve. Overall, steel nets probably accounted for the loss of only six U-boats.[50]

The seabed resembled a junkyard with thousands of sunken ships, tangled steel nets and lost mines. Cruising along underwater, blind to what was ahead, became perilous in some areas along the English coast. The Bruges minelayer *UC-70* had just survived a depth-charge attack when she literally ran into something more dangerous.

> Suddenly, just as we were rounding the headland, we were brought up by a wreck lying at a depth of 31 metres. The boat stopped with a frightful jolt that flung us all to the floor.
> The engines were at once switched off; the boat was slowly sinking by the stern. We then set the engines at full speed and made frantic efforts to jerk ourselves free. We tried to clear the after diving-tank and fill the forward tank, and the crew rushed aft to help to trim the boat. Then we tried to pump out the aft torpedo-tube, and empty the aft ammunition-room and deposit its contents forward. All this took time, and it was all quite useless.[51]

The captain, realizing the ship was nearly out of air, ordered a final desperate maneuver; it would either tear off the bow or possibly free the boat. Using both propellers at full speed astern, he swung the stern from left to right with the crew running from side to side to enhance the momentum, trying to wiggle free of the clutches of the wreck. "While the crew leapt wildly from side to side, there was a sudden snapping sound as though a rope had given way. The boat jerked backwards and lay level on the sea-floor. Saved!"[52]

The sea-floor could also be a death trap as the *UC-47* out of Bruges discovered. Diving hard to escape being rammed by a British destroyer, the boat impaled itself into the sea-floor.

> Examination of the chart, showed the bottom to be mud, and on attempting to move the foremost hydroplanes, the plane motor fuses blew out. This showed that the boat was buried in the mud right up to her foremost planes, which were immovable.[53]

UC-47 tried everything to free herself without uncontrollably rocketing up to the surface. After all, a destroyer might still be lurking about.

> So at 2 a.m. we decided to risk it and we put a blow on all tanks.
> When she had about fifty tons positive buoyancy she suddenly bucketed up,

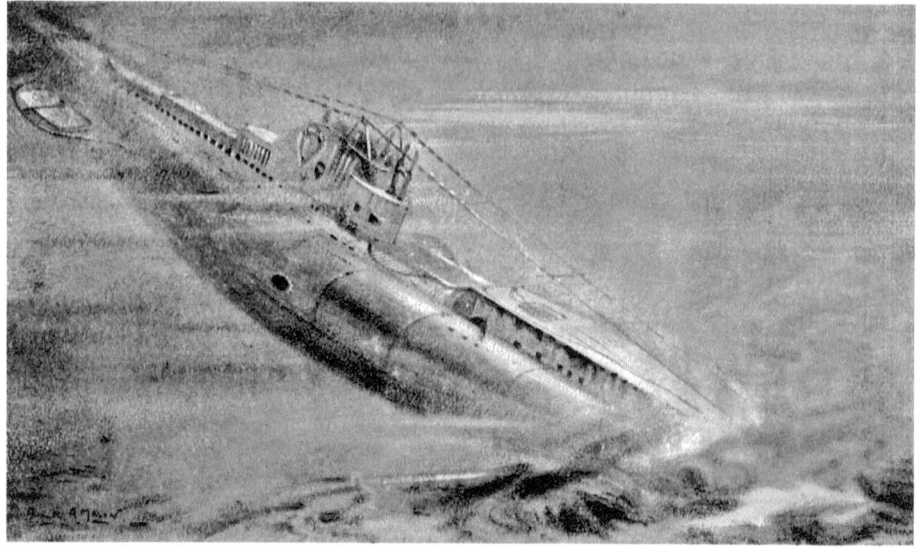

Sub in the mud. A diving U-boat impales itself on the muddy bottom of the North Sea. Cruising around underwater, literally blind to what was ahead, was not without its dangers. Bruges U-boats usually hunted in the relatively shallow southern part of the North Sea where depths were often less than 120 feet (35 m) and where underwater banks were even shallower. Adding to the dangers were steel-net barrages designed to entrap U-boats and uncharted shipwrecks (*The Diary of a U-boat Commander*, 1920).

and, as the motors were running full speed astern at the time, we came up and broke surface stern first.[54]

Fortunately, the destroyer had moved on.

The above are stories of mishaps that U-boats survived; those that did not are dead man's tales. Over 40 U-boats disappeared from unknown causes during the course of the war. Considering all U-boat losses (178), the German navy sacrificed one boat for every 30 Allied or neutral vessels it managed to sink.[55]

In spite of the high totals of Allied and neutral ships sunk, war supplies and food flowed across the Atlantic from the United States to England and France. Britain was not starving and British armies were not short of American-made rifles (American Enfields), field guns, artillery shells or bullets. The U-boat offensive was simply ineffective. Nineteen sixteen was not a good year on the Western Front for the Germans, the French or the British, with massive carnage on both sides at Verdun and the Somme. The German high command advised trying unrestricted U-boat warfare again. Perhaps the war could be won, a starving England might sue for peace before the Americans could enter the fray. In one of his more delusional and misguided decisions of the war, the Kaiser resurrected the no-holds-barred U-boat campaign. With this decision, Germany lost the First World War and the Kaiser his throne. On January 31, 1917, Germany informed Washington that she was resuming an unrestricted U-boat campaign.

> Germany therefore announced that, on or after February 1, she would pursue what was popularly known as the von Tirpitz system of ruthless submarine warfare. Sea traffic was to be stopt "with every available weapon and without further notice," in what she defined as "blockade zones" about Great Britain, France, Italy and the eastern Mediterranean.[56]

On February 3, 1917, President Wilson announced to both Houses of Congress the severance of diplomatic relations with Germany. The German Ambassador, Count von Bernstorff, and the American, James W. Gerard, returned to their respective capitals. America was still not formally at war with Germany, but only just. The U-boat flotillas immediately went on a ship-sinking spree that made war between the two countries all but certain. The Flanders Flotilla probably accounted for 28 percent of this carnage. In February, the offensive accounted for 254 Allied and neutral ships; in March, 310 ships; and in April, 413 ships. The latter number would never be surpassed in any month during the two world wars.[57] The tally included 7 C.R.B. ships carrying a total of 17,000 tons of foodstuffs for occupied Belgium.[58] The most notorious sinking occurred during the night of February 25 when a U-boat torpedoed the Cunard passenger liner *Laconia* without warning off the coast of Ireland. It was winter in the North Atlantic. Some of the life boats sustained damage from swinging into the side of the ship during lowering.

> When we reached the water the sea came over the gunwale, but I got an oar and pushed off about six feet. We were then able to use the oars, but we were full of water.... At times the sea washed over us almost up to our chests.
> There were four women, including Mrs. Hoy and her daughter [Mary E. Hoy and her daughter Elizabeth Hoy of Chicago], who both died from exposure, and had to be thrown overboard in order to lighten the weight in the boat....
> Marshall Highland, a negro American citizen, said he was almost ten hours in an open boat. He thought the Laconia took about one hour and a half to sink. Two other American negroes in his boat died from exposure and were thrown overboard.[59]

Still President Wilson was reluctant to ask Congress for a declaration of war. Except for those living on the east coast, most Americans were very hesitant to enter Europe's bloodbath. The feeling was to let the Europeans butcher each other and America stay out of it; sell the Allies arms and war materiel, make money, but otherwise keep the American Army at home. Regarding Americans who lost their lives to U-Boat attacks, perhaps they should have had more sense than to travel on a British or French ship during wartime.

The most outspoken firebrand advocating American entry into the war was Theodore Roosevelt, even though he was once on friendly terms with the Kaiser. The ex-president and his wife were guests of the Kaiser in Berlin in 1910. Kaiser Wilhelm and Roosevelt were in many senses simpatico; they exchanged letters of advice, both were swashbuckling, provocative, and indiscrete, and each thought the other a bit mad.[60] The invasion of Belgium forced Roosevelt to revise his views of the Kaiser — Wilhelm was still a bit mad, but dangerously so.

> Moreover, it is well for Americans always to remember that what has been done to Belgium would, of course, be done to us just as unhesitatingly if the conditions required it.[61]
>
> I feel in the strongest way that we should have interfered, at least to the extent of the most emphatic diplomatic protest and at the very onset — and then by whatever further action was necessary — in regard to the violation of the neutrality of Belgium; for this act was the earliest and the most important.[62]

Roosevelt published the above in 1915; the "further action" he referred to was the United States entering the war. Two years later, America still remained neutral.

Then the Germans made a foolish mistake. On January 16, 1917, Arthur Zimmermann, German Foreign Minister in Berlin, sent a wireless telegram to Count von Bernstorff, the German Ambassador to the United States. In this communication, Zimmermann outlined a plan to open an American/Mexican front should the United States enter the war. This communication, known as the Zimmermann Telegram, was the final outrage that pushed Wilson to ask Congress for a declaration of war against Germany. Since coded in what the Germans believed was an unbreakable code, it went via wireless. The British obtained a copy of the telegram and set their code breakers to decipher it. While the British were deciphering, Bernstorff received the telegram on January 18 and forwarded it to the German Imperial Minister in Mexico who was to give the decoded message to the President of Mexico. The Mexican president baulked at the plan's audacity and would have nothing to do with it.

After putting in play a suitable cover story to deceive the Germans that their unbreakable code had been broken, the British passed the decoded telegram to the Americans on February 24. Wilson received it that evening. It read as follows:

> On the first of February we intend to begin unrestricted submarine warfare, notwithstanding this, it is our intention to endeavor to keep neutral the United States of America. If this attempt is not successful, we propose an alliance on

the following basis with Mexico. That we shall make war together and together make peace. We shall give general financial support, and it is understood that Mexico is to reconquer the lost territory in New Mexico, Texas, and Arizona. The details are left to you for settlement. You are instructed to inform the President of Mexico of the above in the greatest confidence as soon as it is certain that there will be an outbreak of war with the United States, and suggest that the President of Mexico, on his own initiative, should communicate with Japan suggesting adherence to this plan. At the same time, offer to mediate between Germany and Japan. Please call to the attention of the President of Mexico that the employment of ruthless submarine warfare now promises to compel England to make peace in a few months.[63]

Wilson released the Zimmermann Telegram to the newspapers. The resulting public outcry ended nearly all neutralist, pacifist and pro–German sentiment in America. That Germany planned to take the war to the American southwest, and possibly even to the Pacific coast by involving Japan, was too much![64] Rather than denying the telegram and saying it was a British hoax, and thus defusing the situation, Zimmermann foolishly admitted its validity.[65] As with the violation of Belgium's neutrality, the destruction of Louvain, the sinking of *Lusitania*, the execution of Nurse Cavell, and now the Zimmermann Telegram, it was clear the Germans were curiously insensitive to public opinion outside their borders. Now this blindness came home to roost.

Wilson called Congress in special session on April 2. At eight o'clock in the evening he addressed the assembled; his speech included the lines, "I advise that the Congress declare the recent course of the Imperial German Government to be in fact nothing less than war against the Government and People of the United States; that it formally accept the status of belligerent which has thus been thrust upon it."[66] On April 6, 1917, Congress so declared — America was at war with Germany.

Chapter 11

Americans Going and Coming

> I do not know why we fought. No Archduke's little life was worth the titanic butchery of the world war.... It is all a great slaughter house, legalized by Princes and Kings.[1]— Romeo Houle, an American in the Canadian Army, 1914–1916

With the severing of diplomatic relations between Germany and the United States on February 3, 1917, the American Ambassador to Germany, his staff, and all consular officers received instructions to leave Germany immediately. The American Legation in Brussels as well as the consuls at Antwerp, Liège and Ghent had the same instructions. On February 5, Whitlock received a telegram from the U.S. State Department countermanding the instructions for his immediate departure; the Department was now of the opinion it would be best for the Legation to remain in Brussels if the German authorities did not object.[2] The reason for the change of heart was the American food relief program; the State Department felt that Whitlock's presence was crucial for the continued function of the Commission for Relief in Belgium (and Northern France). It was, of course, in the Germans' interest to keep the relief supplies coming in order to deter civilian unrest. Both General von Bissing, the Governor-General in Belgium, and Baron von der Lancken, head of the *Politische Abteilung* (Political Department), advocated keeping Whitlock in Brussels for as long as possible.

Politische Abteilung
  bei dem
Gouverneur general in Belgien

                                          Brussels, 25 February 1917

My Dear Mr. Brand Whitlock:

    After the rupture of diplomatic relations between the Imperial Government and the Government of the United States of America, I addressed, after having placed myself in accord with the Spanish Minister, Protector of the Work of the *revitaillement*, a letter to him on the 10th February, of which he has told me he sent you a copy. In this letter I suggested to the Marquis de Villalobar that in the interest of the work of the *revitaillement* the continuation of your presence in Brussels would be desirable, and I assured him that in this event the Governor-General would be happy to see you devote to the work of the Commission for Relief your activity, for a long time so useful to that institution.

Lancken[3]

Baron von der Lancken accorded Whitlock every privilege possible, despite the severing of diplomatic relations between their countries. Since the Germans needed Whitlock in Brussels, General von Bissing permitted him to send and receive correspondence, employing the courier of the Spanish Legation. Although now only a private citizen, Whitlock was a distinguished private citizen. Lancken made an additional request concerning the Legation building.

As to the flag, we should prefer that it be removed because we are on the eve of a great battle, the city is full of troops, we do not know what some irresponsible soldier may do, and a regrettable incident might very easily be created.[4]

The key question was the supervision of the C.R.B. when the Americans left the country. There were approximately 50 American delegates in Belgium, assuring that Germany respected her agreements concerning C.R.B. foodstuffs in Belgium and Northern France. Spain and Holland, both still neutral, agreed to send delegates to replace the Americans. The food relief program would continue even after the United States entered the war.

With the C.R.B. assurances in hand, Whitlock was now a man who had lost his job but still came to the office looking for something useful to do. He realized the authorities would soon tell his wife and him to leave Brussels, although he did not know when. He often spent time walking, reminiscing. The weather that February was very frigid. Soldiers crowded the streets on their way to some impending butchery in the west, perhaps at Ypres. Near the Legation coal carts rumbled down Rue Belliard. German soldiers guarded the carts, as the coal was for their use. Behind the carts little children with baskets collected the lumps that dropped on the street. Mostly the soldiers paid no attention to the urchins. Whitlock noted the children wore rags. He visited his favorite bookstalls and antiquarians in the city. The shopkeepers, realizing he was still in Brussels, implored him not to leave, hoping he would stay. "And I knew it was only a postponement; I had not the heart to tell them. Our trunks were indeed all packed, and in our normal attitude of sitting on our boxes; there was no official work to do."[5]

Then, the news of the Zimmermann Telegram arrived in Brussels "like a thunderbolt," as Whitlock described it in his journal.

> March 3, 1917.— 7:45 p.m. ... had sensational news, to the effect that a plot has been discovered in America, evidenced by documents implicating Zimmermann, by which the German Government was instigating revolution in Mexico and *offering Mexico three states of the Union*— Texas and two others.
> Sunday, March 4, 1917.— Everybody laughing at the frightful blunder the Germans made in proposing Mexico to become an ally.[6]

The German response somehow missed the mark; their newspapers attacked President Wilson for having released Zimmermann's plan to the press, implying this was in some way unfair. There were probably more chuckles in Brussels at this inventive response! Whitlock now knew that soon his adventure in Brussels would be history. On March 25, 1917, a telegram arrived from President Wilson instructing Whitlock and his wife Nell, personnel of the Legation and C.R.B. delegates to leave occupied Belgium immediately. The waiting was over. Hearing the news of Whitlock's imminent departure, many friends arrived at the Legation to say their final good-bye. Among the callers was a German officer with whom Whitlock had often discussed the war in terms of Darwinism, the German view of war as a biological struggle between nations, equating nations to biological species. Whitlock countered that this was a "misunderstanding of Darwinism with which they [the Germans] had dosed their muddled philosophy."[7] The officer expressed shock and grief now "that this struggle for life was on between his species and mine."[8]

The first group of C.R.B. delegates left Brussels on March 29. They took the night train from the Gare du Nord, the North Station. Located close by, the Palace Hotel was a convenient place to meet before leaving.

> We were to meet for the last Brussels dinner in the Palace Hotel. We recalled the Palace a few evenings before, when at the entrance of five or six of us, the Belgian orchestra took a long chance, and whispering *"ravitaillement"* [food relief], played *The Stars and Stripes Forever* under the noses of two or three hundred German officers. The Germans suspected the tune, but they were not quite sure, so grinningly the orchestra struck it up again and again.[9]

Finally the day arrived; the Whitlocks would leave Brussels on Monday, April 2, 1917, the same day that President Wilson would address Congress for a declaration of war upon Germany. That Sunday, Brand and Nell took a last look at their beloved Brussels. "I went with my wife for a last walk along the boulevards in the soft spring rain, in the strange sense of realizing one's self as still of a familiar and beloved scene, yet saying sadly all the while within, 'Tomorrow I shall behold all this no more.'"[10]

Whitlock wrote in his journal, "April 2, 1917 — What a day!" There were two official luncheons to attend, both scheduled for one o'clock; fortunately, a German hosted one and a Belgian the other. At one o'clock German time (noon Belgian time) Brand and Nell dined with Governor-General von Bissing and his wife; then at one o'clock Belgian time (two o'clock German time) they lunched again, this meal hosted by the Burgomaster of Brussels. No doubt satiated, they arrived at the Gare du Nord at 4:45 for a scheduled departure at 5:00, having motored there in the Spanish Legation auto driven by Minister Villalobar. In the Place Rogier, at the entrance to the train station and opposite the Palace Hotel, a great crowd had gathered to see the Americans off. Men removed their hats; women cried and held up their children for the Whitlocks to touch. Then the special train arranged by the German authorities to take the Whitlocks to Switzerland drew up along the platform. The party was about 75 persons: 15 members of the Chinese Legation leaving with the Americans, about 25 C.R.B. delegates, American consuls and families, the Whitlocks, various servants and a mountain of baggage. Nell and Brand alone had 15 trunks, 2 great diplomatic pouches containing the Legation records, the diplomatic code book, and, of course, the manuscript of a novel. Adding to the confusion were Kin Kung and Taï Taï, the Whitlocks' Pekingese dogs. Mrs. Whitlock, her arms burdened with flowers and escorted by Villalobar, finally boarded the train. This very long day would soon end. At 5:45, the train slowly left the station; at nearly every railroad crossing, crowds waving handkerchiefs said good-bye.

Three Americans remained on the platform watching the departing train: Prentiss N. Gray, his wife Laura Sherman Gray and their two-year-old daughter Barbara.

> We waved our last farewell to the red tail-lights, which disappeared in the darkness a moment later; then a sense of oppression rushed upon us, and we turned sadly, and with heavy hearts passed out through the throngs of Belgians, none too dry-eyed, who had been allowed to enter the station proper, through the cordon of sentries.[11]

As the Assistant-Director of the C.R.B. in Brussels, Gray would remain behind with three accountants to close the books on the American operation that was handling $15,000,000 worth of foodstuffs per month at that point. He also would facilitate the transition for Dutch and Spanish control of C.R.B. operations in occupied France and Belgium. At Gray's request, while still a delegate in Antwerp, German authorities had permitted his wife and daughter to join him in Belgium. Mother and daughter traveled from San Francisco to New York where they boarded the Holland-America Line Steamer *New Amsterdam* for Falmouth, England, and then Rotterdam in early October 1916. As assurance to the safety-conscious traveler, Holland-America advertised itself as having the largest ships under neutral flag and promised the traveler could make the passage from Falmouth to Rotterdam either through the English Channel or around Scotland, depending upon war circumstances.

In addition to the Gray family, there were six American C.R.B. delegates quarantined in Belgium because they had been near the front recently. The German Army worried they might know military information about pending battles that could be of value to the enemy. The men were initially detained near the front but eventually brought to Brussels. Among those detained was Julius Van Hee, the former American vice consul at Ghent. Van Hee finally arrived in Brussels on April 10, having spent part of the time in a Ghent jail.

By mid–April a new calamity arose; Brussels had sufficient flour for only four days. Food riots were a possibility. The unrestricted U-boat campaign was taking its toll on relief ships; seven sank from either torpedoes or mines with a loss of 28,000 tons of foodstuffs. Consequently, relief ships remained in England, afraid to attempt a passage to Rotterdam. The last hope was to obtain a loan of food from Holland. To effect such a loan, Prentiss Gray and the head of the Belgian relief organization, M. Francqui, required special passes to travel to Holland to plead their cause. The passes could come only from Governor-General von Bissing, who at the time was very ill. On the night before the scheduled trip, they learned of the death of the Governor-General (April 18, 1917).

> When Lancken [Baron von der Lancken] announced "The Governor-General died at nine to-night," I was positively relieved, until I remembered that he was the only one that could sign my pass. After expression of my sympathy, which I fear was not properly lengthy, I hastened to enquire if by any chance I could leave for Holland in the morning.[12]

However, in his last moments of consciousness von Bissing fulfilled his duty; he signed the travel passes. Gray and Francqui traveled to Holland and managed to secure a total of 20,000 tons of wheat from the Dutch as an advance against in-coming relief ship cargos. Although a U-boat torpedoed the next arriving relief ship, tugs managed to bring her to Rotterdam and salvage her cargo of wheat. The unrestricted U-boat offensive probably starved occupied Belgium and France more than its intended target, England.

> Mr. Gray asserted that "if these people are to be kept alive during the coming winter [1917/1918], the relief commission must be supplied with 220,000 tons of shipping, or about 45 steamers of average size." Owing to the loss of ships by submarine warfare, the fleet of relief steamers now numbers less than twenty, he declared.[13]

With the death of von Bissing, Baron von der Lancken, head of the *Politische Abteilung*, became the key German official in charge of food relief and thus the person with whom Gray interacted most.

> We had come to fear this stern, forbidding man during earlier days of our negotiations with him, but by accident I discovered a side of his nature little suspected. One afternoon returning home early I found him at our house for

tea. Could it be the austere Baron whom I saw sprawled on the floor playing blocks with my baby girl?

Often after this I found him at home, building block forts, to be demolished, to the ecstatic joy of my child, with a sweep of his scabbered sword.[14]

Evidently the Baron loved children; before the war, he opened his estates to several hundred orphans every summer. Everyone, including Prussian officers, had more than one side to their personality; this always came as a surprise to the Americans in Belgium.

At the end of April, Prentiss Gray, accompanied by Mrs. Gray, their daughter, three accountants and six delegates, boarded a train for Switzerland. "Every courtesy possible was shown us in our final departure. The German officers had arranged a special car for us, and came to the train with flowers and candy."[15]

As the train left the Gare du Nord, the last official American presence in occupied Belgium ended. However, that did not mean there were no Americans left in the country. Some American businessmen remained even after America declared war. C.C. Clayton, as representative of the Western Electric Company, an American corporation in Antwerp once employing 2,000 people, had resided in Antwerp since 1913. After the Germans took Antwerp (see Chapter 4), life changed for the American abroad.

> While the business life of Belgium is paralyzed, the social life has practically disappeared because people either cannot or do not feel like entertaining, and because one is expected to ask for a permit from the Germans and may find that some would like to be invited. There are no parties, no balls, no festivals. There are no telephones in private use. The railways are run primarily for military purposes and are on only about 20 per cent. of their peace schedule.[16]

As a businessman, Clayton observed and understood how the Germans plundered Belgium, using the ruse of "a legal illegality." German commissions controlled everything: coal, oil, fats, grain, sugar, butter, milk, peas, flour, eggs and meats, everything and anything that one could move or sell. The commission fixed the maximum price above which it was illegal to sell. Belgians who sold above the maximum price went to jail, that is, if they sold to Belgians. At the same time, German agents, prowling the countryside in search of available goods, purchased these at considerably above the maximum commission-set price and promised immunity to the seller. The agents then sent these goods to Germany.

> Like a huge suction pump the maximum price fixer goes about the country, aided and abetted by the clandestine agent, drawing into the German maw every available eatable.[17]

Western Electric had large stocks of brass, copper, and other metals needed by the German war machine. Prior to America's entry into the war, the Germans paid about half value for these materials. The Germans simply confiscated the company's stock of platinum. Clayton spent considerable effort trying to recoup something for his company. After America entered the war, it was hopeless. Clayton also witnessed the Germans rob Belgian banks, again employing "legal" means.

Remarkably, in 1917, Belgian banks were fat with cash. During the invasion in 1914, Belgians who possessed wealth (cash and precious metals) usually buried that wealth to hide it from the invaders. By 1915, people felt it was probably safer to deposit their money in Belgian banks, since the Germans seemed to respect those institutions, rather than worrying about someone chancing upon their buried treasure trove in the back garden. However, the banks could do nothing with these deposits; after all, there were no loans to businesses because there was no business going on. Consequently, the banks became gorged with cash. The German commission in charge of banks devised a clever ruse to withdraw this wealth.

The Hague Convention on Land War permitted an army of occupation to levy taxes to cover its expenses in administering the occupied country, i.e., Belgium. When the collected taxes were insufficient, an indemnity might be levied to supply the balance. Of course, tax collections were always insufficient. To redress this, the German bank commissioner assessed each province an indemnity to cover the additional costs of administering said province. The commissioner issued bonds in the names of the provinces and compelled local banks to purchase the indemnity bonds.

> Of course no one will voluntarily buy these bonds. The next step is to allot to the banks these forced loans. This is done by the German bank commissioner who notifies each bank what portion has fallen its lot, basing his estimate on the capital stock and resources. Unless the banks pay their allotments into the German treasury within a stated time their doors are closed and they are fined.
>
> If the war lasts long enough the resources of the banks will be very largely represented by provincial bonds of which no one can determine the value.[18]

By 1917, these indemnities amounted to 1,680,000,000 francs. Since five francs equaled a dollar, the Germans had robbed Belgian banks of $336,000,000 in 1917 dollars or in today's money, approximately five billion dollars — a record heist!

On August 31, 1917, German authorities permitted Clayton to leave Antwerp and cross into Holland.[19] He traveled to New York aboard a British steamship, arriving on October 21. Also aboard the ship was A.D. Whipple who had represented the Bell Telephone Company in Antwerp. Whipple commented, "Living on a starvation diet in Antwerp I lost 20 pounds in weight before I was able to get away."[20]

While the American population in eastern Belgium diminished in number, western Belgium witnessed the opposite trend. Many Americans enlisted in the Canadian Army and fought in the Ypres Salient. The British actively recruited men who were born in Britain or its empire and who lived in the United States but had not yet become naturalized citizens.[21] In addition to these resident aliens, thousands of American citizens flocked to the British colors.[22] The easiest way to join was to cross into Canada. The Canadian Army readily accepted such recent émigrés, some of whom had only been in their country twenty-four hours. By 1916, there were 16,000 American citizens in various Canadian units.[23] Everyone knew of the ersatz Canadians in uniform, even the King of England.

Captain Alexander Weel, an American in the Thirteenth Royal Highlanders of Canada, was part of an honor guard for King George V. The King asked the captain if he was an American. Captain Weel answered,

"No, your Majesty, a Canadian."

"That's queer," said the King. "I thought you were an American. But you are an American, are you not?"

After a couple more denials, Captain Weel finally admitted,

"Yes, your Majesty, I am an American." The King gave him a gold cigarette case as a souvenir.[24]

Probably one of the first Americans to enlist did so on August 10, 1914. Romeo Houle, of French-Canadian heritage, was an American from New Bedford, Massachusetts. He traveled to Montreal when the war began and joined a French-Canadian Regiment. Shipped to England and then across the English Channel, his regiment boarded London buses that carried them 40 miles (64 km) inland to the lines near Armentières, France. The French-Canadians occupied trenches within calling distance of the enemy. They soon discovered that some of the enemy soldiers were German-Canadians from Ontario. An informal truce developed—fire only when ordered to and then aim high. "Neither side forgot we were both Canadian, and steadfastly kept our treaty of peace."[25] However, the peace soon ended; the British ordered the regiment to the Ypres Salient, just in time for the Second Battle of Ypres (see Chapter 9).

Romeo Houle's Golgotha was at Ypres. The Germans held the high ground and had a clear view of the opposing trenches. Machine guns raked the Canadians mercilessly, causing many casualties. The firing was continuous night and day. Then things got worse. At two o'clock in the morning, a yellow-green fog crept across No Man's Land and into the Canadian defenses. Houle described the effects of the poison gas.

> You breathe fire. You suffocate. You burn alive. There are razors and needles in your throat. It is as if you drank boiling hot tea. Your lungs flame. You want to

scratch and tear your body. You become half blind, half wild. Your head aches beyond description, you vomit, you drop exhausted, you die quickly.[26]

Houle saw horribly wounded men pleading for the release of death, and their friends killing them as a mercy. Of the 500 men in the two French-Canadian companies at Ypres, only 20 survived; the rest were casualties: 480 dead, wounded or missing. Houle was one of the very lucky few to survive.

The sinking of *Lusitania* in 1915 motivated many young men to travel north to Canada and enlist, despite the fact that doing so negated their American citizenship.[27] Alexander McClintock of Lexington, Kentucky, was typical. In October 1915, he traveled to New York, intending to go to France and join the Foreign Legion. After a casual chat with a Canadian recruiter in the bar of his hotel, he traveled to Montreal instead. A couple of days later, he enlisted in the Canadian Grenadier Guards. He noted that discipline "was quite lax." The army gave him a week's leave to settle his affairs in the States; he overstayed by five days. "All that my company commander said to me when I got back was that I seemed to have picked up Canadian habits very quickly."[28] At a review during training camp, his major addressed the troops, "Boys, for God's sake don't call me Harry or spit in the ranks. Here comes the general!"[29]

Discipline tightened considerably in England where combat training occurred. Because he was an American and, therefore, must be a baseball player, the Brits sent him to bombing school.

> The average British soldier is not an expert at throwing; it is a new game to him, therefore the Canadians and Americans, who have played baseball from kindergarten up, take naturally to bomb throwing and excel in this act. A six-foot English bomber will stand in awed silence when he sees a little five-foot-nothing Canadian out-distance his throw by several yards.[30]
>
> The standard bomb used in the British Army is the "Mills." It is about the shape and size of a large lemon,... The Mills bomb is made of steel, the outside of which is corrugated into forty-eight small squares which, upon the explosion of the bomb, scatter in a wide area, wounding or killing any Fritz who is unfortunate enough to be hit by one of the flying fragments.[31]

The Mills bomb (hand grenade) had a lever that extended half way around its circumference, held in place at the bottom by a fixed pin. In this pin was a small metal ring for extracting the pin. With the pin pulled, and the bomb thrown, the lever flew off, forcing the firing pin into a percussion cap that ignited the bomb's fuse. The fuse burned down and set off the detonator, which exploded the bomb. Hopefully the bomb reached the enemy and exploded before he could pitch it back. For three weeks, McClintock threw bombs, studied bombs and took apart bombs. As he said, he did everything that you could do with a Mills bomb, except eat it.

McClintock, along with the Grenadier Guards, arrived in Belgium in the early summer of 1916, coming by train from Le Havre to Poperinghe, and then to the front line trenches the following day. They were to defend a position known as "The Graveyard of Canada," where during the Second Battle of Ypres (1915) the Canadians had withstood one of the first gas attacks of the war. After a couple of weeks at the front, McClintock and 60 others volunteered for a bombing raid in which they would sneak into enemy lines at night, pitch a few Mills bombs and, hopefully, capture a prisoner or two.

> A bombing raid — something originated in warfare by the Canadians — is not intended for the purpose of holding ground, but to gain information, to do as much damage as possible, and to keep the enemy in a state of nervousness.[32]

Such actions in the First World War were usually a pointless waste of lives, and McClintock's bombing raid confirmed expectation. Of the sixty, only seven returned, the rest being wounded or killed. McClintock was one of the lucky returnees; he came back without a scratch. He then made four return trips to No Man's Land under heavy machine gun fire, searching for wounded comrades. He brought two back alive and one who soon died. For bravery, King George V conferred the Distinguished Conduct Medal on the American.[33]

In 1916, a Unitarian clergyman from the United States, C. Seymour Bullock, founded the American Legion, a Canadian brigade (5,000 men) made up of American citizens.[34] The brigade as envisioned by the Reverend Bullock would be unique in the British forces as it advocated total abstention from demon rum or any other booze. When British officers toasted the King with an alcoholic libation, "the American officers rise and drink the toast 'The King' in cold water."[35] American officers with the smell of liquor on their breath had to resign from the Legion. Officers were to lead their men by booze-free example; whether their men followed is a moot point. What the British and Canadians thought of Bullock's prohibition is left to the imagination; they saw Bullock raising more cannon fodder, so no one cared about his Puritanical beliefs. The British Army always had its rum ration, the French Army drank wine rather than water, and the German soldiers were serious beer drinkers; none of these libations seemed to impair their fighting abilities. If the Americans wanted to drink cold water, so be it. The first regiment (97th Canadian Regiment made up of Americans recruited in Toronto) of the so-called American Legion sailed aboard the White Star liner *Baltic* from Canada in mid-March 1916,[36] its ultimate destination Flanders. Presumably, there was no liquor on board, at least none visible to the Reverend Bullock.

In addition to ground soldiers, the Royal Flying Corps recruited hundreds of flyers in the United States. The requirements included good reflexes, keen eyesight and hearing and weighing under 14 stone (196 pounds).

> Only part of the aviator's time has to be devoted to routine work and "stunts." He has his social life, and a merry time it is, with a full dose of the *joie de vivre*. "Bird-men" are the best company in the world; they are the cream of society, and yet modest.[37]

What the recruiting pamphlet omitted was the low probability of surviving the "Birdman" experience.

> That is one of the saddest things connected with service in the R.F.C. [Royal Flying Corps] You don't care much what happens to you, but the constant casualties among your friends is very depressing.[38]

Patrick O'Brien of San Francisco succumbed to the British recruiting campaign; in the fall of 1916, he traveled to Canada and enlisted in the Royal Flying Corps. Nine months later, having completed pilot training and now Leftenant O'Brien, he was aboard ship heading for England. There were eighteen pilots in his group, nine of whom were Americans. By the end of 1917, of the nine Americans, four would be dead, two seriously wounded, and Leftenant O'Brien seriously wounded and a prisoner of war. The *joie de vivre* of being a "Birdman" often was of short duration. In the summer of 1917, O'Brien joined a fighter squadron near Ypres.

> My squadron was one of four stationed at an aerodrome about eighteen miles back of the Ypres line. There were eighteen pilots in our squadron, which was a scout-squadron, scout-machines carrying but one man.
>
> A scout, sometimes called a fighting-scout, has no bomb-dropping or reconnoitering to do. His duty is just to fight, or, as the order was given to me, "You are expected to pick fights and not wait until they come to you."[39]

His first flight acquainted him with the battlefield: forests, lakes, buildings, roads and other landmarks that might help if he became lost. Hospitals were of key importance; if ever wounded, he should do his best to land or crash as near as possible to a hospital, either English or German. O'Brien's first forced landing was near the British trenches nowhere near a hospital; he watched from a shell hole as German artillery destroyed his airplane. A few weeks later, he remembered the advice about hospitals. In a dog-fight behind German lines on August 17, 1917, his plane shredded with bullet holes and spinning out of control from 8,000 feet, O'Brien somehow managed to crash near a German hospital.

> I glanced at my instruments and my altitude was between eight and nine thousand feet. While I was still looking at the instruments the whole blame works disappeared. A burst of bullets went into the instrument board and blew it to smithereens, another bullet went through my upper lip, came out of the roof of my mouth and lodged in my throat, and the next thing I knew was when I came to in a German hospital the following morning at five o'clock, German time.[40]

In the hospital his first visitors were German flying officers who congratulated him on his miraculous landing. There was a chivalry among pilots. Later a German flyer dropped a message O'Brien wrote over his British aerodrome behind Ypres. In it O'Brien explained his situation and how to contact his mother.

Located near the front lines in a house, the hospital had four rooms; O'Brien was in a room for officers. A German officer occupied the bed next to him. The fellow also turned out to be from San Francisco. Responding to Germany's need, he had taken a ship to South America where he had obtained a false passport and had booked passage to New York and then to England. From there he had traveled to Italy, which was neutral at the time, and then to Austria and finally to Germany. The two Californians became chums and had long discussions. They both had traveled a long distance to meet in a hospital in Ypres. The German had some radical views about what should happen in Germany. "If I had my way about it, I would make her a republic to-day and hang the damned Kaiser in the bargain."[41]

After he had recovered somewhat, O'Brien traveled by auto about an hour's ride east to the town of Courtrai (Kortrijk). Located in the town center, the civil prison was now a prison camp for captured officers. O'Brien remained there for two weeks. One of his interrogators was a German-American from Jersey City, New Jersey. O'Brien got the impression that the man would have preferred serving in the American Army and was only in Germany because of family. "The Kaiser himself visited Courtrai while I was in the prison, I was told by one of the interpreters, but he didn't call on me and, for obvious reasons, I couldn't call on him."[42]

From Courtrai, O'Brien traveled on a train bound for a prison camp in Germany, locked in a coach with seven other British prisoners, guarded by four old soldiers. Somewhere in Germany, as the train slowed for some reason, O'Brien jumped from the coach's window. It was four o'clock in the morning, September 9, 1917. For the next 72 days, the American escaped capture, walking across Germany, occupied Luxembourg and occupied Belgium before reaching safety in Holland. He traveled at night guided by the North Star and slept in the woods in the day. He foraged in farm fields for food, eating mostly beets and turnips. He drank water where he thought it clean. He stayed away from roads and houses, traveling cross-country away from people, floundering through marshes, swimming across canals and small rivers. Before he crossed into Belgium, O'Brien had been cold, wet and very hungry for 18 days. In Belgium, he chanced knocking on the doors of isolated peasant cottages asking the inhabitants for help. They shared a hot meal with him, often only thin potato soup, let him warm himself by their fire and urged him on, fearful of German retribution. Sometimes they gave him old clothing. Dressed as a local, he occasionally chanced walking during the day down roads, past German guards at checkpoints. No guard ever stopped the emaciated dirty traveler dressed in rags, probably assuming he was just another down and out Belgian. Nevertheless, even in Belgium he mostly traveled cross-country, foraging for food in farm fields.

> The cabbage that I got in Belgium consisted of the small heads that the peasants had not cut. All the strength had concentrated in these little heads and they would be as bitter as gall. I would have to be pretty hungry to-day before I could ever eat cabbage again, and the same observation applies to carrots, turnips, and sugar-beets — especially sugar beets.[43]

After eight weeks of wandering around Belgium, O'Brien finally made it to the Dutch frontier. There he made a depressing discovery. A nine-foot-high electrified fence separated Belgium and Holland. Parallel and on either side of the electrified fence were six-foot-high barbed wire walls. German sentries patrolled the barrier. The principal reason for such a robust barrier was to prevent German deserters from reaching sanctuary in neutral Holland. O'Brien managed to get under the barbed wire wall and tried to cross the fence with a crude ladder he fashioned. The ladder collapsed and he received a nasty electric shock. Finally, he managed to burrow under the fence.

> To dig the hole must have taken me more than two hours, and I had to stop frequently to hide while the sentry passed.... I certainly suffered enough that night to last me a lifetime. With a German guard on one side, death from electrocution on the other, and starvation staring me in the face, my plight was anything but a comfortable one.
> It was the 19th of November, 1917, when I got through the wires.[44]

After 72 days on the run, he was in Holland.

When the United States finally entered the war, there was considerable concern about the country's "preparedness." Dr. Harvey Cushing, Professor of Surgery at Harvard University Medical School, was one of those most concerned about the lack of war experience in the medical profession. As a remedy, he founded the Harvard Unit, a medical team organized into a base hospital unit, known as Base Hospital No. 5. Cushing's first idea was to set up Base Hospital No. 5, a rather large tent city, on the Boston Common as a way of drawing public attention to wartime medical needs. However, the town fathers of Boston rejected the proposal; Boston Common was open public space and should remain so. Although Cushing lost the "Battle of the Common," as he described it, another opportunity soon arose for his Harvard Unit. Mobilized into the U.S. Army Medical Reserve Corps, the Harvard Unit received sailing orders for the Western Front. On May 4, 1917, it boarded *Saxonia* in New York harbor. The Unit consisted of 26 officers (mostly physicians), 185 enlisted men,

81 nurses, 1 dietitian, and 3 secretaries. In addition to passengers, *Saxonia* carried a cargo of munitions. Dodging U-boats, the ship made it to Falmouth, England. After a couple of weeks in England, the Harvard Unit crossed the English Channel and traveled to Royal Army Medical Corps No. 11 General Hospital in Camiers, France. Approximately 60 km (37.2 miles) south of Calais, the R.A.M.C. hospital was near a huge British Army depot known as Etaples Camp, which supplied the Flanders front. Cushing described No. 11 as "a shockingly dirty, unkempt camp."[45] He learned that in wet weather No. 11 was under water. German aircraft frequently bombed the hospital; such attacks would kill six Americans and severely wound six, including a nurse.

In addition to the Harvard Unit, five other American medical schools and hospitals sent staff for war experience in R.A.M.C. hospitals in France: Presbyterian Hospital, New York City; Lakeside Hospital, Cleveland; Pennsylvania Hospital, Philadelphia; Northwestern University Medical Department, Chicago; Washington University School of Medicine, St. Louis. All of these units arrived in France in late May 1917 and joined R.A.M.C. hospitals near the Channel ports. When the Third Battle of Ypres began later that summer, the R.A.M.C. sent many of these Americans to Ypres to help deal with the flood of wounded.

The Third Battle of Ypres originated from the failed attempts by the British Navy and Royal Air Corps to destroy the German submarine bases at Zeebrugge, Ostend, and Bruges. Sir Douglas Haig, the British Commander-in-Chief, thought that the army might prove to be more successful. He planned to breach the German defenses in the Ypres Salient and then push east 40 miles (64 km) to Bruges. His plan was the inverse of the earlier German plans, which attempted to breach the Allied defenses in the Salient to reach the Channel ports. Haig's plan failed for pretty much the same reason the German plans had — Flanders mud. However, as many plans do, it sounded promising.

> This was an offensive against the enemy forces in Flanders, with the aim of clearing the Belgian coast and turning the northern flank of the whole German defence system in the West. It was a scheme which, if successful, promised the most profound and far-reaching results. It would destroy the worst of the submarine bases; it would return to Belgium her lost territory, and thereby deprive the enemy of one of his cherished bargaining assets.[46]

An arch of low hills bordered Ypres to the east. Playing key roles in the battle were the villages of Wytschaete (Wijtschate) and Messines (Mesen), located on a ridge in the south, and the village of Passchendaele (Passendale), on the high ground in the north. The Germans held all the high ground and thus had observation points commanding the entire British line within the salient. To break out of the salient and drive for Bruges required breaking through the German positions on the high ground, positions the Germans had reinforced with concrete blockhouses and other defensive works since the last battle in 1915.

The British offensive began in the south at the Wytschaete and Messines ridge. The British lines were just to the west of the ridge, while the Germans held the ridge. To reach the main enemy line on the ridge, British forces had to fight across two and a half miles of skillfully sited trenches and redoubts, designed to bring flanking fire on the attackers. At 3:20 in the morning of June 7, 1917, the British set off their surprise. They had tunneled under the German front line and packed the ends of the tunnels with over a million pounds of explosive.

> With a shock that made the solid earth quiver like a pole in the wind, nineteen volcanoes leaped to heaven. Nineteen sheets of flame seemed to fill the world.... In most places the German front lines had been blown out of existence.[47]

By June 12, after five days of fighting, with fewer casualties than expected, the Wytschaete and Messines ridge was in British hands. Now came the hard part, to win the high ground east of the Salient, especially in the direction of the village of Passchendaele, which lay seven miles distant. Following a massive artillery barrage, the initial British attack on July 31 made substantial gains, achieving most of its first day's objectives. However, at midday on August 1, it began to rain. During the following months, rain was the dominant weather event. Because of the heavy bombardment of a battlefield underlain with impervious clay (see Chapter 9), the water did not drain through the soil; shell craters became ponds disguising pits of quicksand, the entire battlefield became a nearly impassable huge swamp.

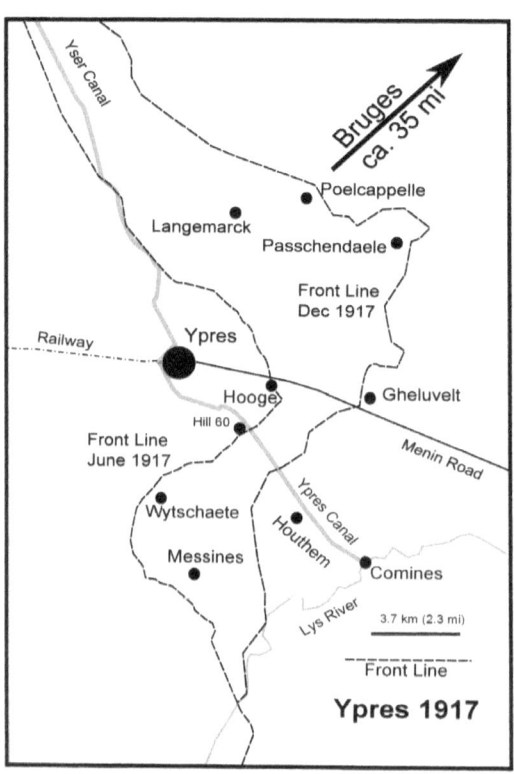

A few days after the battle began the rains began, and hardly ceased for four months. Night after night the skies opened and let down steady torrents, which turned all that country into one great bog of slime.... The hurricanes of artillery fire which our gunners poured upon the enemy positions for twenty miles in depth churned up deep shell-craters which intermingled and made pits which the rains and floods filled to the brim. The only way of walking was by "duck-boards," tracks laid down across the bogs under enemy fire, smashed up day by day, laid down again under cover of darkness.[48]

In the week prior to the attack on July 31, the Royal Army Medical Corps moved teams of American physicians and nurses from their base hospitals in France to Casualty Clearing Stations (C.C.S.s) west of Ypres (often military cemeteries identify former C.C.S. locations in Belgium and northern France). The wounded initially were stabilized at field dressing stations (*postes de secours*) near the fighting, then moved to C.C.S.s a few miles west of Ypres, later moved to a base hospital near the English Channel, and finally to a convalescent hospital in England. American C.C.S. teams consisted of a surgeon, an anesthetist, an operating room nurse and an orderly. The Presbyterian Hospital Unit sent at least five different teams, possibly as many as eight.[49] Some of the stations had humorous slang names mixing English and Flemish, e.g. Mendinghem, Bandagehem and Dosinghem. At one time, there was even an Endinghem; however, that name was dropped as being too insensitive. The Harvard Unit occupied Mendinghem and found it soon overwhelmed with wounded.

Aug. 1
The preoperative hut is still packed with untouched cases, so caked in wet mud that it's a task even to strip them and find out what they've got.

Aug. 2
2.30 a.m. Pouring cats and dogs all day — also pouring cold and shivering wounded, covered with mud and blood....
Something over 2000 wounded have passed, so far, through this one C.C.S. There are fifteen similar stations behind the battle front.[50]

The teams worked sixteen-hour days for weeks at a time. Sometimes 200 wounded would arrive at once, keeping 7 operating tables continuously occupied. An American nurse in the New York Presbyterian Hospital Unit, Louise Marsh, described the scene:

The pre-operation tent defies description after a drive, the most ghastly and pathetic spectacle I ever hope to see.... In the theater, amputation after amputation, many double; lads of nineteen and twenty; abdominal wounds with cavity full of free fluid and rapidly spreading peritonitis.[51]

Wounded men were just so much flotsam, left where they dropped. Some of the wounded who arrived at the clearing stations had lain in flooded shell craters for days, soaked from the constant rain and with maggots in their wounds. An American surgeon, Dr. F.F. Callahan of Minnesota, serving with a British division at the Messines ridge during July 1917, remembered one unfortunate.

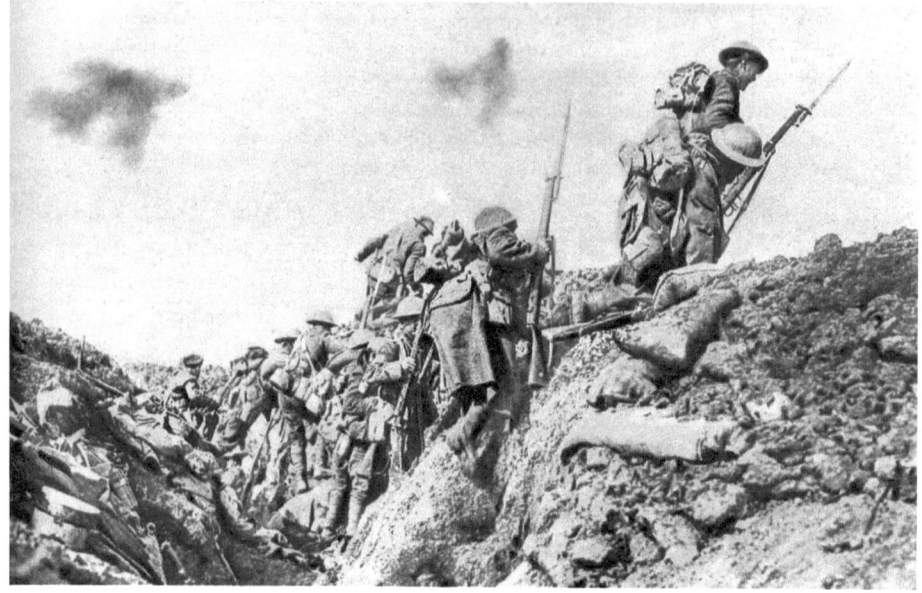

Canadian troops going over the top during the third battle of Ypres, Passchendaele. The dark puffs in the sky are exploding shrapnel shells. Each shell sent a hail of hundreds of lead bullets downward. Shrapnel shells were particularly effective against troops in the open (*Le Miroir*, 1918).

> Wounded were coming in all the time, but the big rush was over. Six days after the attack one poor fellow was brought in who had been marooned in a shell hole in "No Man's Land" since the morning of the 31st. His wounds were not serious but they were full of maggots and his general condition was terrible.[52]

Often after a successful surgery, patients succumbed to infection. Adding to the insanity, the Germans bombed the clearing stations.[53] Another New York Presbyterian Hospital Unit nurse, Jane Rignel, only two years out of nursing school, had her C.C.S. bombed by German aircraft.

> Night before last we were trying to operate on a patient when Fritz came over, and three times in the next hour we fell flat on our abdomens, with steel helmets on our heads, and held our breath while our operating theatre was shaken with the vibrations of eight huge bombs dropping uncomfortably close.[54]

Sir Douglas Haig acknowledged the courage of American nurses in those first six American medical units assigned to the British Expeditionary Force (B.E.F.), listing their names as deserving special mention in a dispatch he sent to London newspapers.[55] In September, more American medical help arrived. By the end of the war, 1,427 American physicians were medical officers in the B.E.F. Of this number, 1,200 saw service with combat troops, 30 were captured,

18 killed, 250 wounded and 163 decorated for bravery by King George V.[56] Nearly all were in the Ypres battles of 1917 and 1918. The number of American nurses with the B.E.F. probably exceeded the number of physicians. In fact, the first American wounded was Nurse Beatrice MacDonald. On August 17, 1917, at 61 C.C.S. a bomb fragment struck her and she lost her right eye.

The offensive into the Salient continued in surges for three months: a cycle of an all-out attack, carnage, some attempt to retrieve wounded, resupply, and perhaps a week later another try. The cycle continued for three months as the British clawed their way east through the mud. For the German Army, the Third Battle of Ypres was also a horror.

> Enormous masses of ammunition, such as the human mind had never imagined before the war, were hurled upon the bodies of men who passed a miserable existence scattered about in mud-filled shell-holes.... It was no longer life at all. It was mere unspeakable suffering . And through this world of mud the attackers dragged themselves, slowly but steadily, and in dense masses. Caught in the advanced zone of our hail of fire they often collapsed, and the lonely man in the shell-hole breathed again. Then the mass came on again. Rifle and machine gun jammed with the mud. Man fought against man, and only too often the mass was successful.[57]

> The enemy charged like a wild bull against the iron wall which kept him from our submarine bases.... Only one thing we did not know — how long the battle would continue. The enemy must tire at some time.[58]

During the many frightful assaults made on Passchendaele ridge, there were occasional instances of live and let live. For example, in September 1917, the British captured a German dressing station. Stoutly constructed of concrete, the station had one great flaw for its new tenants; its doorway faced east toward the German line. This stout concrete structure, with its doorway facing the enemy, would become a death trap should the Germans target the door. An American medical officer, Dr. Rufus Crane, spent a nervous time there, never entirely sure of the duration of the enemy's good will.

> The advanced dressing station, which was one that had been captured from the enemy, was a snug affair built of concrete within which one felt quite secure against anything but a direct hit, tho the door faced the enemy. The Germans in most instances respected the Red Cross flag here, for with their observation from the ridge they could easily have wiped this aid post out at will.[59]

To enable the British to move against the Flanders submarine bases before winter, the high ground around the village of Passchendaele should have been under British control two weeks from the beginning of the offensive on July 31. The distance from the British front line to Passchendaele was about seven miles. On November 6, the Canadians finally took Passchendaele. It had taken three months and probably half a million British and German casualties to cover the distance. No one mentioned going on to Bruges!

> After the first heavy rains had fallen the offensive ought to have been abandoned, and that it was a frightful error of judgment to ask masses of men to attack in conditions where they had not a dog's chance of victory, except at a cost which made it of Pyrrhic irony.[60]

Chapter 12

Final Acts

> Poor fellows! As they lay outside in a row so young and innocent looking, frozen hard as boards, one thinks and ponders on the awfulness of this war. There is a little graveyard just by our aid post growing rapidly in size. Each morning finds a score or more laying beside the little cemetery waiting to be buried. A blanket or a piece of burlap is wrapped about them and they are buried in cold ground. The value of a life out here seems practically nothing.[1]— Dr. Chas. C. Crouse, American medical officer, B.E.F., December 1917

On March 3, 1918, Germany and Russia signed the Treaty of Brest-Litovsk,[2] a peace treaty ending the war in the east. On the Eastern Front, Germany had won the war and now had nearly a million soldiers available to move to the Western Front. Germany finally had an advantage in numbers with which to defeat the British and French. However, that numerical advantage would continue for only several months, until combat-ready American divisions entered the fray that summer. Thus, the German High Command had to strike, and strike fast, to end the war successfully before the full strength of the American Army made itself felt on the Western Front.

The first German offensive, Operation Michael (March 27–April 5), took place in the French region of Picardy. Covering approximately 50 miles (80.5 km) of front, from the river Scarpe near Arras to the river Oise south of St. Quentin, this attack pushed a salient 40 miles (64.4 km) deep into the British line before it ran out of steam. The Germans captured 1,200 square miles of territory, more than the Allies had taken since the beginning of the war. Although the Germans captured nearly 90,000 British soldiers and the Allies suffered over a quarter of a million casualties, Operation Michael did not result in a strategic breakthrough. The stalemate of the Western Front was shaken but not broken.[3]

If at first you do not succeed, try another offensive somewhere else and hope for success. And that is what the German High Command did, launching Operation Georgette into Flanders and northern France. Georgette began on

April 9 and continued until April 29. It had been a dry spring, ideal for war in Flanders. The German Army's motto of *Gott mit uns* (God is with us) seemed self-fulfilling — the weather god was cooperating. The Allied front retreated from Dixmude to the Passchendaele ridge and then to La Bassée, France, 30 miles (48.3 km). The river Lys, the boundary between Belgium and France in this area, divided the battlefield, thus the English refer to Operation Georgette as the Lys Offensive. The major German thrust in the south went through Armentières, driving northwest about 15 miles (24.2 km); in the north the main thrust was against the Messines ridge, which was taken. These were old battlefields well fertilized with recent dead from the fighting in 1917.

> When we occupied the battle-field in the spring of 1918 we encountered the horrible spectacle of many unburied corpses. They lay there in thousands. Two-thirds of them were enemies, one-third German soldiers.[4]

The British fell back toward Ypres, withdrawing "approximately to the old position a mile east of the town from which the Third Battle of Ypres had started."[5] On April 17, the Germans attacked the Belgian line north of the salient. The Belgians drove the attackers into marshy ground and soundly defeated them, killing 2,000 and taking 700 prisoners. It was "perhaps the most successful counterstroke so far in the Lys battle."[6]

The German Army pushed deep into Flanders and northern France but at great cost to itself, suffering 20 percent casualties. For the first time their troops often seemed more interested in looting Allied camps for food and drink than in fighting. Seeing the wealth of supplies in the enemy camps convinced many that the war was pointless. Finally, the British blockade was affecting the fighting morale of the German soldiers. German officers in the field warned the High Command, "The troops will not attack, despite orders [to do so]. The offensive has come to a halt."[7] This reluctance to attack was perhaps one of the first indications that something was amiss in the vaunted German Army. In his memoir, Kaiser Wilhelm grumbled how the soldiers of 1918 were no longer willing to sacrifice themselves for their War Lord.

> The army, to be sure, was no longer the old army. The new 1918 troops particularly were badly tainted with revolutionary propaganda and often took advantage of the darkness at night to sneak away from the firing and vanish to the rear.[8]

When the battle finally closed at the end of April, it became clear to the German Army that although it was a tactical success, it was a strategic failure. The Channel ports were still in British hands and the German Army had squandered some of its best reserves. Since Operations Michael and Georgette were strategic disappointments, the German High Command decided to throw the dice again and launch another offensive somewhere else — something was bound to work. That something occurred in France on May 27. A German offensive crossed the Chemin des Dames ridge and rapidly pushed west toward the city of Château-Thierry on the Marne, bringing the Germans to within 56 miles (90 km) of Paris. At Belleau Wood, near the apex of the drive, a brigade of U.S. Marines helped stop the drive. The counterattack by the French Army and nine divisions of the U.S. Army, known as the Second Battle of the Marne, was not a positive experience for the German Army. The Germans had lost their gamble to beat the Allies before the Americans arrived in force. By the summer of 1918, American soldiers were disembarking in French ports at the rate of 250,000 per month. The unrestricted U-boat campaign begun in January 1917 was now bearing fruit; however, not the harvest the German High Command had sought.

In Belgium, the Flanders submarine bases were still very much on the mind of the British. The U-boats, torpedo boats and destroyers based at Bruges accounted for one third of the shipping lost in the unrestricted campaign of 1917–1918. The failure of the Third Battle of Ypres to reach Bruges, and the loss of territory after Georgette, made it clear that a land assault was impossible. Only two avenues of attack remained: from the air and from the sea. Bombing missions over Ostend, Zeebrugge and Bruges intensified.

A young American, Harry Bruno from Montclair, New Jersey, took part in one of the Ostend bombing missions. Bruno's parents had been aboard *Lusitania* on their "second honeymoon" when a German U-boat sank her in 1915. Both perished. In revenge, and when he was old enough, Bruno traveled to Toronto and joined the Royal Flying Corps in the spring of 1917. Several months later, in September, Bruno and his squadron took off from an aerodrome somewhere in northern France for Ostend.

> A little before 7 a.m. we got under way. At the four-thousand-foot level, obedient to a signal from the Commander, we formed into raiding formation. The scouts [fighter planes] were above, the leader in front, two others behind and the other brought up the rear. Just below them I flew with the other two reconnaissance planes at the same level, but a little bit behind. Below us were the four bombers, their powerful twin motors drumming away fiercely.[9]

Bruno piloted a heavily armed two-seat reconnaissance plane. In this plane, the pilot fired a Vickers machine gun through the propeller arc. Seated behind him, his observer had a Lewis machine gun with six fully loaded drums for the gun on each side of his seat. Half the drums contained explosive bullets. Bruno's aircraft had two jobs: reconnaissance and protecting the bombers. As soon as the squadron crossed into Belgium, it came under nearly continuous fire from anti-aircraft batteries. Approaching a German aerodrome near Courtrai, about 30 miles (48 km) south of Ostend, enemy fighter aircraft greeted the R.F.C. raiders.

Suddenly an "Archie" [anti-aircraft shell] caught one of the fighters, tore off a wing and sent plane and gallant pilot crashing down to death. There were only three "fighters" left and one was already opening fire on the two Huns.[10]

One of our "bombers" was out — I saw it sagging and slowly dropping. Not content with the damage already done to it, two Huns swooped together and sent it crashing below.[11]

As things heated up, the R.F.C. commander signaled the bombers to attack the aerodrome. He probably felt if they continued to Ostend, there would be no bombers left to mount an attack! The bombers successfully dropped their bombs. However, as all prepared to return home, 15 German fighters appeared in the distance. In the ensuing air battle, the R.F.C. lost 2 more planes. Just getting to Ostend was dangerous! During the 6 weeks in which Bruno flew with Reconnaissance Squadron No. 680, it lost 19 pilots.

Since the Royal Flying Corps was not getting anywhere with its bombing campaign, perhaps the Royal Navy might be more successful, at least that was the hope. In April 1918, two daring amphibious raids attempted to close Bruges from the North Sea. The idea was to sink concrete-filled block ships in the entrances to the Zeebrugge and Ostend canals, essentially land locking Bruges. However, to reach the canals, ships had to pass through a gauntlet of artillery fire from German coastal batteries sited to protect the ports. Unless the German gunners could be distracted, in all probability they would destroy any British block ships attempting a run for the canals. The British plan for Zeebrugge had two components: to launch a surprise amphibious attack on the Zeebrugge mole and, while German defenses focused on the attackers, sneak three block ships into the harbor behind the mole and steam hell-bent for the Bruges canal. Motor boats would rescue the crews after they scuttled their ships. The plan might just work — if the Germans were asleep.

On April 23 at 12:10 a.m., various small Royal Navy craft approached the Zeebrugge mole and laid a dense smoke screen to hide the approaching amphibious raid. Unfortunately, at 12:50 a.m. the wind shifted, blowing the artificial fog away; what the Germans first saw was the cruiser *Vindictive* heading for the mole. Tucked behind her were two ferry boats, *Iris* and *Daffodil*. All three vessels carried troops who would stage the diversion by attacking the defenses on the mole. German gunners, seeing *Vindictive* crammed with British soldiers, raked the ship with gunfire. Somehow, the British captain brought the ship alongside the mole but missed the landing area; the withering fire of the German batteries killed three of four of the officers who were to lead the assault and knocked the remaining one unconscious. For a while confusion reigned among the attackers. In addition, only two of the landing bridges especially built to convey the troops from the ship to the mole survived, the top of the mole was fifteen feet above the deck of the *Vindictive*.

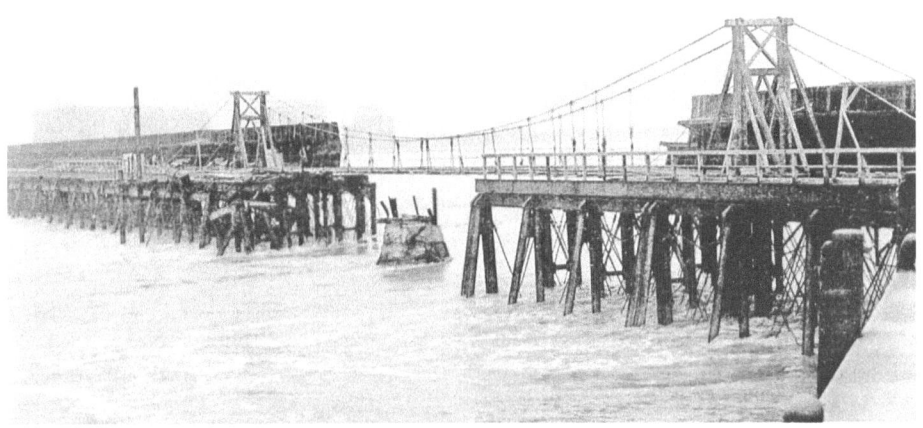

A breach in the Zeebrugge trestle bridge that connected the shore and the mole. The obsolete British submarine *C-3*, loaded with tons of explosive in its bow, wedged itself between the piers. After the crew abandoned the ship, she exploded, ripping a 66 m breach in the bridge and isolating the mole from German reinforcements. The photograph shows a suspension bridge constructed afterward to span the breach. The structure sticking out of the water in the gap may be the conning tower of the submarine (Klekowski collection).

> Only a few German shells hit our hull because it was well protected by the wall of the mole, but the upper structure, masts, stacks and ventilators showed above the wall and were riddled. A considerable proportion of our casualties were caused by splinters from these upper works.[12]

After getting into position, *Vindictive* began to drift away from the mole. *Daffodil* pushed her back into position against the mole. The ferry's troops crossed through *Vindictive* to reach the mole — not many made it. The other ferry, *Iris,* could not be secured to the mole so its troops played only a small role in the attack. During this mêlée, only one thing went according to plan. One obsolete British submarine, *C-3,* packed with explosives, reached the viaduct that connected the mole to land and managed to jam itself among the girders. The crew abandoned *C-3,* which then exploded, cutting the viaduct and isolating the mole garrison.

Hoping that German attention remained focused on the mole attack, three old cruisers, the concrete-filled block ships, entered the harbor. *Thetis* entered first, followed by *Iphigenia* and *Intrepid*. *Thetis* was to enter the Bruges canal and steam up to the locks where her crew would scuttle her. In reality, *Thetis* came under heavy fire immediately, including hits below the waterline, and veered to port into a steel net barrage guarding the canal mouth. With her screws entangled and engines stopped, she scuttled herself there, well short of her goal. The remaining two block ships were successful; they entered the canal, turned sideways and sank themselves, successfully blocking the canal.

Seeing the block ships in the harbor, the British captain ordered *Daffodil* to sound the recall order on her whistle. It was 2:00 a.m. Motor launches took off the crews of the block ships. As the raid was winding down, a British destroyer, *North Star*, entered the harbor to give help. The mole battery sank her, but not before she sank the harbor dredger — an event not without later consequence. With their raiders on board, the British ships made their escape. German batteries tore into the ships, reducing *Iris* to a flaming wreck and seriously damaging *Vindictive* and *Daffodil*. Nevertheless, they escaped, and *Vindictive* would fight again. The British suffered 170 killed, 400 wounded and 45 missing out of the 800 raiders. German losses were 8 dead and 16 wounded.

The Ostend raid was unsuccessful. The block ships were the old cruisers *Sirus* and *Brilliant*. Because the Germans had moved a light buoy that marked the channel, the block ships ran aground one mile east of the Ostend-Bruges canal entrance. Motor launches rescued their crews. On May 10, in the early morning, the British made a second attempt to block the canal. A refurbished and concrete-filled *Vindictive* served as the block ship. The ship reached Ostend harbor but initially failed to locate the canal's mouth. She sailed along the coast searching as German batteries riddled her. Finally trying for the canal, the crippled ship ran aground east of the entrance to the shipping channel. This second, and last, attempt to block the canal failed.[13] The bow of *Vindictive* is now a war memorial in Ostend.

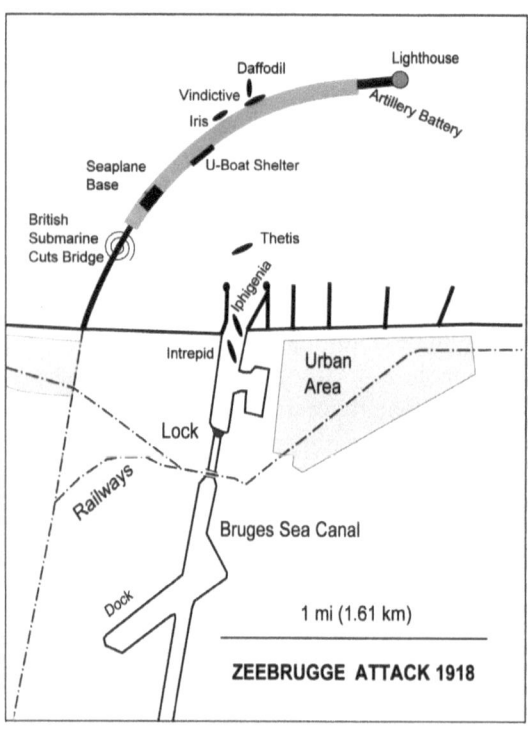

ZEEBRUGGE ATTACK 1918

Regardless of the results of this attempt to block the canal, American newspapers presented the final voyage of

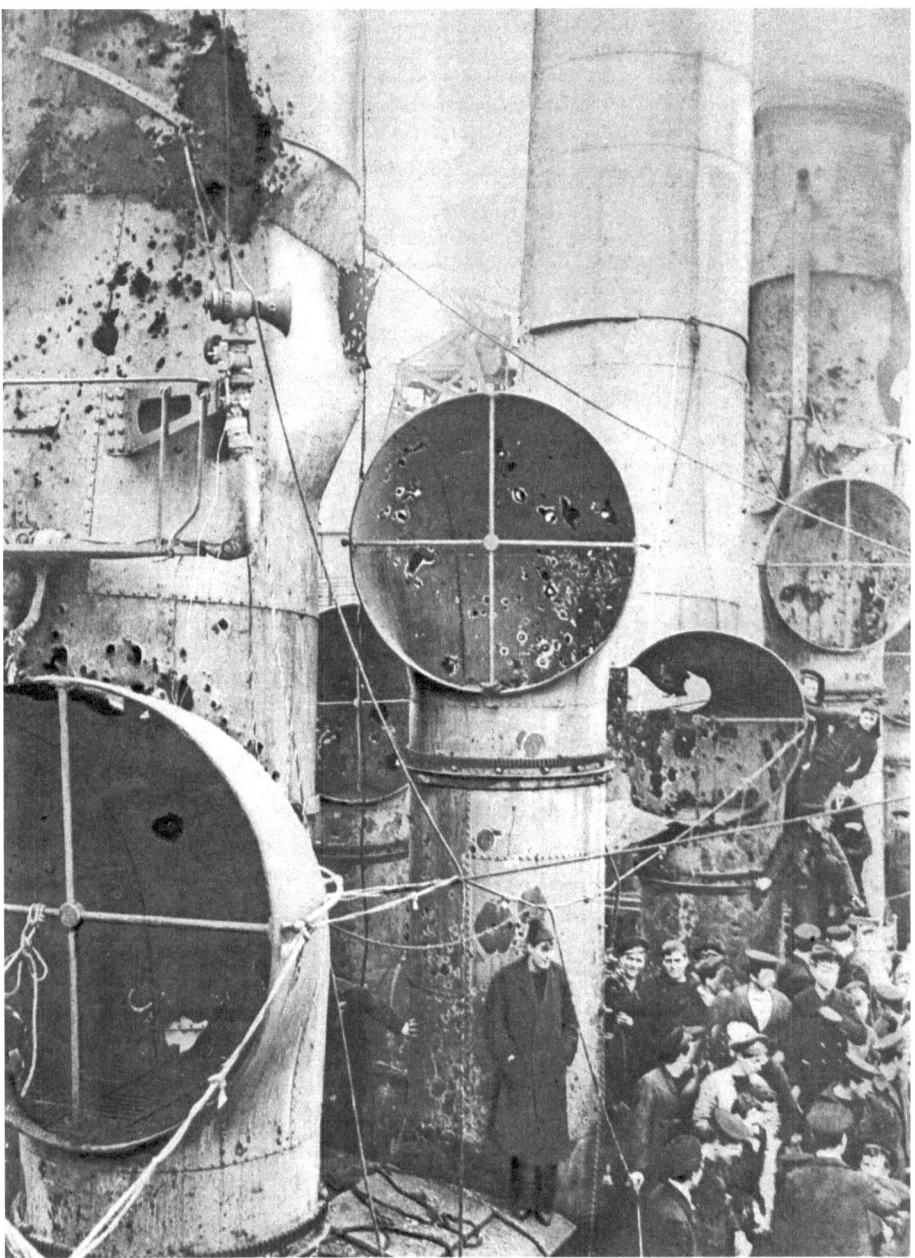

The British cruiser *Vindictive* in England after the Zeebrugge raid. Although raked by German gun fire and suffering a huge number of casualties, the ship made it home. The photograph shows what appears to be visitors touring the ship (*Le Miroir*, 1918).

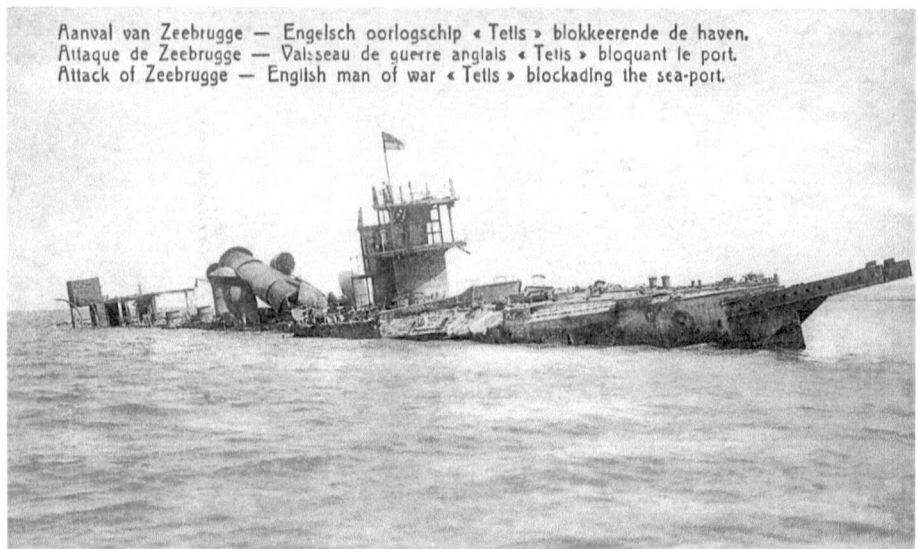

Aanval van Zeebrugge — Engelsch oorlogschip « Tetis » blokkeerende de haven.
Attaque de Zeebrugge — Vaisseau de guerre anglais « Tetis » bloquant le port.
Attack of Zeebrugge — English man of war « Tetis » blockading the sea-port.

The wreck of the British block ship *Thetis*. The mission of *Thetis* was to enter the Zeebrugge-Bruges canal and scuttle itself against the lock. The ship never even reached the mouth of the canal; she entered the harbor and sank from German gun fire after her screws became entangled in a net barrage (Klekowski collection).

Vindictive as a success. On May 11, the *Boston Daily Globe* headlined: British Block Ostend U-Boat Channel by Sinking Vindictive

The article conceded the ship seriously obstructed only the entrance to Ostend harbor, which evidently it did not. With the raids touted as such brilliant successes, the question arose as to why the British waited until April 1918 to launch them. A feeble answer was that the British wanted the port facilities intact, believing that they would soon take Ostend and Zeebrugge.[14] More probably, British leaders thought that such raids would be ineffective and a waste of lives.

So the question remained: Did the raids impede the operation of the Flanders submarine bases? Obviously, the Ostend raids had no military consequence. At the time, much was made of the Zeebrugge raid. However, the high tide following the raid saw the passage of torpedo boats around the block ships at Zeebrugge. The following day a small UB class U-boat navigated around the block ships. Nevertheless, the larger U-boats and destroyers were bottled up in Bruges. Attempts to dredge a channel around the block ships depended upon the availability of a dredger; unfortunately for the Germans, of the two Zeebrugge dredgers, the destroyer *North Star* sank one and the block ship *Intrepid* rammed and damaged the other. Once a functional dredger was

12. Final Acts

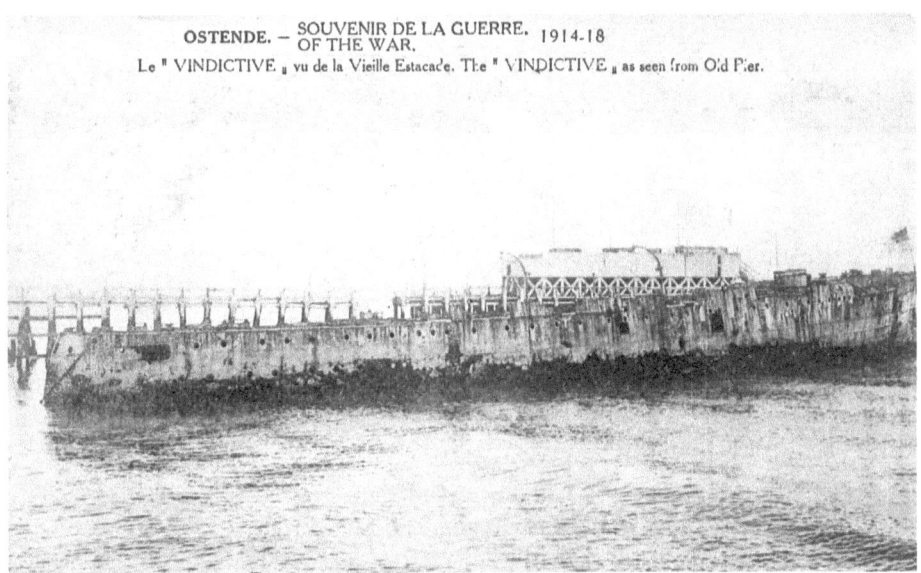

The wreck of *Vindictive* run aground in Ostend harbor (Klekowski collection).

finally at hand, a channel around the block ships was dredged. On May 4, the first ocean going UC-II class submarine passed through the canal. On May 14, four destroyers passed through the canal. Three weeks after the raid, it was business as usual. "The long-term effects of the raid on the course of the naval war, therefore, were minimal."[15]

In early March 1918, the German High Command moved its headquarters to the Belgian resort city of Spa. The city offered three advantages: it was closer to the German border if escape became necessary; neutral Holland was also relatively close if sanctuary became necessary; and the Kaiser and his generals could take the cure in Spa waters if stress relief became necessary. All of these hypothetical situations materialized during the course of 1918.

The Kaiser first occupied the Château La Farineuse, now a sports center; later he moved to the more spacious Château du Neubois, today a Foyer de Charité, a place for religious retreat. In rooms that once echoed with the Kaiser's orders, now silence and religious contemplation prevail. In the cellar of Neubois is a concrete *abri* or bomb shelter, the Kaiser's refuge from the attentions of Allied airmen. While in Spa, when not pretending to be in command of the German war machine, the Kaiser pursued his favorite pastime, cutting firewood. "The Emperor was harmlessly busy in the solitudes of the woods of Géronstère, where his person was guarded by a good number of policemen."[16]

Field-Marshall von Hindenburg and General Ludendorff were actually in charge of all things pertaining to the war; the Kaiser was only a figurehead.

Hindenburg lived in the Château Sous-Bois; his *abri* was also in a cellar. The workaholic Ludendorff lived less pretentiously in Hill Cottage.

> The new headquarters had in the mean time been established at Spa. We got very good accommodation there. The offices were in the Hôtel Britannique, in which I [Ludendorff] had been billeted before, during our invasion of Belgium in the autumn of 1914.[17]

As more and more American divisions arrived on the Western Front, the normally anxious Ludendorff experienced greater and greater angst. Reports from senior officers at the front did little to alleviate his anxiety. "These Americans are terrible. For every ten you kill there are a hundred in their place, seeming to spring from the ground. Nothing seems to stop them, and we — we are weary of war."[18]

Ludendorff probably availed himself of the Spa cure, or at least he should have. As the Western Front literally imploded that autumn, he suffered a nervous breakdown. The Kaiser accepted Ludendorff's resignation on October 27.

In the summer of 1918, 2 American divisions, approximately 55,000 men, arrived in Belgium — the 27th Division made up of National Guard companies from the state of New York and the 30th Division formed of National Guard companies from the states of North Carolina, South Carolina and Tennessee. The divisions served under the British, holding parts of the line south of Ypres established at the end of Operation Georgette in April 1918. The Lys River divided the salient the Germans had pushed into the Allied line during Operation Georgette. The British assigned much of the area north of the Lys and south of Ypres to the American arrivals. They got there just as the German Army was beginning to leave.

> For the sake of economizing men we simultaneously evacuated the salient north of the Lys which bulged out beyond Mount Kemmel and Merville. All these were disagreeable decisions which had been carried out by the end of the first week of September. These movements did not ease the situation, as we had hoped.[19]

The U.S. 27th Division entered the trenches July 25, the U.S. 30th Division on August 16. Both relieved British divisions. It soon became apparent the German lines opposite the Americans were hollow shells compared to earlier periods in the war; the German Army was withdrawing. Often American patrols sent out at night to capture prisoners found German positions undermanned or even unmanned. On August 30, artillery observers from the 30th Division reported dense clouds behind the German lines.

> This smoke, at first thought to be from a gas attack by our own troops, was later confirmed as coming from burning enemy dumps. On the night of August 30th–31st, a prisoner captured near Kemmel Hill reported the enemy to be

retiring to the WYTSCHETE-MESSINES RIDGE. He said that Kemmel Hill was held very lightly, having only one machine gun per company front in place.[20]

The 27th Division also witnessed the enemy vacating its lines.

Information of an enemy withdrawal was received on August 31, and on the same day the division advanced its front line about 1 kilometer against weak resistance. The attack was renewed and the line advanced on the right during the morning of September 1. Another attack was made in the afternoon, but some of the ground gained was lost as the result of a local German counterattack.[21]

Nevertheless, even as it fell back the German Army was still a dangerous foe. Before the 27th Division left Belgium in early September (September 7), it suffered 1,336 casualties, including 250 killed.[22] The 30th also left Belgium on September 7, after sustaining 777 casualties, including 156 killed.[23] The British sent both divisions south into the Somme Offensive, where alongside the Australians they breached the Hindenburg Line. American casualties at the Somme were ten times greater than those they sustained in Belgium.

In early October, the Western Front in Belgium began to collapse. The German Army withdrew east, attempting to save what it could. On the morning of October 14, King Albert attacked on the entire front in Belgium. From Dixmude to the Lys River, Belgian, French and British armies crossed the defenses of the Ypres Salient and literally flowed as an unstoppable tsunami wave into the previously occupied territories beyond. The wave flowed around the Yser inundation and spread to the coast. The goal of four years of bloodshed, a breakout to open ground beyond the trenches, had finally happened. "In spite of the difficulties of the Flanders autumn, the Allies moved fast, for they were beyond the area which had been tortured by four years of incessant war."[24]

By October 16, the Allied armies had penetrated about 15 miles (24.2 km) inland, nearly reaching Ostend on the coast. The German Army evacuated the French city of Lille on October 17. That same day the Royal Navy staged a raid on Ostend but found the place empty; the enemy had fled.

A German officer riding a train from Charleville to Brussels on October 16 noted that the train overflowed with soldiers, despite the fact that Headquarters had stopped all furloughs. Soldiers were leaving by the droves regardless of orders. No one wanted to be the last martyr for the Fatherland. The train stopped at the Namur station. The waiting hall was a sea of field-gray uniforms, soldiers sleeping side by side on the floor, all waiting for a train bound for Germany. The officer commented in his diary, "Where do those gray crowds come from, since leaves are forbidden?... One would believe that the great evacuation of the territory occupied by us had already started."[25] What the German High Command in Spa had not yet realized, the men in the field already knew — Belgium was lost; it was time to get out.

King Albert and his army entered Bruges on October 19. Across the central square flew the Stars and Stripes. The American artist S. Arlent Edwards, who with his wife had lived in Bruges throughout the German occupation, hung out the flag as the Belgian Army entered the city. "I was awakened at 6:30 o'clock Saturday morning by tremendous cheering, and, looking out of the window, saw a Belgian private surrounded by an excited crowd. I dashed across in a dressing gown and had the flag up five minutes later."[26]

October 20 saw the entire Flanders coast liberated; the Allies reached the Dutch frontier in the north and were approximately 10 miles (16.1 km) west of Ghent. By the Armistice, November 11, the Allied line had advanced about another 10 miles (16.1 km) to include Ghent.[27]

Behind the lines in still-occupied Belgium, the German Army began to disintegrate as a military organization. The American novelist Julia Helen Twells[28] resided in Brussels throughout the war. Even though in her seventies, she pedaled around the city on her bicycle, which sported a small American flag. When rubber became unavailable, she used tires made of rope. Ms. Twells witnessed the haughty entrance of the German Army into Brussels on August 20, 1914, and now she watched its retreat.

> Often small detachments passed through, not in line, but trudging along as best they could under heavy burdens — probably the sorry remnants of once-proud regiments. These had no commander and evidently no interest save the one fixed purpose to get back to their homes. They carried their belongings either on their backs, or in heavy carts which they dragged along, four or five together straining at the ropes. These cumbrous country carts, probably bought or stolen from peasants, were piled high with bulging knapsacks, boxes, French and English helmets, and other trophies of the battlefield. And, in strange contrast to these, were bits of furniture, coops containing live hens, and often a cow or two tethered behind.[29]

In the Belgian city of Charleroi that October, one saw the same strange wagon convoys of goods being hauled to Germany. The Belgian mayor of the city described the wagon train to an American journalist; it was like a scene from an apocalyptic-themed motion picture.

> They had been in flight for the last three weeks without order, loading their wagons with loot, often of the most useless character, such as dog kennels, birdcages, and chairs or tables with a leg missing, collected anywhere or anyhow.[30]

In Brussels, in spite of the rush to get out with what one could, there seemed to be a surprising lack of bitterness between the soldiers and Belgian onlookers. Julia Twells noted an almost congenial attitude between them, as if the soldiers were happy to have escaped taking up permanent residence in Belgium — in a shallow grave.

> While standing, one day, at the Porte de Namur watching a battered regiment pass by on its slow, foot-weary way to Liège and Germany, I was amazed to hear what an amount of good-natured taunting they received from the crowd, not only without resentment, but often with responsive levity. One man near me cried out in Flemish: "They are bound to get to Paris, but have decided the shorter and best route is by way of Berlin!"
> "*Ja, ja!*" returned laughingly a haggard-faced youth seated on a cannon-wagon, "*Sie haben recht!* The road to Berlin is the best of all roads!"[31]

A common joke among German soldiers at the time poked fun at Marshal von Hindenburg, the hero of the Eastern Front: "Hindenburg is like the sun, he rose in the east and is going to sink in the west."[32]

To Ms. Twells, the soldiers seemed more a pack of travel-worn peddlers than an army. Nevertheless, it was an army, one seething with the virus of social revolution. The communist contagion from Russia had spread to the rank and file soldiers. The Prussian officer class was now the enemy rather than the Belgians. The red flag of revolt appeared in the streets as throngs of enlisted men confronted officers, stripping them of their symbols of rank.

> The more aristocratic officers, despisers of the red flag, fled as best they could. Occasionally a high-power automobile tore through the city, bearing three or four of these outraged gods toward the German frontier. But soldiers, with leveled rifles, checked their course, two of whom mounted the car, and, dragging the shining epaulettes from their superiors' shoulders, threw them to the crowd.[33]

A body of officers and some loyal followers took possession of the Gare du Nord, hoping to deny the railway to the revolutionaries. A party of revolutionaries along with hundreds of Belgian citizens converged on the Place Rogier in front of the station and next to the Palace Hotel. Added to the crowd was a mass of troops recently returned from the front, with cannon, machine guns, field kitchens and armored cars. Suddenly shots rang out; machine gun fire from the station sprayed the Place Rogier. Chaos followed as everyone broke for cover.

> Rushing blindly from a menace so little expected, the people crowded into shops or fled up side-streets for protection. Meanwhile the roar continued until the officers, surprised by troops (who, I believe, entered the building unperceived from the rear), were obliged to capitulate, and the irrational conflict was brought to an end.[34]

Episodic local skirmishes between revolutionaries and officers occurred in various parts of the city during all of October as troops passed through on their way home.

Later on, the troops strode through in regimental order under command of revolutionary leaders, but bearing, even then, little resemblance to the brilliant legions that had marched so haughtily through Brussels on the 20th of August 1914.[35]

While the pot simmered in Brussels, it boiled at G.H.Q. in Spa, coming to a roaring boil during the first ten days of November. Pressured to abdicate as a prerequisite for peace negotiations, Kaiser Wilhelm prevaricated. In Berlin, Prince Max of Baden, the Imperial Chancellor, decided for the Supreme War Lord. On November 9, Prince Max announced to the Berlin press that the Kaiser had abdicated. Kaiser Wilhelm, not the most stable of leaders, now had to decide between numerous distasteful choices: whether to surrender himself to the Allies, to die at the front with his soldiers, to return to Berlin and lead still loyal troops to quell revolution, or just to run. Never a physically brave man, he chose the last option. He ran. In his post-war memoir he rationalized the decision.

> I went through a fearful internal struggle. On the one hand, I, as a soldier, was outraged at the idea of abandoning my still faithful, brave troops. On the other hand, there was the declaration of our foes that they were unwilling to conclude with me any peace endurable to Germany, as well as the statement of my own Government that only by my departure for foreign parts was civil war to be prevented.
>
> In this struggle I set aside all that was personal. I consciously sacrificed myself and my throne in the belief that, by so doing, I was best serving the interests of my beloved fatherland.[36]

At Château La Farineuse in Spa on November 9, he made preparations for his "departure to foreign parts," the "foreign parts" being in nearby neutral Holland. A train loaded with Hohenzollern treasures waited at the Spa station to take the Kaiser and selected officers to sanctuary. Warned by Marshall von Hindenburg that revolutionaries might intercept the train, the Kaiser left Spa that night for the Dutch frontier. He and his party traveled by fast automobiles. He was truly a man on the run. He arrived at Esyden railroad station on the Dutch-Belgian frontier at 8:00 in the morning. Seeing a Dutch soldier loitering nearby, the Kaiser walked up to the surprised fellow, announced that he was the German emperor, gave him his imperial sword and asked for asylum. The astonished soldier probably looked at the old man as some kind of a screwball. The soldier pondered whether to admit into Holland a man many considered to be the most notorious war criminal in Europe — after all the German had no passport! As the Kaiser nervously puffed cigarettes on the station platform, his treasure train rolled in. Eventually the Queen of the Netherlands intervened and granted asylum. The Kaiser boarded his train and rolled into Holland. He would never leave.

Even after the signing of the Armistice on November 11, the German Army still occupied Brussels. It was only on November 18 that the last German troops left the city. During that final week, no longer constrained by any authority, some German soldiers thieved and looted, even robbing banks, anything to get cash. Some individuals, desperate for money, sold their rifles and boots. On the outskirts of Brussels soldiers held open-air bazaars with their looted goods. Julia Twells described the shopping.

> At Forest and other suburban parts of the city, great car-loads of material, looted from shops and private houses probably months or years ago,—for the dry-goods shops of Brussels had been cleaned out quite two years before,—were offered at absurdly trivial prices. Silk-velvet, which could not be had in Brussels for less than two hundred francs, went at a mark a yard; warm woolen stuffs, which the shivering population, thinly clad in dyed cotton, could not obtain at any price in the shops, were sold — to such as deigned to buy — for an equally small sum ... all manner of other things, as if from some pirates' cave, were bartered back to those who had been robbed of them.[37]

The formal liberation of the recently occupied territory began November 19. In October 1914, the Belgian Army had escaped from Brussels to Antwerp and then west for the final stand on the Yser. The liberation of these cities came in the reverse order.

> The King and Queen of the Belgians arrived at Antwerp, and that afternoon attended a *Te Deum* in the Cathedral. The last Belgian troops had left it on the night of October 9, 1914, when smoke and flames made a pall like some city of the Inferno. They returned to streets bright with flags and crowded with cheering citizens whose long torment was over.[38]

On November 20, Brand and Nell Whitlock left Le Havre, France, where they had resided since leaving Brussels in the spring of 1917. Now, traveling in two automobiles followed by two great trucks piled high with their luggage, the Whitlocks were returning home to Brussels. The following day the party crossed into Belgium through the desolate remains of the front, navigating on an improvised road through mud flats of the now receding Yser inundation. The party stopped at Bruges, then pushed on to Ghent, arriving in Brussels after dark. As they approached the outskirts, they joined a procession of military vehicles entering the city. Crowds filled the city's thoroughfares and lights illuminated the boulevards. The city had a pre-war atmosphere — normalcy had returned quickly, to Minister Whitlock's astonishment. The party finally entered rue Belliard and reached the Legation. At the door, the old servants of 1917 greeted the Americans. The house was warm, filled with flowers and with heaps of cards and notes of welcome.[39]

The Whitlocks had raced across Belgium for one goal, to be present for

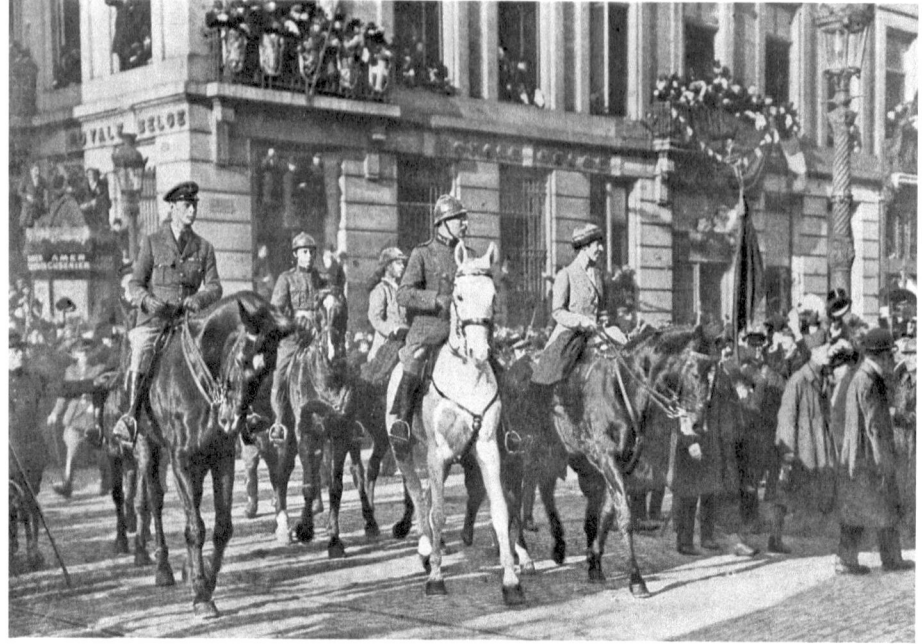

The royal entry into Brussels on November 22, 1918. King Albert rides a white horse. At his side is Queen Elizabeth and far to the left in a British uniform is Prince Albert, the future George VI of England. King Albert died in 1934 in a mountaineering accident. He fell while climbing a cliff along the Meuse River north of Namur (*Album de la Guerre*, 1922).

the royal entry into Brussels on November 22. At ten o'clock that morning, they took their seats in the gallery reserved for the diplomatic corps.

November 22, 1918, was a glorious day, the sky blue and cloudless, the air crisp and transparent with a flutter of a breeze. Brussels prepared to welcome King Albert and Queen Elizabeth. From the windows and balconies of Brussels "floated the colours of the Allies: Belgian, English, Italian, Russian, Japanese, and the stars and stripes."[40] Twells noted that although most of the flags were homemade, some were of German manufacture.

> A German merchant of Bonn, with the opportunist cleverness of his race, had prepared a vast number of Allied flags, in time to meet, more or less, the eager demand all through Belgium. But (a fact which suggests the enterprising Teuton must have formed his scheme before America came in) there was a great dearth of American flags.[41]

Hundreds of thousands packed the city to welcome their heroic King and Queen. All work ceased. Trains and trams stopped service. As horses or private vehicles had long ago vanished, pedestrians packed the roads leading into the city. Some walked nearly the entire night to secure a vantage point to see the royal entry. People jammed the sidewalks, which became impassable; they packed close on church steps, climbed trees, hung out of windows and perched on roofs. They seemed dazed and overwhelmed, as if after four years of German occupation they had forgotten the meaning of joy. Julia Twells was in the crowd, presumably waving her American flag.

> However, when King Albert appeared, riding, and beside him his young wife — who looked rather worn after her hospital labours — tremendous acclamations arose from the massed crowds. These were repeated for Mayor Max, just returned from imprisonment, and for General Leman, the hero of Liège. Then, after a brief pause, the acclamations rose again to salute the American troops, — which were honoured with first place behind the royal cortège, — the British, French, and Belgians.[42]

Whitlock noted that leading the parade after the royals was an American Army band playing Sousa's *Washington Post*. Then followed a regiment of American infantry; Whitlock learned that they were troops from Ohio, some from his own city of Toledo; it was all unbelievable for the ex-mayor of that city.

That night Brussels erupted into delirium. Drunken masses filled the streets, joyfully singing and dancing. The streets lights were on for the first time in four years. Cafés opened their hidden stocks of champagne; glasses sparkled with bubbles; drunken revelers gave endless toasts to the King, the Queen, the Allies, to everyone. English, French and other just released Allied prisoners of war somehow stumbled into the party; street dancers formed rings hand in hand around them; the former prisoners of war, skinny and with hollow eyes, stood or sat, contentedly drunk. On the main boulevards Belgians sang, danced and shouted themselves hoarse. The party lasted all night. For Belgium and the Belgians, the war was finally over.

Chapter 13

After the War

> If the sons and daughters of our race ever forget that sacrifice or remember it otherwise than with gratitude and respect, the world which Belgium saved will be unworthy of its deliverance.[1]— Senator Albert B. Cummins, U.S. senator from Iowa, 1919

Probably one of the most farcical post-war actions was an attempt by a small group of rogue American soldiers to kidnap Kaiser Wilhelm II from his sanctuary in Holland. Using a U.S. Army Cadillac limousine, which they had commandeered, they planned to take the ex–War Lord to Paris. Their intention was to make a gift of the Kaiser to President Woodrow Wilson, who was attending the Paris peace conference. If the Kaiser's Cadillac were stopped en route, the kidnappers vowed, "He would never have been taken from it alive."[2]

The story begins in Holland, Kaiser Wilhelm's place of asylum. The Kaiser escaped Spa, Belgium, on November 9 and traveled at night by automobile, arriving at the Belgian-Dutch frontier village of Eysden at 8:00 a.m. on November 10, 1918. Denied entry by a puzzled Dutch border guard, the Kaiser waited anxiously for permission to enter Holland, permission that finally came on November 11. In the meantime, Germany signed the Armistice; a momentous event in which the Kaiser seemed surprisingly uninterested. His focus was only on escape. After some pressure from the Dutch Foreign Office, Count Godard Bentinck agreed to house the Kaiser and his retinue at his castle in Amerongen, but for only three days. The visit lasted until May 1920.

Immediately after the Armistice, there were calls to bring the Kaiser to justice, justice meaning a hangman's noose. However, Holland, his place of asylum, honored its commitment for his protection. At the end of 1918, some Americans decided to take the law into their own hands and kidnap the Kaiser. The kidnappers were from Tennessee, members of the U.S. 30th Division, a National Guard division from Tennessee and North Carolina (See Chapter 12). There were eight, led by Colonel Luke Lea of Nashville, a former U.S. Senator, newspaper publisher and, much later, a convict in a North Carolina prison. In December 1918 and January 1919, the would-be kidnappers made two attempts to capture the Kaiser, both originating from Luxembourg, the postwar base of their regiments as part of the Allied Army of Occupation. The first trip to capture the Kaiser took place from December 24 to 28. On Christmas Eve, they traveled from Luxembourg in a seven-passenger Winton, the regimental car. Considered the Achilles heel of the regiment, the Winton was forever breaking down. "It always needed repairs but never twice in the same place until a complete cycle of repairs had been passed."[3] Once, in the Meuse-Argonne, it suffered sixteen punctures in one night. Adding to their woes, the jinxed auto had a voracious appetite for gasoline, which then cost $5.00 per gallon. They made it to Liège, where they spent the night. The next day, Christmas, they motored toward the Dutch frontier, stopping at an inn just inside Germany. They tried crossing into Holland the following day but found that without the proper passports it was impossible to gain entry. Having failed in their first kidnap attempt, they turned the Winton for their base in Luxembourg. Somehow, perhaps a good omen, the auto made it back to base without problems.

Not deterred by failure, the Tennesseans made another attempt on December 31. Running true to old form, 30 km (18.6 miles) into their journey the Winton broke down. Flagging a passing American truck for a ride, one of the kidnappers returned to division headquarters for another auto. He returned with an eight-cylinder Cadillac limousine, described as a splendid vehicle, especially in comparison to the Winton. By then the Winton was again running and both autos continued the mission. The Winton had a fifty-gallon drum of gasoline strapped to it to feed its hungry carburetor. Again, they stopped at Liège, to fill the cars' fuel tanks and enquire about passports to enter Holland. Told that such passes would require at least six weeks, Colonel Lea remembered an old acquaintance from his Senate days, Minister Brand Whitlock. Perhaps he could cut the red tape. Lea had supported Whitlock during the Minister's confirmation in the Senate when some opposed him. Off the would-be kidnappers went to Brussels. Fudging the truth, Colonel Lea told Whitlock that he and his men intended to visit Holland as civilian tourists. Reluctantly, Whitlock issued their passports and arranged for them to have special passes from the Legation of Holland. The Americans had dinner at the American Legation and returned to their kidnapping mission the following day. Later, when the kidnapping attempt became a small scandal, Whitlock wondered what passports had he viséd?

They traveled to Liège through a snowstorm, with the Cadillac pushing the Winton up slippery grades. They arrived after dark, spent the night in the city and then crossed into Holland without problem. Over the border they breakfasted; their resident linguist determined the meal was cheap, so they each ordered double breakfasts washed down with whiskey highballs—a Tennessee breakfast. Unfortunately, the bill was in gold guilders rather than Belgian francs (1 guilder equaled 2.1 francs) and nearly bankrupted the enterprise. Realizing they could not afford any more mistakes, they hired a Dutch boy, about 15 years old, as an interpreter. He sat in front with the driver of the Cadillac and asked directions from the locals, roughly translated as, "Where is the residence of the damn crazy German Kaiser?" The party reached Amerongen at 8:00 p.m. on January 5, 1919, and soon found the castle of Count Bentinck. Surrounded by a double moat, the castle seemed the perfect place to protect the most wanted man in Europe. In winter, when the moat froze, the ice was broken up every night as part of the castle's security.

> A strong military guard had been posted at Amerongen before the fugitive's arrival, and from that time no one was allowed to pass unless furnished with a special "permit."
> At the outer entrance, where the walls meet the gates, there is a large brick-floored orangery, and this was used as a guard-room. Here an authorized visitor was given a white card with his or her name written in full on it (no card being given unless the name had been "passed" by Count Godard). Passing up the avenue and over the outer moat, the visitor yielded the white card at the inner gate to the officer in charge of the second detachment of soldiers, and received a blue one in exchange. This was the last formality before entering the Castle. On returning, the visitor gave up the blue card, and was then free to leave the grounds.[4]

Leaving four men to watch the cars, Colonel Lea and three other officers somehow managed to circumvent the compound's security and bluff their way into the castle. A butler showed them to the library where Count Bentinck asked in precise English what was the purpose of their visit. Colonel Lea prevaricated, attempting to think of something to say. "Count von Bentinck then again asked what the purpose of the visit was. 'I can reveal the object of our visit only to the Kaiser,' replied Colonel Lea."[5]

And so the conversational sparring went, until a new player entered the library, the Amerongen burgomaster (mayor). The Americans attempted to communicate with him in high school German; he, a Harvard graduate, answered in Boston English. The verbal sparring continued, the Americans asking to see the Kaiser but not saying why. Finally, at eleven o'clock that night the count and burgomaster ushered them out. In the courtyard, a surprise awaited them. Illuminated by two search lights mounted on the castle walls, 150 Dutch troops surrounded the autos. With their tails between their legs, the Americans slowly drove through the cordon of soldiers. Their only achievement was an ashtray from the library with the Kaiser's monogram, which one of the men had pilfered.

European and American newspapers loved the story, which they wildly embellished.[6] In Brussels Brand Whitlock heard that American officers in an armored car tried to kidnap the Kaiser. Surprisingly, the American Army only mildly censured Colonel Lea, describing the kidnap attempt as "amazingly indiscreet."[7] Colonel Lea's luck sailing close to the legal wind ran out in 1931. Convicted of defrauding a North Carolina bank of over a million dollars, a court sentenced him to a term of six to ten years in prison.[8] On the other side of the Atlantic the man Lea had attempted to kidnap, the man responsible for the invasion of neutral Belgium, for being instrumental in starting a war that killed millions, that man remained free, indulging his favorite hobby with axe and saw.

> The rest of the morning would be spent in cutting and sawing wood. We have often heard that this was his favorite pastime at Amerongen, but I did not realize with what zest he applied himself to it or the great amount of work he got through till I saw his handiwork myself. In the whole of his stay he cut down several thousands of trees....
>
> Here, in his serge suit, collarless, with his shirt slightly open at the neck, would the fallen monarch spend most of his time when not in the house — sawing, sawing, sawing![9]

It was how he kept physically fit, and no doubt was a release from stress. In May 1920, the Kaiser moved from Amerongen Castle to Huis Doorn, a Dutch manor house he purchased in the village of Doorn. A determining factor at the time of the purchase of the estate was its large woodland. He soon got to work cutting it down. The Kaiser lived at Huis Doorn until his death in 1941 at age 82. A mausoleum on the grounds contains his remains; the woodland he cut down has grown back.

While the Kaiser busied himself chopping wood, in Belgium there was a building boom repairing the damage caused by his army. The most famous reconstruction occurred in Louvain. The Louvain University Library, today the Leuven University Library, burned during the night of August 25–26, 1914, with the loss of approximately 300,000 books (See Chapter 2). The following month in Holland and France, initiatives began for the collection of books and money for a new library. Eventually, 25 Allied and neutral countries formed committees to aid in the library's reconstruction. At the war's end, the Treaty of Versailles (1919) included a provision that German libraries donate books to help replace those burned in 1914.

The American aid effort had its headquarters in the Pierpont Morgan Library in New York. The National Committee of the United States for the Restoration of the University of Louvain (a.k.a. the American Committee) focused its efforts on raising funds for the construction of a new library building to house the collections of donated books. The American Committee included a galaxy of the prominent, including ex-presidents William Taft and Theodore Roosevelt, the Chief Justice of the Supreme Court, the presidents of Harvard, Yale, Columbia and the University of Pennsylvania, important religious figures, as well as sundry politicians. The American Committee launched its first public appeal for funds on November 11, 1918. The appeal targeted school children and their teachers, students and faculty of colleges, universities, academies and preparatory schools, police departments, fire houses, professional associations, civic associations and women's clubs. Donations ranged from pennies to thousands of dollars. Funding appeals continued throughout the early nineteen twenties.

Since the American Committee was paying for the building, its opinion counted in selecting the building's location. The site it selected, a block of burned-out houses along a large open public space, was the most prominent in the city.

> The location of the new library upon the *Place du Peuple* [now Mgr. Ladeuzeplein (Mgr. Ladeuze Square)] could not have been equalled anywhere else. The site was intended for the *Palais de Justice*, which is now nearing completion in one of the backstreets north of the City Hall. The *Place du Peuple* is the highest tract in the town and is at the junction of four streets.[10]

In addition to the site, the American Committee also selected an American architect, the well-known Whitney Warren of New York. Warren was one of the architects who designed New York's Grand Central Station. In partnership with Charles D. Wetmore, the firm Warren and Wetmore was responsible for many significant buildings in Manhattan, including the Biltmore and Ritz-Carlton hotels.

> The inhabitants of Leuven nor the academics were entirely at ease with the choice of an American architect. The University administration was no less traditionally minded. In their horrified imaginations they could already see a skyscraper rising up on the Leuven skyline or a colossal temple in the style of the Greek Revival in which American libraries have been built until the 1930s.[11]

The citizens of Louvain (now known by its Flemish name, Leuven) need not have worried. Whitney Warren had trained in Paris at the École des Beaux-Arts; he was aware of the importance of designing a building to fit its historical context.[12] His design "harked back in an atavistic reflex to the domestic tradition of the Flemish, Dutch or Netherlandish Renaissance."[13] He designed a new/old library. A beautiful structure that easily fit in with buildings reconstructed in Louvain after the war.

The laying of the corner stone on July 28, 1921, was an occasion of great ceremony and one Brand Whitlock remembered as a hot affair. Brand and Nell Whitlock were among the honored guests, which included King Albert, Queen

Elizabeth, Cardinal Mercier, the Prince of Monaco, the chairman of the American Committee, Nicholas Murray Butler (the money man), and a galaxy of other notables. Brand Whitlock sarcastically described the event in his journal, setting the tone by describing Louvain as a particularly unattractive town. The ceremony took place in a packed stuffy auditorium on a very hot day. With nearly everyone attired in heavy woolen robes denoting ecclesiastical or academic affiliation, and with nearly everyone sweating profusely under their garments regardless of how attired, Whitlock described the *odeur* as appalling and thought he might faint from the heat and stink. The orations seemed endless, everyone seemed to be melting, the King bored and wilting. Afterward, all 400 of the participants adjourned to a banquet hall for the typical Belgian *banquet de province,* an agony consisting of heavy meats and old burgundy — Whitlock thought he would choke; it was too hot to eat such fare; he recalled he spent most of the time eating a crumb of bread. Then finally, worst of all, the speeches began. Numb from the food, heat and very long speeches, Whitlock daydreamed, wondering why American Protestants should build up a Roman Catholic seat of learning. Protestant Whitlock, perhaps stifling a yawn, noted that Cardinal Mercier was a dear, anyway.[14]

As construction progressed, the cost of the building rose faster than the building itself; Whitney Warren's Flemish architectural marvel was going to come in at a million dollars. The American Committee had managed to raise only $500,000. There was only one person to turn to, the man controlling a hoard of cash left over from the Committee for Relief in Belgium, Herbert Hoover. After the war, Hoover had established a Belgium educational foundation with these monies; this foundation contributed $382,500 to the library building fund. The Carnegie Endowment for International Peace contributed $157,000.[15] These two donors made the library a reality and work began again.

The architect and his American underwriters conceived of the library building as a monument to American generosity. To that end, the walls and pillars incorporated more than 300 memorial stones inscribed with the names of benefactors written in gold letters and in over a hundred different styles of calligraphy. Benefactors ranged from world famous American universities such as Harvard and Yale to less well known institutions such as Mississippi State College for Women, Tennessee College and the New York State College for Teachers. In addition to institutions of higher learning, memorial stones acknowledged donations from elementary and high schools as well as academies: Greenfield High School (Massachusetts), Northern High School (Detroit), Public Schools, Hackensack (New Jersey), Miss Hopkins School (New York) and Vermont Academy. The names of other donors also have inscriptions: Women's Clubs, Police Department of the City of New York, American Library

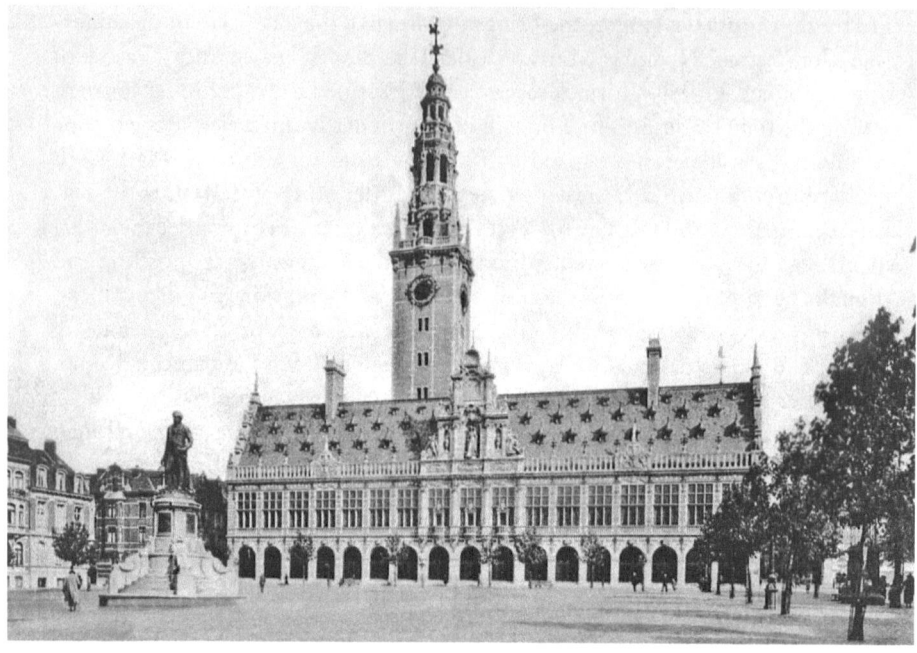

The new Louvain University Library. The New York architect Whitney Warren designed the building; large and small contributions from American donors funded its construction. To acknowledge this generosity, the American flag flies from the tower every July 4 (Klekowski collection).

Association, Porto-Rican School Teachers. Wall inscriptions acknowledge a total of 320 American benefactors.[16]

The library also grew to be a war monument with stone iconography representing all the Allied countries. In many respects, the building resembled a Gothic cathedral, with nearly every nook and cranny inhabited by an inscription or carving symbolizing the Allied war victory rather than an Old or New Testament story. However, being a library for a Catholic university, the religious motif always held center stage. The most dominant element in the front façade of the library was a four and a half meter tall statue of the Virgin Mary; flanking her were statues of Saint George and the dragon and Saint Michael with the devil. The statue of Mary carries the infant Jesus on her left arm and in her right hand, she wields a sword whose point is piercing the head of a Prussian eagle. She wears a Belgian style helmet and a breastplate.

> The breastplate and helmet are covered by the gold beaten from a five-dollar gold luck piece found upon the body of an American soldier killed in the war, returned with his effects to his mother and by her subscribed to the fund gathered to construct the Library.[17]

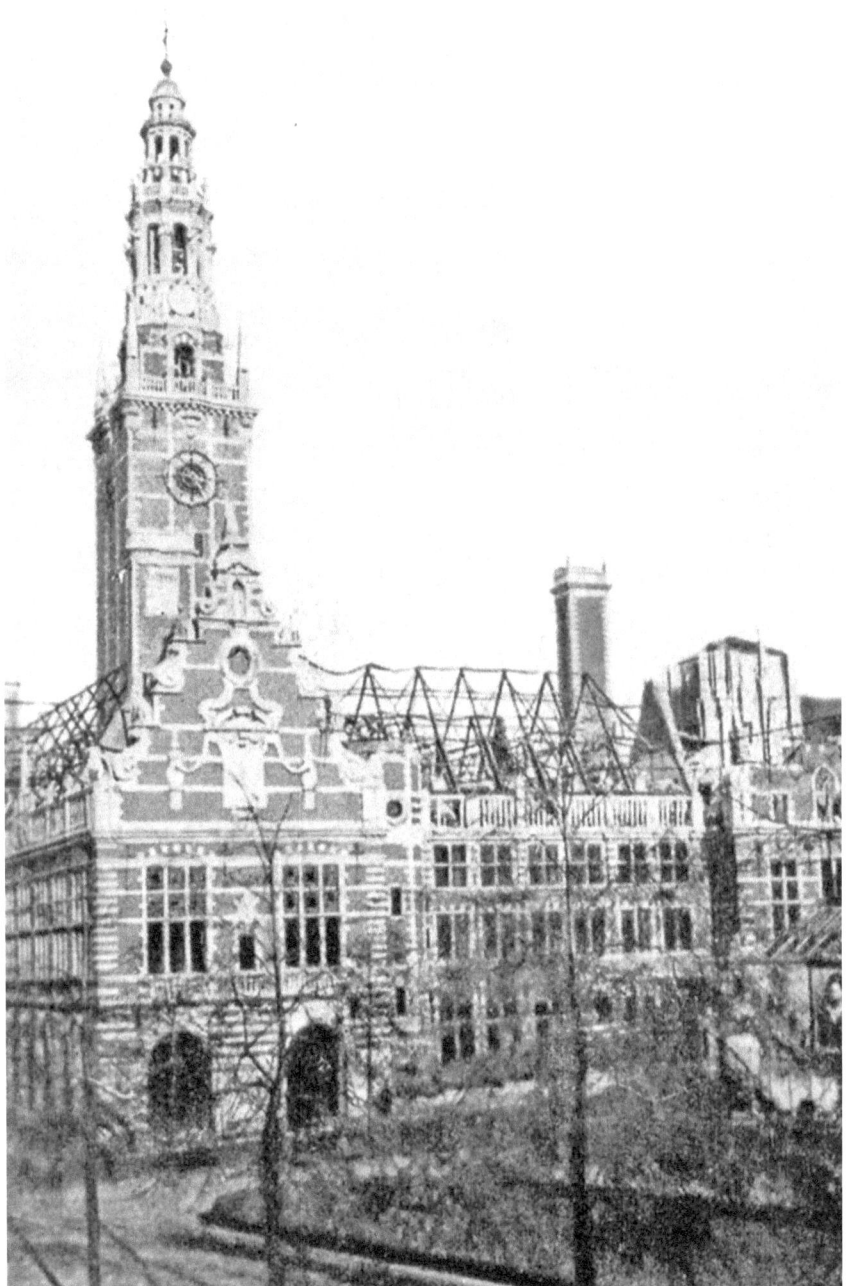

The destroyed library. On the night of May 16–17, 1940, repeating history, the Louvain University Library burned. Inside the fire-gutted building, the steel beams that supported the roof are visible. The library tower escaped damage and, fortunately, the walls with their inscriptions did not come down (*Kingdom of Belgium War Crimes Commission*, 1946).

The Virgin of Louvain is certainly not depicted as the Queen of Peace. Critics thought the statue a better representation of the pagan goddess of war, Pallas Athena or Minerva, rather than the mother of Jesus.[18] The Armed Virgin[19] was only mildly controversial when compared to another aspect of the library's iconography — the infamous anti-German inscription. In 1921, Whitney Warren met with Cardinal Mercier and other clerics to discuss the new library's design.

> The Cardinal had voiced his desire to see upon the monument such an inscription as would constitute for the future *a safeguard against the recurrence of similar destructions* and desired that it be sufficiently in evidence to avoid the possible result of insignificance. Discussion took place how in few words to embody history, teach a lesson, safeguard the future and testify to Belgium's gratitude.[20]

One of the learned clerics devised a Latin six-word inscription that satisfied the spirit of the Cardinal's idea.

Furore Teutonico Diruta: Dono Americano Restituta
"Destroyed by German Fury, Restored by American Generosity"

The anti-German Latin inscription incited a storm of protests both for and against its incorporation into the library façade. "Immortalizing hatred in stone," was a common description.[21] The idea was to incorporate the carved letters of the inscription into the stone balustrade along the roof of the building "that like a giant advertisement banner was to run over the whole length of the front of the building."[22] Since the stone letters were over a meter high, the inscription would dominate the front of the building; there was nothing subtle in Warren's architectural conception for placement of the inscription.

By early 1926, as the feeling of hate engendered by the war evolved into a desire to bring Germany back into the community of European nations, the Louvain inscription seemed counter-productive. Pressure from American donors, especially Herbert Hoover, from the Louvain University administration and even from the Vatican pushed to have the inscription omitted. It seemed a revival of the war spirit of 1914–1918, rather than the hoped for era of European peace. On the other hand, the architect Whitney Warren and the inscription's sculptor, the Belgian/American Pierre de Soete, argued they had the right to insist the library must follow the construction plan, including the balustrade with the offending inscription. Belgians soon divided into those for or against the inscription. It became a political issue, with most newspapers in Brussels attacking the anti-inscription folks. University students, socialists, and anti-Catholics seized the pro-inscription cause; other university students were just as hysterically anti-inscription. In Louvain, public sentiment was split equally on the subject. As the date for the formal dedication of the library on July 4,

1928, approached, the controversy heated up. On June 23, the architect and sculptor arrived at the library site with vans carrying some of the huge inscription stones. The police blocked their installation.[23] The university rector Monsignor Ladeuze had a stone balustrade, without the offending inscription, ready for installation; on June 27, in a pelting rain, a mob attacked the inscriptionless balustrade as it was being erected and destroyed it.[24] Architect Warren, wearing a student cap, rabble-roused his faithful. Things were getting insane!

King Albert and Queen Elizabeth opted out of participating in the July 4 dedication. Herbert Hoover did not attend; he was too busy campaigning for the American presidency. Hugh Gibson, then American Ambassador to Belgium, represented the United States at the dedication. Gibson ended his oration with the following: "This monument will ever remind us both that a friendship which has passed through the crucible of war must be refined and pure. The building should ever symbolize peace."[25]

Although architect Warren and Rector Monsignor Ladeuze asked for a truce during the dedication ceremony, it was not to be.

> An airplane, which during the Ambassador's speech had hovered about the outskirts of the audience and dropped handbills containing the hateful words of an inscription banned from the library balustrade, now grew bolder and threw down masses of the material close to the second speaker while his address was in progress. But the aerial offender created only a temporary diversion.[26]

The hoped for European peace and brotherhood of the nineteen twenties degenerated into the fascism of the nineteen thirties. The Second World War began in 1939 with Germany's invasion of Poland. On May 10, 1940, Germany invaded Belgium. During the night of May 16–17, as British troops withdrew from Louvain and German troops were about to enter, the university library went up in flames.[27] Very likely the German Army targeted the building because of the anti–German inscription controversy of the nineteen twenties. Many German officers believed that the building still carried the inscription.[28] Although nearly one million volumes went up in flames, the fire gutted only the building; it did not bring down its walls. The Great War iconography and symbolism incorporated into the building in Whitney Warren's design survived. Restored after the war, the library is one of the most beautiful buildings in Leuven and should be on the itinerary of American visitors coming to Belgium.

The Whitlock post-war odyssey began soon after America entered the war on April 6, 1917. In mid–April, Brand and Nell Whitlock (and their two dogs) arrived in Le Havre, France, the location of the Belgian government in exile. During the war, the population of this city had doubled and accommodations were scarce. The couple booked two rooms in a rundown hostelry pretentiously named the Grand Hôtel des Regâtes and situated on a rocky beach, which to

Whitlock's nose was foul-smelling with the sewage of all the cities and towns along the Seine from Paris to Havre. The meals the proprietor served were poisonous concoctions that tasted and smelled of chemicals. Minister Whitlock described Le Havre as a filthy hole, probably the filthiest city in Christendom. He thought it probably a good place for a penal colony. Unfortunately, he had to live there as he was a member of the diplomatic corps. The Whitlocks stayed at the most execrable of all hotels until mid-July. After much searching, the couple rented a pleasant house surrounded by a high wall. The place had a large kitchen, a fat chef and a small garden for the dogs.[29] Even after they left the hotel, when he walked the dogs Whitlock complained. He wished that his neighbors would at least occasionally take a bath, and why was there so much garbage in the streets? If the city had possessed a golf club with showers, he probably would have been more positive about the port on the mouth of the Seine.

Days became routine; Nell Whitlock volunteered at the British Y.M.C.A. hut most mornings and spent her afternoons cheering up wounded soldiers in nearby hospitals. Brand Whitlock began his day walking the dogs, usually in the rain, and then spent time at his desk doing diplomatic tasks followed by lunch with visitors, who often included government officials, Belgian politicians, and journalists. In the afternoon and evening, Minister Whitlock worked on his two-volume treatise *Belgium*, the expurgated story of his experiences in Brussels.[30] Writing to his old friend of Ohio politics

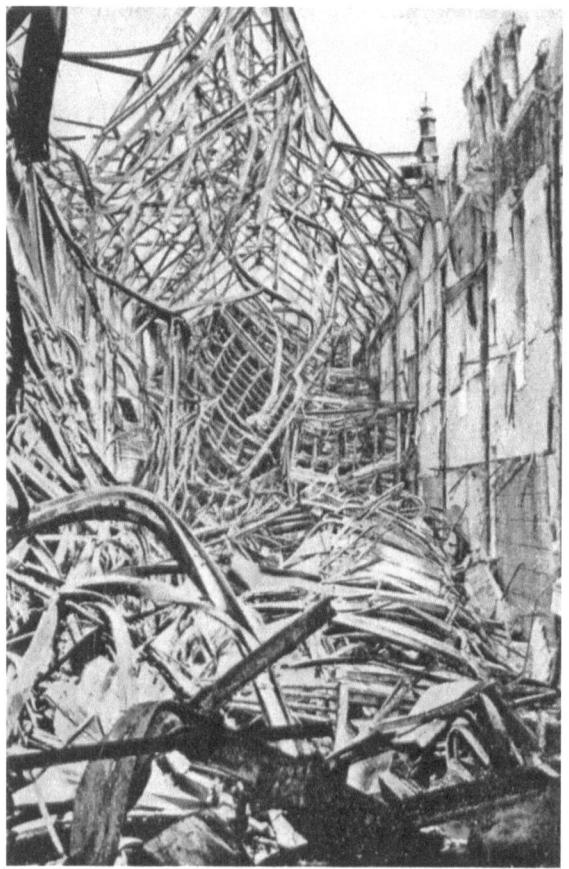

Interior view of the burned library. The heat of the burning books was so intense that the steel beams supporting the roof softened and collapsed (Kingdom of Belgium War Crimes Commission, 1946).

and then U.S. Secretary of War Newton D. Baker, Whitlock assured Baker that *Belgium* would not tell all.

> I think the book will be not without its patriotic value, not without its value to all of our ideals, and I shall try to be as discreet as possible. I promise you to report no private conversations, to violate no confidences and to be untrue to no obligations of hospitality.[31]

One of Whitlock's most welcome visitors was Colonel House, friend and foreign policy advisor to President Woodrow Wilson. From Colonel House he caught up on Allied infighting and gossip. One particularly unpleasant story concerned Hugh Gibson, Herbert Hoover and Whitlock himself.

The story began in November-December 1915, when Whitlock was in the United States on a recuperative break from the stress of dealing with events in occupied Belgium (See Chapter 6). Hugh Gibson, Secretary of the Legation, was chargé during Whitlock's absence. Head strong and brash, Gibson continually ruffled the feathers of German authorities. Upon Whitlock's return to Brussels, Baron von der Lancken (*Politische Abteilung* [Political Department]) and Governor-General von Bissing met with him and requested Gibson's dismissal. They charged Gibson with unpleasant incidents with border guards during his frequent trips to Holland on Legation business, his lack of tact in dealing with officials at meetings, and for joy riding with a Belgian girl "showing off his diplomatic prowess to her by defying German sentries."[32] Eventually, with a very positive letter of recommendation from Whitlock, Gibson left Brussels and joined the embassy in London. There he became a close friend and acolyte of Hoover. Gibson and Hoover conspired to influence the British government to pressure Belgium to ask for Whitlock's recall. Presumably, Hoover wanted someone in Brussels who would literally jump at his commands and Gibson wanted some kind of revenge for an imagined slight. Unfortunately, for the conspirators, the Belgian Government wanted Whitlock where he was, so the plan miscarried. When Whitlock learned of the conspiracy at the end of November 1917, he was deeply hurt. "It is hard to work with snakes and cads like Gibson," he wrote, "after all the kindness I showed, or tried to show him ... and, while I was recommending him for promotion to the Department, he was conspiring against me, or trying to — it is hard to keep down bitterness."[33]

At regular intervals, the American novelist Edith Wharton and her good friend Walter Berry came up from Paris.[34] Both shared Whitlock's political prejudices and Wharton always had much to say about writing. Not all visitors were as charming as Wharton and Berry. Minister Whitlock's duties included entertaining sanctimoniously dull clergy, hack journalists wanting stories of German atrocities, and hick congressmen from the Midwest who demanded and got an audience with King Albert. Even though the King thought them charming and was ever the gracious royal, their dress and "Howdy King" behavior mortified Whitlock. It was all so embarrassing. On November 9, 1918, Whitlock's old friend Clarence Darrow visited for an afternoon. An erudite conversationalist with a "witty and agreeable pessimism," Darrow was someone special. Whitlock wrote in his journal, "On the whole, the happiest two hours I have spent in a year, an oasis in the midst of the wide and arid desert of dullness in which I live."[35] Le Havre was turning Whitlock into a bitter old man of forty-nine. He and Nell finally managed to escape on November 20, returning to Brussels for the royal entry into the city (see Chapter 12).

Things picked up for Whitlock when he was "home" in Brussels. He caught up on the experiences of colleagues who had remained in Brussels after the Americans left. He renewed his friendship with King Albert now that the stresses of the war were behind them. A major event was the visit of President Woodrow Wilson on June 18, 1919. Wilson traveled by train from Dunkerque to Adinkerke, a village about two miles inside Belgium.

Since Adinkerke was not far from La Panne, King Albert and Queen Elizabeth had flown to La Panne from Brussels the day before. Whitlock, traveling less adventurously, went by auto, meeting them in La Panne for dinner. The following morning the King took an early morning swim in the sea before the party left to meet Wilson and his entourage, which included Herbert Hoover. After ceremonies at the Adinkerke station, the party clambered into automobiles for the trip to Brussels, with a few tourist stops along the way. The King, driving his large Renault with Wilson as his passenger, roared off at high speed, leaving the other cars in its dust. The King was passionate about driving fast. One wonders what Wilson thought as King Albert roared across Flanders.

After brief stops at Nieuport and Dixmude to allow the American guests to scramble about the ruins, the motorcade continued its fast pace, with, of course, the King in the lead. The cavalcade soon reached a large tent erected near the road; inside, servants were setting a long table with palace china for a memorable picnic luncheon hosted by the King and Queen. As the guests sat, an army of journalists, photographers, cinema cameramen and secret service agents surrounded the illustrious luncheon guests. Soon a six-legged army descended from the air; clouds of biting black flies attacked everyone, regardless of their rank or status. While the guests had cold chicken, bread, salad, coffee and red wine, the insects feasted as well. Whitlock found the ordeal terrible. President Wilson thought it funny and laughed a great deal; in fact, he was the life of the party.[36] After everyone ate, the caravan proceeded to Ypres and then motored to Ostend and Zeebrugge to catch a train for Brussels. It must have been a very long day.

The following day was just as hurried: a morning touring destroyed factories, luncheon at the Royal Palace in Brussels, coffee and a reception with members of the American colony, off to the Belgian Parliament where Wilson delivered an address, then by fast motorcade, the King in the lead, to Louvain. There, in the ruins of the famous library, the university rector, with great ceremony, conferred an honorary degree, *Doctor honoris causa,* on President Wilson. Then all raced back to Brussels for a reception at the Royal Palace. It was now early evening. The notables soon dispersed into their respective automobiles for rides home to dress for the grand banquet at the Palace at 8:15; that is, all except Brand Whitlock who somehow missed his ride! In great stress, Whitlock ran all the way home (about a half mile), just managing to bathe and dress before being driven back to the palace. When the President finally boarded his train that night for Paris, Whitlock was near collapse.

Later that summer, Whitlock received permission for a leave of absence from Brussels to return to the United States for a couple of months. Brand and Nell Whitlock and their two dogs arrived in New York August 29. Things were afoot in Washington that needed Whitlock's attention. President Wilson had proposed to Congress the raising of the American Legation in Belgium to the rank of an embassy. Whitlock very much wanted to be the first ambassador. It would be best to be in Washington to smooth the appointment. Wilson agreed to nominate Whitlock after the presidential railroad trek to the western states, a speaking tour promoting the League of Nations. Whitlock relaxed and played golf waiting for the President's return. After nearly 10,000 miles and numerous speaking engagements, President Wilson suffered a complete physical and nervous breakdown in Kansas on the return leg of the trip. He returned to Washington on September 28, a broken man.[37] Nevertheless, on October 1, 1919, the President sent to the Senate the nomination of Brand Whitlock to be Ambassador to Belgium; later in the day the Senate confirmed the appointment.[38] Taking the official oath of office in New York on October 2, Minister Whitlock was now Ambassador Whitlock — just in time to rush to the dock to greet the Belgian royal family on its American tour.

King Albert, Queen Elizabeth and their son Prince Leopold arrived in New York mid-day on October 2. Brand and Nell Whitlock were among the notables who welcomed them to America. The Whitlocks were to travel with the Belgian royals on their month-long American tour. After ceremonies greeting the royals in New York, the party traveled to Boston where they visited Harvard University, which conferred the Doctor of Laws on King Albert. Meanwhile, Prince Leopold, then nearly 18, went on a special tour of the campus.

> Except for the fact that Prince Leopold ran away from the exercises in University Hall, and went off with a pretty girl in a motor to have the Harvard Stadium explained to him — the day was purely formal.[39]

After Boston, the train with the royal party headed west to Toledo, Ohio, where Whitlock had been mayor, then on to California. Stops included Los Angeles, San Francisco, Reno, Yosemite and the Grand Canyon. Unfortunately, for the Belgians, they were traveling through a country where Prohibition was the law and ice water the national beverage.

> During the journey the King easily bore this privation from all wine and liqueur.... But such was not the case with the members of his suite.[40]
>
> Can you imagine a banquet, a sumptuous banquet without the smallest drop of wine or liqueur? It was, nevertheless, the gloomy reality. As I write these lines I still see placed in front of the King that solitary glass filled with hopelessly limpid water on which a few small pieces of ice floated sadly about. That endless ice water during this long journey![41]

The American tour ended in Norfolk, Virginia, where on October 31 the royal party boarded the steamship *George Washington* for their return home. Interestingly, although bearing an American name, the ship was originally German, having been part of the Norddeutscher Lloyd fleet for the Germany-America trade. The United States commandeered the ship, which had been caught in New York harbor in August 1914, after entering the war in 1917.[42] Brand and Nell Whitlock sailed with the royals, arriving in Brussels November 13, which the ambassador described as cold, and drab and dull.[43]

Whitlock, with time on his hands, restarted his career as a novelist. Warren G. Harding won the presidency in 1920 and Whitlock's tenure as ambassador was over (he was a Wilson man); he tendered his resignation, serving his last day in office on December 31, 1921. For the remainder of his life he and Nell lived in Europe. Whitlock never adjusted to post-war America; in his view it had become the land of philistinism and of prohibition. The Roaring Twenties were all too much for the ex-mayor of Toledo. The couple became part of the American expatriate colony: winter in Cannes, spring or fall in Brussels or Paris, summer at Vichy, always living in hotels, always writing. Whitlock had seven novels published in the nineteen twenties and thirties, as well as a highly regarded two-volume biography of Lafayette.[44] Nevertheless, he was very pessimistic about his achievements as a writer. Edith Wharton's critique of his writing during a visit to Cannes in the fall of 1931 did little to restore his confidence. He described her as hard as nails. Whitlock's insecurity as a writer in the nineteen thirties matched the decline in his health. Finally, after a second operation for an enlarged prostate, Brand Whitlock died on May 24, 1934. Burial was at Cannes.[45] "He died overwhelmed by a sense of failure. His great novel, which he wished so much to write, remained unwritten."[46] However, the people of Belgium, especially those in Brussels, knew otherwise — Brand Whitlock was anything but a failure.

Chapter Notes

Introduction

1. Gustave Le Bon, *The Psychology of the Great War* (London: T. Fisher Unwin, 1916), 20, 170.
2. G.J. Meyer, *A World Undone* (New York: Delacorte, 2006), 609.
3. Wythe Williams, *Dusk of Empire* (London: Charles Scribner's Sons, 1937), 41.
4. Le Bon, 20.
5. Both names refer to springs in the city. Aachen derives from the Old High German word for water, *aha*. Aix evolved from the Latin *aquis* and la-Chapelle refers to the church where Charlemagne is interred. Adrian Room, *Placenames of the World* (Jefferson, NC: McFarland, 2006), 17.
6. A. de Gerlache de Gomery, *Belgium in War Time*, translated by Bernard Miall (New York: George H. Doran, 1916), 25.
7. Emile Waxweiler, *Belgium Neutral and Loyal* (New York: G.P. Putnam's Sons, 1915), 42.
8. Francis Whiting Halsey, *The Literary Digest History of the World War* (New York and London: Funk and Wagnalls, 1919), 1:255.
9. de Gerlache de Gomery, 25.
10. Count Bernstorff, *My Three Years in America* (New York: Charles Scribner's Sons, 1920), 58.

Chapter 1

1. Hugh Gibson, *A Journal from our Legation in Belgium* (Garden City, NY: Doubleday, Page, 1917), 33.
2. Glenna Lindsley Bigelow, *Liége—On the Line of March* (New York and London: John Lane, 1918), 20.
3. In 1878, the French Academy changed the spelling of Liége to Liège, from a closed é to an open è. This change applied to place names only within France. Belgium formally adopted this new spelling of Liège in 1946, 68 years later. The authors will use the 1946 spelling.
4. G.H. Perris, *The Campaign of 1914 in France and Belgium* (New York: Henry Holt, 1915), 4.
5. A graduate of the Columbia School of Nursing (1902).
6. Bigelow, 34–35.
7. L. Mokveld, *The German Fury in Belgium* (New York: George H. Doran, 1917), 40.
8. Bigelow, 61.
9. Herbert Jäger, *German Artillery of World War One* (Marlborough, UK: Crowood, 2001), 34–39.
10. Bigelow, 38–39.
11. Mokveld, 65.
12. Bigelow, 46.
13. Bigelow, 46–47.
14. Bigelow, 47–48.
15. Bigelow, 49.
16. Elected 1905, 1907, 1909, and 1911; Whitlock declined to run in 1913, saying he had had enough of politics.
17. David D. Anderson, *Brand Whitlock* (New York: Twayne, 1968), 47.
18. Brand Whitlock, *The 13th District: A Story of a Candidate* (Indianapolis, IN: Bowen-Merrill, 1902).
19. Belgium was so insignificant it did not rate ambassadorial status.
20. Alan Nevins, *The Letters and Journal of Brand Whitlock: The Letters* (New York: D. Appleton-Century, 1936), 175, from a letter written to Marshall Sheppy, February 22, 1914.
21. Previously Gibson had been Secretary of Legation in Honduras and then in Cuba.
22. Gibson, 3.
23. The Palace Hotel still survives in Brussels but much of the Quartier Léopold has been destroyed, not by war but by peace. The Quartier Léopold metamorphosed into the Quartier des Institutions Européennes, housing the bureaucracies of the European Union as well as the

countless offices of lawyers, lobbyists, and businesses feeding from the Union trough. The beautiful nineteenth-century buildings, including the old American Legation, stand no longer and soulless office blocks now replace them. European peace is big business.

24. Also spelled Below-Saleske.

25. Brand Whitlock, *Belgium, A Personal Narrative* (New York: D. Appleton, 1919), 1:3.

26. "Won't Violate Belgium," *New York Times*, August 3, 1914. How much did Bellow-Saleski know? Bellow-Saleski, German minister in Brussels, received a sealed envelope on July 29 with instructions not to open before receiving a telegram from Berlin. Such a telegram arrived on Sunday, August 2, with instructions to deliver an ultimatum to the Belgium government by 8 p.m. that evening. The German ultimatum demanded Belgium grant right of free passage for the German Army across Belgium; if not, the German Army would fight its way across. Barbara W. Tuchman, *The Guns of August* (New York: Bantam, 1976), 120; Larry Zuckerman, *The Rape of Belgium* (New York: New York University Press, 2004), 13. Did Bellow-Seleski give the interview before the telegram arrived?

27. Whitlock, *Belgium, A Personal Narrative* 1:72.

28. Whitlock, *Belgium, A Personal Narrative* 1:75.

29. Richard Harding Davis, *With the Allies* (New York: Charles Scribner's Sons, 1919), 156.

30. "Cunarder Slips Out; Will Pick up British Cruisers as Escorts," *New York Times*, August 5, 1914.

31. "Lusitania Nears Goal" *New York Times*, August 8, 1914.

32. "The Lusitania Safe," *New York Times*, August 12, 1914.

33. Davis traveled in first class luxury with his wife who was pregnant at the time. She remained in England. In a letter to his brother Charles, Davis described the *Lusitania* experience: "They gave me a 'regal' suite which at other times costs $1,000 and it is so darned regal that I hate to leave it. I get sleepy walking from one end of it to the other; and we have open fires in each of the three rooms. Generally when one goes to war it is in a transport or a troop train and the person of the least importance is the correspondent. So, this way of going to war I like." Charles Belmont Davis, editor, *Adventures and Letters of Richard Harding Davis* (New York: Charles Scribner's Sons, 1918), 367–368.

34. Davis reported on the war between Cuba and Spain in 1897, the Spanish-American War in 1898, the Boer War in 1900, the Japanese-Russian War in 1904; he also reported on atrocities in the Congo in 1907 and the U.S.-Mexican conflict in the spring of 1914.

35. Gibson, 74–75.

36. Charles Belmont Davis, 369.

37. Frederick Palmer, *My Year of the Great War* (New York: Dodd, Mead, 1916), 21.

38. Irvin S. Cobb, *Paths of Glory* (New York: George H. Doran, 1915), 38.

39. *Twice in a Lifetime, Belgium 1914–1940* (London: Evans Brothers, 1943), 38.

40. Gibson, 101–102.

41. Richard Harding Davis, 24–25.

42. Richard Harding Davis, 25.

43. Richard Harding Davis, 26.

44. Cobb, 77.

45. The Gaiety had a notorious reputation during the war. "That city boasted a famous pimp and bully called Macro, one of the leading dancers at the Gaiety, for whom many women sold their bodies to Germans." Magnus Hirschfeld, *The Sexual History of the World War* (New York: Falstaff, 1937), 157–158. The Gaiety Theater still stands in Brussels' theater district.

46. "Dancers Saw Real War," *New York Times*, January 31, 1915, 14.

47. "Dancers Saw Real War," *New York Times*, January 31, 1915, 14.

48. E. Alexander Powell, *Fighting in Flanders* (New York: Charles Scribner's Sons, 1915), 112–114.

49. A special dance performance for German officers in a nearby castle raised additional funds.

50. Gibson, 107.

51. Gibson, 108–109.

52. Gibson, 126.

53. John T. McCutcheon, *Chicago Tribune*; Will Irwin, *New York Tribune*; Irvin S. Cobb, *The Saturday Evening Post*.

54. Gibson, 122.

55. Richard Harding Davis, 36.

56. Richard Harding Davis, 40–41.

57. Richard Harding Davis, 69.

58. Richard Harding Davis, 74–77.

59. Whitlock, *Belgium, A Personal Narrative*, 1: 148.

Chapter 2

1. Foster Watson, "The Humanists of Louvain," *Nineteenth Century and After*, October 1914, 76:765.

2. Now known by its Flemish name, Leuven.

3. The cartographer Gerardus Mercator matriculated from the university in 1530. He worked and lived in Louvain from 1534 until 1552.

4. P. Delannoy, "The Library of the University of Louvain," *Nineteenth Century and After*, 1915, 77: 1062.

5. Arno Dosch, John T. McCutcheon, Will Irwin and Irvin S. Cobb.

6. Will Irwin, "Detained by the Germans," *Collier's*, October 3, 1914, 54(3):5.

7. Irwin, "Detained by the Germans," *Collier's*, October 3, 1914, 54(3):5.
8. Irwin, "Detained by the Germans," *Collier's*, October 3, 1914, 54(3):6.
9. Will Irwin, "Wreckage of War," *The American Magazine*, 1914, 78:49.
10. Irwin, "Detained by the Germans," *Collier's*, October 3, 1914, 54(3):24.
11. Irvin S. Cobb, *Paths of Glory* (New York: George H. Doran, 1915), 94.
12. Cobb, 95–96.
13. In 1915, fifty bodies were discovered near the Railway Yard. Mark Derez, "The Flames of Louvain: The War Experience of an Academic Community," in *Facing Armageddon: The First World War Experienced*, eds. Hugh Cecil and Peter Liddle (London: Cooper, 1996), 618.
14. Irwin, "Detained by the Germans," *Collier's*, October 3, 1914, 54(3):26.
15. Cobb, 99.
16. Irwin, "Detained by the Germans," *Collier's*, October 3, 1914, 54(3):27.
17. L. Mokveld, *The German Fury in Belgium* (New York: George H. Doran, 1917), 115.
18. Mokveld, 116.
19. Delannoy, "The Library of the University of Louvain," *Nineteenth Century and After*, May 1915, 77:1061–1062.
20. Derez, 626.
21. "Louvainers Crazed by Their Troubles," *New York Times*, September 6, 1914, 3; "Attack on Louvain Told by Refugee," *New York Times*, September 4, 1914, 3.
22. Spelled Uttebroick in the *New York Times* article cited below.
23. "American Girl's Bravery," *New York Times*, September 10, 1914, 4.
24. Doctrine of the Roman Catholic Church that the Virgin Mary was conceived without sin.
25. Kevin A. Codd, "The American College of Louvain," *The Catholic Historical Review*, 2007, 93:47–83.
26. Hugh Gibson, *A Journal from Our Legation in Belgium* (Garden City, NY: Doubleday Page, 1917), 128.
27. Gibson, 140.
28. "German March Is Like Tidal Wave," *Morning Oregonian*, August 24, 1914, 1.
29. Richard Harding Davis, *With the Allies* (New York: Charles Scribner's Sons, 1919), 79.
30. Razed in 1955 and replaced with a modern station.
31. Irwin, "Wreckage of War," *The American Magazine*, 1914, 78:76.
32. Irwin, "Wreckage of War," 78:76.
33. Irwin, "Wreckage of War," 78:77.
34. Irwin, "Wreckage of War," 78:77.
35. Richard Harding Davis, "Night of Dread Marked the Sack of Louvain," *Boston Daily Globe*, August 31, 1914, 1.
36. "Miss O'Reilly Back from Her Daring Tour," *Boston Herald*, February 15, 1917.
37. "Fired to Back a German Lie," *Boston Daily Globe*, January 12, 1915, 8.
38. Gibson, 157–158.
39. Gibson, 159.
40. Gibson, 162.
41. Gibson, 165.
42. Gibson, 170.
43. Gibson, 162.
44. "Ruins of Louvain Visited by Crowds," *New York Times*, November 13, 1914, 4.
45. George B. McClellan, *The Heel of War* (New York: G.W. Dillingham, 1916), 73.
46. McClellan, 74.
47. Cobb, 409–410.
48. Cobb, 411.
49. Geoffrey Wawro, *The Franco-Prussian War* (Cambridge University Press, 2003), 309.
50. Brand Whitlock, "Belgium: The Atrocities," *Everybody's Magazine*, 1918, 38 (4):16.
51. Whitlock, "Belgium: The Atrocities," 38(4):16.
52. Whitlock, "Belgium: The Atrocities," 38(4):16.
53. Whitlock, "Belgium: The Atrocities," 38(4):18.
54. George B. McClellan, "How I Found Belgium Under German Rule," *New York Times*, October 10, 1915.
55. McClellan, "How I Found Belgium Under German Rule," 46.
56. McClellan, "How I Found Belgium Under German Rule," 46.
57. George B. McClellan, *The Heel of War* (New York: G.W. Dillingham, 1916), 81–82.
58. Larry Zuckerman, *The Rape of Belgium* (New York University Press, 2004), 30–37.

Chapter 3

1. Brand Whitlock, "Belgium: The Reign of Terror," *Everybody's Magazine* 38 (5), May 1918, 18.
2. L. Mokveld, *The German Fury in Belgium* (New York: George H. Doran, 1917), 151.
3. Whitlock, 18.
4. The Meuse flows from south to north; facing downstream the right bank is the east bank.
5. *Handbook for Travellers in Holland and Belgium* (London: John Murray, 1876), 207.
6. Fortescue was the illegitimate son of Robert Roosevelt, President Theodore Roosevelt's uncle. Robert had established a satellite family with an Irish immigrant named Marion Theresa O'Shea, inventing the surname Fortescue. When Robert's wife died, Robert married Ms. O'Shea and adopted their three children. Granville and Teddy Roosevelt were first cousins.

7. Granville Fortescue, *Frontline and Deadline* (New York: G.P. Putnam's Sons, 1937), 63.
8. Fortescue, 67.
9. Fortescue, 72.
10. Fortescue, 76.
11. Whitlock, 11.
12. Mokveld, 164.
13. Whitlock, 11.
14. Mokveld, 164.
15. Camille David, "Dinant la Morte," *The Contemporary Review*, 1915, 108: 215.
16. Holger H. Herwig, *The Marne, 1914* (New York: Random House, 2009), 166.
17. Herwig, 168–169.
18. David, 212.
19. Mokveld, 168.
20. Mokveld, 167.
21. Irvin S. Cobb, *Paths of Glory* (New York: George H. Doran, 1915), 380.
22. Karl Baedeker, *Belgium and Holland, Handbook for Travelers* (Leipzig, Germany: Karl Baedeker, 1910), 222.
23. Handbook for Travellers in Holland and Belgium, 175.
24. Mokveld, 147–148.
25. Mokveld, 148–149.
26. Mokveld, 151.
27. Whitlock, 13.
28. Fortescue, 59.
29. Francis Whiting Halsey, *The Literary Digest History of the War* (New York and London: Funk and Wagnalls, 1919), 1:308.
30. Brussels was still in Belgian hands at this time.
31. The Technical Academy at Karlsruhe conferred on Professor Otto Rausenberger, designer of the famous 42-centimeter Krupp gun, the degree of Doctor of Engineering *honoris cause*. "Honor For Designer of 42-Centimeter Gun," *New York Times*, September 2, 1915, 1.
32. The next fortified city defending the Sambre River corridor, 50 miles (30 km) west of Namur.
33. Halsey, 1:314.
34. G.H. Perris, *The Campaign of 1914 in France and Belgium* (New York: Henry Holt 1915), 38–39.
35. Perris, 85.
36. Mokveld, 154.
37. Herwig, 319.
38. "Huge Losses at Maubeuge," *New York Times*, September 20, 1914, 1; "Wounded German Here: First Man to Arrive Says Losses Have Not Been Exaggerated," *New York Times*, November 1, 1914, 5.
39. "Maubeuge Won Mercy Through French Nurse," *New York Times*, December 24, 1914, 2.
40. Cobb, *Paths of Glory*, 306.
41. Cobb, *Paths of Glory*, 308.
42. Cobb, *Paths of Glory* 312.
43. Anita Lawson, *Irvin S. Cobb* (Bowling Green, OH: Bowling Green State University Popular Press, 1984), 116.
44. Hugh Gibson, *A Journal from Our Legation in Belgium* (Garden City, NY: Doubleday Page, 1917), 127–128.
45. Lawson, 117.
46. Cobb, *Paths of Glory*, 111.
47. Cobb, *Paths of Glory*, 111–112.
48. Irvin S. Cobb, "The Funniest Thing That Ever Happened to Me," *The American Magazine*, October, 1923, 172.
49. Court photographer to the Belgian king.
50. "American Writers Escape to Holland" *New York Times*, September 11, 1914, 6.
51. Cobb, *Paths of Glory*, 137.
52. John McCutcheon (*Chicago Tribune*), Irvin S. Cobb (*Saturday Evening Post*), Harry Hansen (*Chicago Daily News*), James O'Donnell Bennett (*Chicago Tribune*), Roger Lewis (Associated Press), Maurice Gerbeault, Victor Hennebert and Lawrence Sterne Stevens.
53. Cobb, *Paths of Glory*, 164–165.
54. Cobb, *Paths of Glory*, 174.
55. "Americans Saw No Cruel Acts," *New York Times*, September 7, 1914, 1.
56. John T. McCutcheon, *Drawn From Memory* (New York: Bobbs-Merrill, 1950), 280–281; Lawson, 121.
57. Lawson, 121.
58. Cobb, *Paths of Glory*, pages 198–414, are based on his experiences as a guest of the German Army in 1914.
59. "Finds German Army Polite and Kindly," *New York Times*, September 17, 1914, 5; "Saw No Atrocities Says Irvin S. Cobb," *New York Times*, October 17, 1914, 3; James O'Donnell Bennett, "Sir A. Conan Doyle's Statement on Belgium Attacked by American Correspondent," *New York Times*, January 17, 1915, 2.
60. Irvin S. Cobb, "Punitives Versus Primitives," *The Saturday Evening Post*, November 14, 1914, 14.
61. Whitlock, 20.
62. John Horne and Alan Kramer, *German Atrocities, 1914* (New Haven: Yale University Press, 2001), 4.
63. Horne and Kramer, 77.
64. Cobb, "Punitives Versus Primitives," 14.
65. Horne and Kramer, 77.

Chapter 4

1. Francis Whiting Halsey, *The Literary Digest History of the World War* (New York and London: Funk and Wagnalls, 1919), 1: 326.
2. Herbert Jäger, *German Artillery of World War One* (Marlborough, UK: Crowood, 2001), 34–35.
3. In 1911, there was a chance to negotiate Belgian/Dutch co-sovereignty of the Scheldt to

its mouth, but negations failed. Demetrius C. Boulger, "The Truth about Antwerp," *The North American Review*, February 1916, 203:236. With co-sovereignty, the course of the war might have been very different. British warships in Antwerp constituted Germany's worst nightmare. With a British naval base and consequent Allied stronghold almost astride German supply lines in Belgium, the northern part of the Western Front would probably have been unsustainable if not impossible.

4. Edmond Dane, *Hacking Through Belgium* (London: Hodder and Stoughton, 1914), 16–17.

5. John Horne and Alan Kramer, *German Atrocities, 1914* (New Haven: Yale University Press, 2001), 42.

6. Horace Green, *The Log of a Noncombatant* (Boston and New York: Houghton Mifflin, 1915), 23–24.

7. A Corps consisted of 1,500 officers and 40,000 noncommissioned officers and men. Holger H. Herwig, *The Marne, 1914* (New York: Random House, 2009), 46.

8. Herwig, 124.

9. Horace Green was not included in the list of reporters active on the Western Front. Emmet Crozier, *American Reporters on the Western Front, 1914–1918* (Oxford University Press, 1959).

10. Green, 61.
11. Green, 5–6.
12. Green, 7.
13. Green, 8.
14. Belgian ministers that left Brussels as the German Army approached resided in the Grand Hotel about 600 meters from the Royal Palace.

15. E. Alexander Powell, *Fighting in Flanders* (New York: Charles Scribner's Sons, 1915), 12.

16. Powell, *Fighting in Flanders*, 23.
17. Powell, *Fighting in Flanders*, 26.
18. Powell, *Fighting in Flanders*, 14.
19. David Mould, "Donald Thompson: Photographer at War," *Kansas History*, September 1982, 5 (3): 156–157.

20. Supposedly, he paid her 250 francs, and the rest in cigar coupons, convincing her they were American money, but Thompson was known to embellish his tales.

21. "Paid a War Bribe in Cigar Coupons," *New York Times*, November 16, 1914, 4.

22. Mould, 158.
23. Mould, 158.
24. Powell, *Fighting in Flanders*, 46.
25. Green, 119.
26. After surviving numerous air battles in World War I, Captain Lehmann died from burns when the Nazi Zeppelin *Hindenburg* burst into flames on May 6, 1937, over Lakehurst, New Jersey.

27. Ernst A. Lehmann and Howard Mingos, *The Zeppelins* (New York: J.H. Sears, 1927), 25–26.

28. Lehmann and Mingos, 28.
29. Powell, *Fighting in Flanders*, 57.
30. Powell, *Fighting in Flanders*, 62–63.
31. Powell, *Fighting in Flanders*, 64–65.
32. "Forty German Zeppelins and Ten Parsevals Lost Since the War Began, Says Geneva Report," *New York Times*, September 25, 1915, 1.

33. Wilbur Cross, *Zeppelins of World War I* (New York: Paragon House, 1991), 60–61.

34. Vernon Kellogg, *Headquarters Nights* (Boston: Atlantic Monthly Press, 1917), 38–39.

35. "Haul Big Guns in Pieces," *New York Times*, September 24, 1914, 4.

36. Powell, *Fighting in Flanders*, 81–82.
37. Powell, *Fighting in Flanders*, 84.
38. Brand Whitlock, "Belgium: The Reign of Terror," *Everybody's Magazine*, 38 (5), May 1918, 14–16.

39. Whitlock, 14.
40. John Horne and Alan Kramer, *German Atrocities, 1914* (New Haven: Yale University Press, 2001), 26–30.

41. Powell, *Fighting in Flanders*, 85–88.
42. Powell, *Fighting in Flanders*, 101–102.
43. E. Alexander Powell, *Slanting Lines of Steel* (New York: Macmillan, 1933), 72–73.

44. W. Van Lede, "An Eyewitness's Impressions of the Fall of Antwerp," *The National Review*, November 1915, 66: 442.

45. Boulger, 241.
46. "Antwerp Guarded by German Sailors," *Boston Daily Globe*, October 20, 1914, 9.

47. Gladys Hughes Appleton was married to Captain Archibald Winterbottom.

48. E. Alexander Powell, "Boston Woman's Act of Heroism in War," *Boston Daily Globe*, October 2, 1914, 1, 8.

49. Van Lede, 444–445.
50. Van Lede, 445–446.
51. His friend Willard Luther had returned to Boston.

52. Green, 71–72.
53. Powell, *Fighting in Flanders*, 187.
54. Powell, *Fighting in Flanders*, 181.
55. Powell, *Fighting in Flanders*, 183.
56. Winston S. Churchill, *The Great War* (London: George Newnes, 1933), Part 5: 300–302.

57. After the war, Churchill argued that the idea for the Antwerp expedition was not his but imposed upon him by his superiors. Churchill, 302–304.

58. W. Van Lede, "An Eyewitness's Impressions of the Fall of Antwerp," *The National Review*, November 1915, 66: 454.

59. Arthur Ruhl, *Antwerp to Gallipolli* (New York: Charles Scribner's Sons, 1916), 50.

60. "Saved by Whitlock," *Boston Daily Globe*, October 29, 1914, 11.

61. Sven Hedin, *With the German Armies in*

the West (London and New York: John Lane, 1915), 218.

62. During World War One, shrapnel shells burst in the air and released a hail of lead balls. In today's usage, shrapnel refers to shell splinters or fragments from high explosive shells; this was not so in World War One.

63. "Antwerp Guarded by German Sailors," *Boston Daily Globe*, October 20, 1914, 9.

64. Halsey, 1:336–337.

65. Cooper C. Graham and Ron van Dopperen, "Edwin F. Weigle: Cameraman for the *Chicago Tribune*," in *Film History* (New Barnet, Herts., UK: John Libbey, 2010), 22: 391–396.

66. Edwin F. Weigle, *My Experiences on the Belgian Battlefields* (Chicago: Hamming, 1914), 52.

67. Weigle, 53.

68. Weigle, 54–55.

69. Green, 91.

70. Green, 94.

71. *A War Nurse's Diary* (New York: Macmillan, 1918), 31.

72. Powell, *Slanting Lines of Steel*, 105.

73. Powell, *Slanting Lines of Steel*, 106.

74. Green, 105–106.

75. Powell, *Slanting Lines of Steel*, 120.

76. Powell, *Slanting Lines of Steel*, 125.

77. Powell's action scandalized the U.S. Department of State. Consul-General Diederich tried to have Powell arrested. Powell, *Slanting Lines of Steel*, 128–129, 140.

78. Powell, *Slanting Lines of Steel*, 130.

79. Powell, *Slanting Lines of Steel*, 139.

80. Powell, *Slanting Lines of Steel*, 142–143.

81. George F. Porter, "The Germans in Antwerp," *Harper's Weekly*, 1914, 59: 511–512.

82. Frank H. Simmonds, *The Great War: The Second Phase* (Kennerly, NY: Mitchell, 1915), 19.

83. Swen Hedin, 226.

84. Swen Hedin, 227.

Chapter 5

1. Emile Joseph Galet, *Albert King of the Belgians in the Great War* (Boston and New York: Houghton Mifflin 1931), 234.

2. Emile Cammaerts, *Albert of Belgium* (New York: Macmillan 1935), 182.

3. Anonymous, *A War Nurse's Diary* (New York: Macmillan 1918), 29–30.

4. Cammaerts, 182.

5. *A War Nurse's Diary*, 36.

6. May Sinclair, *A Journal of Impressions in Belgium* (London: Hutchinson, 1915), 146.

7. E. Alexander Powell, *Italy at War* (New York: Charles Scribner's Sons, 1917), 242.

8. Powell, 243.

9. "American Couple Under German Fire," *New York Times*, October 1, 1914.

10. "Kentucky Hunter Fought Germans," *New York Times*, November 24, 1914, 3.

11. "Kentucky Hunter Fought Germans," 3.

12. *The New York Times*, November 24, indicated his name as Edward, but Cantrell often gave his name as Ed, so very likely the reporter assumed it was foreshortening of Edward. Edgar played banjo and teamed up with Richard Williams, a mandolin player, to form the Ragtime Duo in 1894, which toured London in 1902. Banjoist and singer Edgar Cantrell made over 70 disc records and cylinders between October 1902 and February 1907, over 40 of them with his mandolin-playing partner Richard Williams. Williams was born in Germany, immigrating to the United States in 1887, and died in London in late 1906 after a short illness. Cantrell applied for a passport at the American Legation in Brussels in 1899, giving his occupation as musician, residing in Antwerp. Email 27 July 2012: Mark Berresford, editor, VJM's Jazz & Blues Mart.

13. Arthur H. Gleason and Helen Hayes Gleason, *Golden Lads* (New York: A.L. Burt, 1916), 197–198.

14. Philip Gibbs, *The Soul of the War* (New York: Robert M. McBride, 1915), 198–199.

15. Gleason and Gleason, 203.

16. Cammaerts, 182.

17. Paul Van Pul, *In Flanders Flooded Fields* (Barnsley, South Yorkshire, UK: Pen and Sword, 2006), 58–74, for the military considerations and politics of this decision.

18. Cammaerts, 187.

19. *Ypres, 1914* (London: Constable 1919), 16; translation of a report to the German General Staff prepared by Otto Schwink, 1917.

20. These vessels had nothing in common with the American Civil War *Monitor*.

21. Ian Buxton, *Big Gun Monitors* (Annapolis, MD: Naval Institute, 1978), 81.

22. Francis Whiting Halsey, *The Literary Digest History of the World War* (New York: Funk and Wagnalls, 1919), 2: 211–212.

23. Part of the German III Reserve Corps, the 4th *Erzatz* Division fought along the coast between Ostend and Nieuport.

24. *Ypres, 1914*, 22.

25. *Ypres, 1914*, 33.

26. G.H. Perris, *The Campaign of 1914 in France and Belgium* (New York: Henry Holt, 1915), 303.

27. Newspaper Man Wounded, *New York Times*, October 31, 1914, 2.

28. Gibbs, 180.

29. Gibbs, 183.

30. Philip Gibbs, "Seeking Wounded on Battle Front," *New York Times*, October 26, 1914, 1.

31. H.S. Souttar, *A Surgeon in Belgium* (New York: Longmans, Green, 1915), 189.

32. Now a bikeway.

33. Gleason and Gleason, 204, 207.
34. Souttar, 196.
35. Also decorated were Mrs. Elsie Knocker, Miss Mairi Chisolm and Lady Dorothie Fielding. "A Gallant Work May Stop," *New York Times*, March 27, 1915, 10.
36. Gleason and Gleason, 207–208.
37. Gleason and Gleason, 209.
38. *Handbook to Belgium and the Battlefields*, 8th ed. (London: Ward, Lock, 1935), 86–87.
39. Gleason and Gleason, 214.
40. Gleason and Gleason, 213.
41. *Ypres, 1914*, 50.
42. Van Pul, 153–218 for the hydrology of the inundation.
43. Because the inundation was so successful in stopping the German advance, there were many claimants for the idea. The French maintained it was Marshal Ferdinand Foch's suggestion, *The Yser and the Belgian Coast* (Clermont-Ferrand, France: Michelin, 1920), 14. The Belgians attributed it to Henry Geeraert.
44. *Ypres, 1914*, 51.
45. Arno Dosch, "The Last Ditch in Belgium," *World's Work*, 1915, 269.
46. Nothing remains of Albert's and Elizabeth's La Panne except the church where they worshiped. The idyllic little village behind the dunes is now a phalanx of high-rise vacation accommodations facing the North Sea.
47. Dosch, 272.
48. Dosch, 272.
49. The submarine cable to Dover began at La Panne. Karl Baedeker, *Belgium and Holland* (Leipzig: Karl Baedeker, 1910), 18.
50. Her first mystery, *The Circular Staircase*, published in 1908, sold over a million copies.
51. His wife, Marie Depage, was then in Brussels working as a nurse in Edith Cavell's clinic (see Chapter 6).
52. Mary Roberts Rinehart, *Kings, Queens and Pawns* (New York: George M. Doran, 1915).
53. Rinehart, *Kings, Queens and Pawns*, 39.
54. Rinehart, *Kings, Queens and Pawns*, 68.
55. Rinehart, *Kings, Queens and Pawns*, 67.
56. Mary Roberts Rinehart, "The Queen of the Belgians," *The Saturday Evening Post*, July 3, 1915, 188: 23.
57. Charles Le Goffic, *Dixmude* (London: William Heinemann, 1916), 146–147.
58. Walter Austin, *A War Zone Gadabout* (Boston: R.H. Hinkley, 1917), 10.
59. Austin, 33.
60. Austin, 51.
61. Austin, 53.
62. Austin, 55–56.
63. Austin, 56.
64. Walter Austin was not the screwball he comes across as in his book. A Harvard graduate (A.B. 1887, LL.B. 1890), he was a noted Boston lawyer. His favorite recreations were golf, swimming and, of course, adventurous travel. He died in 1929. His fellow gadabout, Edwin B. Hotchkiss, had a shorter life; on May 7, 1915, he went down with the *Lusitania* when it was torpedoed.
65. Anonymous, *Ypres, 1914*, 71–72.

Chapter 6

1. Adolf von Bachofen, "German Civil Administration in Belgium," *Current History*, October 1916, 5:136.
2. Ernesta Drinker Bullitt, *An Uncensored Diary from the Central Empires* (Garden City, NY: Doubleday, Page, 1917), 127.
3. Larry Zuckerman, *The Rape of Belgium* (New York University Press, 2004), 90–91.
4. Von Bachofen, 138.
5. Von Bachofen, 138.
6. Von Bachofen, 139.
7. P.P.F., "Incidents of German Rule in Belgium," *Outlook*, 1915, 111: 407.
8. Edward Eyre Hunt, *War Bread* (New York: Henry Holt, 1916), 242–243.
9. "German Crowds Enliven Brussels," *New York Times*, November 22, 1914, 3.
10. Frank Hoyt Gailor, "A Rhodes Scholar in Belgium," *Littell's Living Age*, 1915, 285:721.
11. "German Crowds Enliven Brussels," *New York Times*, November 22, 1914, 3.
12. Gailor, 285:721.
13. Magnus Hirschfeld, *The Sexual History of the World War* (New York: Falstaff, 1937), 158.
14. "As far as the occupied districts in the west were concerned, Lille can be regarded as the chief center of prostitution." Hirschfeld, 156.
15. "German Crowds Enliven Brussels," *New York Times*, November 22, 1914, 3.
16. Albert Rhys Williams, *In the Claws of the German Eagle* (New York: E.P. Dutton, 1917), 95.
17. Williams, 87.
18. Williams, 90.
19. "Whitlock as King in Belgian's Minds," *New York Times*, November 5, 1915, 3.
20. "Bookings to Europe Since Jan. 1 Cut 70%," *New York Times*, April 25, 1915.
21. Will Brownell and Richard N. Billings, *So Close to Greatness* (New York: Macmillan, 1987), 49–61.
22. Bullitt, 85.
23. Bullitt, 123.
24. Bullitt, 147.
25. "Mrs. Beaux Bride of S.L.M. Barlow," *New York Times*, March 11, 1928, 26.
26. Kenneth S. Davis, "For the President," *New York Times*, December 17, 1972.
27. Bullitt, 139.
28. Brand Whitlock, *Belgium* (New York: D. Appleton, 1919), Volume I: 499.
29. "Whitlock as King in Belgian's Minds," *New York Times*, November 5, 1915, 3.

30. "Belgians Thank America," *New York Times*, January 23, 1915, 4.
31. "Brussels Celebrates on Washington's Day," *New York Times*, February 25, 1915, 2.
32. The Imperial German Embassy in Washington received the warning two months earlier, but delayed its publication until ordered to do so at once. Diana Preston, *Lusitania* (New York: Walker, 2002), 415.
33. "Disaster Bears out Embassy's Warning," *New York Times*, May 8, 1915, 3.
34. "German Embassy Issues Warning," *New York Times*, May 1, 1915, 1.
35. Preston, 130–131.
36. Preston, 171.
37. Preston, 168.
38. "Disaster Bears out Embassy's Warning," *New York Times*, May 8, 1915, 3.
39. Preston, 185.
40. Preston, 441.
41. Preston, 442.
42. Preston, 447.
43. Preston, 210.
44. What happened on *Lusitania* was very different from the gallantry aboard *Titanic* when she sank in1909. On *Lusitania* selfish behavior dominated, whereas on the *Titanic* social norms and social status dominated. It is hypothesized that because *Lusitania* sank quickly the impulse was to escape (short-run flight impulse). The slowly sinking *Titanic* (two hours and forty minutes) allowed socially determined behavioral patterns to take hold. Bruno S. Frey, David A. Savage, and Benno Torgler, "Interaction of Natural Survival Instincts and Internalized Social Norms Exploring the *Titanic* and *Lusitania* Disasters," in *Proceedings of the U.S. National Academy of Sciences*, March 16, 2010, 107:4862.
45. Preston, 303.
46. Bullitt, 159.
47. "Aid for Belgian Wounded," *New York Times*, April 27, 1915, 4.
48. Renamed rue Franz Merjay, in the commune of Ixelles.
49. A.E. Clark-Kennedy, *Edith Cavell* (London: Faber and Faber, 1965), 58–75.
50. Helen Judson, *Edith Cavell* (New York: Macmillan 1941), 227.
51. "Worked with Miss Cavell," *New York Times*, November 1, 1915, 5.
52. Hugh Gibson, "The Last Hours of Edith Cavell," *World's Work*, October 1917, 34:650.
53. The confession is given in Clark-Kennedy, 159–160.
54. Clark-Kennedy, 160.
55. Brand Whitlock, *Belgium* (New York: D. Appleton, 1919), Volume 2: 94.
56. Gibson, 34: 653.
57. In the Belgian senate chamber, a plaque commemorates those convicted there in World War One.
58. De Laval became persona non grata to Germany for his connection to the Cavell affair and the Germans ordered his expulsion from Belgium. "Whitlock Will Return," *New York Times*, November 12, 1915, 3.
59. Gibson, 34: 657.
60. On the front wall of the prison is a plaque listing those inmates shot during the First World War; Cavell's name is on that list. Next to it is another plaque listing those shot in the Second World War—it is even longer.
61. The Tir National is absent from contemporary Brussels maps. It is now the site of the state television, Radio-Télévision Belge Francophone (RTBF). There is a monument to those martyred at the old shooting range near the entrance of the station complex at the suitably named Place des Carabiniers. Nearby are the Boulevard Brand Whitlock and Avenue Herbert Hoover.
62. Gaston de Laval, "Trial and Death of Edith Cavell," *Current History*, July 1919, 10: 142.
63. Whitlock, *Belgium*, Volume II: 180.
64. "Denies Political Move in Whitlock's Return," *New York Times*, November 5, 1915, 3.
65. "Whitlock Leaves Holland," *New York Times*, January 11, 1916, 2.

Chapter 7

1. Francis A. March, *History of the World War* (Chicago: United Publishers of the United States and Canada, 1919), 88 for a translation of the *Kriegsbrauch im Landkriege [The Usages of War on Land]* (Great General Staff of the Imperial German Army, 1902).
2. J.H. Morgan, *The German War Book*, an English translation of the entire *Kriegsbrauch im Landkriege*, 1902 (London: John Murray, 1915), 52.
3. Vernon Kellogg, "The Belgian Wilderness," *Atlantic Monthly*, 1916, 117: 411–412.
4. Vernon Kellogg, "Getting England and Germany to Agree," *World's Work*, August 1917, 409.
5. George H. Nash, *The Life of Herbert Hoover: The Humanitarian* (New York: W.W. Norton, 1988), 2:28.
6. Vernon Kellogg, "Getting England and Germany to Agree," 405.
7. Nash, 2:18–19.
8. Allan Nevins, *The Letters and Journal of Brand Whitlock, The Journal* (New York: D. Appleton-Century, 1936), 55.
9. Vernon Kellogg, *Fighting Starvation in Belgium* (Garden City, NY: Doubleday, Page, 1918), 20–25 for the founding and a list of early members of the C.R.B.
10. Vernon Kellogg, "Getting England and Germany to Agree," 406.

11. Lewis R. Freeman, "Hoover and the Belgians," *Outlook*, September 8, 1915, 111: 82.
12. Freeman, 82.
13. Vernon Kellogg, "Getting England and Germany to Agree," 406.
14. Kellogg, "Getting England and Germany to Agree," 410.
15. "This Man Fed 6,000,000 Belgians," *New York Times Magazine*, February 28, 1915, 7.
16. "This Man Fed 6,000,000 Belgians," 7.
17. "Admits $1,000,000 Theft for Belgium," *New York Times*, September 25, 1915, 3.
18. "Admits $1,000,000 Theft for Belgium," 3.
19. "Admits $1,000,000 Theft for Belgium," 3.
20. Vernon Kellogg, *Fighting Starvation in Belgium*, 119.
21. Frank Hoyt Gailor, "A Rhodes Scholar in Belgium," *Littell's Living Age*, 1915, 285: 720.
22. Vernon Kellogg, "Feeding Belgium via Canals," *World's Work*, 1917, 98.
23. Vernon Kellogg, "Getting England and Germany to Agree," 412.
24. Kellogg, "Getting England and Germany to Agree," 412.
25. 126 Avenue Louise.
26. Edwin W. Morse, *The Vanguard of American Volunteers* (New York: Charles Scribner's Sons, 1919), 196.
27. Edward Eyre Hunt, *War Bread* (New York: Henry Holt, 1916), 217.
28. "Belgium Honors New Englanders," *Boston Globe*, March 11, 1919, 3.
29. Robert Withington, *In Occupied Belgium* (Boston: Cornhill, 1921), 75.
30. Tracy B. Kittredge, *The History of the Commission for Relief in Belgium 1914–1917* (London: Crowther and Goodman, 1918), 234.
31. J.H. Twells, Jr., *In the Prison City* (London: Andrew Melrose, 1919), 76–77.
32. Twells, Jr., 78.
33. Morse, 194–195.
34. "Regulations Governing Personal Correspondence," regulation #3. No reference may be made directly or indirectly to matters concerning war or war conditions, nor to operations or affairs of the C.R.B. Withington, 30.
35. Vernon Kellogg, *Herbert Hoover, The Man and his Work* (New York: D. Appleton, 1920), 184.
36. Nash, 2:77.
37. "Reservists Flock to the Consulates," *New York Times*, August 5, 1914, 6.
38. "Take Reservists Off Ships," *New York Times*, August 26, 1914, 5.
39. "German Reservists Held," *New York Times*, September 6, 1914, 2.
40. Hunt, 1–33 for the full story of the voyage of *Nieuw Amsterdam*.
41. Hunt, 85.
42. Hunt, 85–86,109–110 for a description of life in Thompson's Fort.
43. Hunt, 114.
44. Hunt, 202.
45. Now named Tolstraat.
46. Hunt, 207.
47. Hunt, 224.
48. The Christmas Ship for Russia sailed to Archangel and there a special train transported the gifts inland.
49. "5,000,000 Gifts Off Today on Xmas Ship," *New York Times*, November 14, 1914, 13.
50. "Christmas Ship Off to Soften War Woe," *New York Times*, November 15, 1914, 3.
51. The Kaiser hosted a reception and public dinner honoring America when the gifts arrived. "Berlin to Greet Americans," *New York Times*, December 18, 1914, 5.
52. Hunt, 226.
53. Hunt, 201.
54. His son, Lindon Bates, Jr., perished on *Lusitania*, his body washed ashore on the Irish coast. "Lindon Bates's Body," *New York Times*, July 25, 1915, 1.
55. The Commission for Relief in Belgium, General Instructions, 1915, 23.
56. Vernon Kellogg, "How Belgium Was Fed," *World's Work*, September 1917, 34: 533–534.
57. Kellogg, "How Belgium Was Fed," 535.
58. Kellogg, "How Belgium Was Fed," 538.
59. Walter S. Hiatt, World's Biggest Commissary Job, *Technical World Magazine*, April 1915, 23: 141.
60. Vernon Kellogg, *Fighting Starvation in Belgium*, 162.
61. Mabel Hyde Kittredge, "Taking Care of Belgium," *The New Republic*, July 31, 1915, 8.
62. Arno Dosch, "A Day in the Belgian Relief Stations," *World's Work*, 1915, 29: 555.
63. Charlotte Kellogg, *Women of Belgium* (New York: Funk and Wagnalls, 1917), 44–45.
64. Charlotte Kellogg, 129.
65. Charlotte Kellogg, 153.

Chapter 8

1. Vernon Kellogg, *Headquarters Nights* (Boston: Atlantic Monthly, 1917), 84–85.
2. Jacques Loeb, "Biology and War," *Science*, January 26, 1917, 45: 75.
3. Tracy B. Kittredge, *The History of The Commission for Relief in Belgium, 1914–1917* (London: Crowther and Goodman, 1918), 135.
4. "Ghent Yields Peacefully," *New York Times*, October 14, 1914, 2.
5. Kittredge, 152.
6. Allan Nevins, *The Letters and Journal of Brand Whitlock, The Journal* (New York: D. Appleton-Century, 1936), 78.
7. Brand Whitlock, *Belgium* Volume 1 (New York: D. Appleton, 1919), 362–363.

8. Whitlock, 368–369.
9. Frederick Palmer, *My Year of the Great War* (New York: Dodd, Mead, 1916), 117–127.
10. Hugh Gibson, *A Journal from Our Legation in Belgium* (Garden City, NY: Doubleday, Page, 1917), 340.
11. Gibson, 341.
12. Whitlock, 413.
13. Whitlock, 414.
14. Gibson, 342–343.
15. Kittredge, 138.
16. Kittredge, 143.
17. Kittredge, 144.
18. Kittredge, 147.
19. Kittredge, 150.
20. Kittredge, 151.
21. Kittredge, 152.
22. Henri Domelier, *Behind the Scenes at German Headquarters* (London: Hurst and Blackett, 1919), 66.
23. See Introduction and the German violation of a treaty guaranteeing Belgium's neutrality. Chancellor Bethmann-Hollweg described the treaty as only a scrap of paper.
24. Domelier, 20.
25. "At the Kaiser's Headquarters," *New York Times*, November 15, 1914, 1.
26. Domelier, 24–25.
27. Domelier, 99.
28. "At the Kaiser's Headquarters," 1.
29. Domelier, 41.
30. Domelier, ix.
31. Kellogg, *Headquarters Night*, 19.
32. Matthis Krischel, "Perceived Hereditary Effect of World War I: A Study of the Positions of Friedrich von Bernhardi and Vernon Kellogg," *Medicine Studies*, 2010, 2: 146.
33. Vernon Kellogg, "How North France Has Been Fed," *World's Work*, 1918, 303.
34. Kellogg, *Headquarters Nights*, 29–30.
35. Friedrich von Bernhardi, *Germany and the Next War* (New York: Chas. A. Eron, 1914), 18.
36. Von Bernhardi, 20.
37. Von Bernhardi, 27–28.
38. Kellogg, *Headquarters Nights*, 32.
39. Vernon Kellogg, "Eugenics and Militarism," *The Atlantic Monthly*, 1913, 112: 101.
40. Vernon Kellogg, "War for Evolution's Sake," *The Unpopular Review*, July 1918, 10: 158.
41. The Bavarians were commanded by Crown Prince Rupprecht, son and heir of King Ludwig III of Bavaria. The Crown Prince was a descendent of the British Royal House of Stuart, a royal line that included Bonnie Prince Charlie, leader of the 1745 Scottish rebellion. Before the war, Scottish Jacobites recognized Rupprecht as Prince Rupert of England, Scotland, France and Ireland. After the war, with the death of his mother, he succeeded to all her British rights and was recognized by Jacobites as King Rupert (Robert) of Britain. Ironically the most costly battles fought by the British — the Somme, Arras, Lille and Ypres — were against armies commanded by the Crown Prince. After the war, the Crown Prince, who was an ardent anti–Nazi, was on Hitler's most wanted list. He escaped death in 1939 by hiding in Italy. When he died in 1955 at the age of 86, the *New York Times* published a laudatory obituary. Ed Klekowski and Libby Klekowski, *Eyewitnesses to the Great War* (Jefferson, NC: McFarland, 2012), 20.
42. Vernon Kellogg, "The Capture of Charleville," *The Atlantic Monthly*, September 1918, 297.
43. James W. Gerard, *My Four Years in Germany* (New York: Grosset and Dunlap, 1917), 236.
44. Gerard, 241.
45. Kittredge, 319.
46. Gerard, 241.
47. *The Deportation of Women and Girls from Lille* (New York: George H. Doran, 1916), 10–11.
48. "Memorandum by L.C. Wellington," in George I. Gay, *Public Relations of The Commission for Relief in Belgium: Documents* (Stanford, CA: Stanford University Press, 1929), 2: 77.
49. *The Deportation of Women and Girls from Lille*, 16.
50. Kittredge, 322.
51. George H. Nash, *The Life of Herbert Hoover: The Humanitarian* (New York: W.W. Norton, 1988), 2:362.
52. Lewis R. Freeman, "Hoover and the Belgians," *Outlook*, September 8, 1915, 111:81.
53. Herbert C. Hoover, "Bind the Wounds of France," *National Geographic*, 1917, 31:439.

Chapter 9

1. *History of the American Field Service in France* (Boston: Houghton Mifflin, 1920), Volume 1: 85.
2. Douglas Wilson Johnson, *Battlefields of the World War* (New York: Oxford University Press, 1921), 29.
3. *Handbook to Belgium and the Battlefields*, 8th ed., (London: Ward, Lock, 1935), 92.
4. Karl Baedeker, *Belgium and Holland: Handbook for Travelers* (Leipzig, Germany: Karl Baedeker, 1910), 44.
5. Francis Whiting Halsey, *The Literary Digest History of the World War*, Volume 2 (New York: Funk and Wagnalls, 1919), 238–239.
6. *Handbook to Belgium and the Battlefields*, 93–94.
7. The Yser Canal linked Nieuport, Dixmude and Ypres.
8. John Buchan, *Nelson's History of the War* (London: Thomas Nelson and Sons, 1919), Volume 4, 92.
9. Halsey, Volume 2, 236.

10. Will Irwin, "Kaiser's Chances Buried in Shambles of Ypres," *New York Tribune*, March 18, 1915, 4.
11. John Keegan, *The First World War* (New York: Alfred A. Knopf, 1999), 132.
12. "Ypres Cost Huns War," *New York Times*, May 4, 1919, 16.
13. Halsey, Volume 2, 230.
14. Irwin, "Kaiser's Chances Buried in Shambles of Ypres," 4.
15. Buchan, *Nelson's History of the War*, Volume 4, 103.
16. Irwin, "Kaiser's Chances Buried in Shambles of Ypres," 4.
17. Irwin, "Kaiser's Chances Buried in Shambles of Ypres," 4.
18. "An American War Correspondent," *The Literary Digest*, April 24, 1915, 50:954–955.
19. Irwin, "Kaiser's Chances Buried in Shambles of Ypres," 4.
20. Buchan, *Nelson's History of the War*, Volume 4, 112.
21. Irwin, "Kaiser's Chances Buried in Shambles of Ypres," 4.
22. Moore had made a fortune in Detroit in street railway companies. Robert V. Hudson, *The Writing Game: A Biography of Will Irwin* (Ames: Iowa State University Press, 1982), 88.
23. George H. Cassar, *The Tragedy of Sir John French* (Newark: University of Delaware Press, 1985), 181–183.
24. Lois Gordon, *Nancy Cunard* (New York: Columbia University Press, 2007), 30.
25. Cassar, 181.
26. "French's Chum in U.S.," *Washington Post*, June 27, 1915, 4.
27. Cassar, 244.
28. Hudson, 89.
29. "An American War Correspondent," 50: 954.
30. For the complete story behind Will Irwin's article see: Hudson, 88–92.
31. Halsey, Volume 2, 247.
32. Karl N. Llewellyn, "An American Private in the German Army," *The Saturday Evening Post*, May 8, 1915, 187:28.
33. Llewellyn, 29.
34. Buchan, *Nelson's History of the War*, Volume 4, 112.
35. Buchan, Volume 4, 113.
36. Buchan, Volume 4, 114.
37. Winston Groom, *A Storm in Flanders* (New York: Atlantic Monthly, 2002), 70–71; Keegan, 132.
38. Hugh B.C. Pollard, *The Story of Ypres* (New York: Robert M. McBride 1917), 61.
39. Mary Roberts Rinehart, *Kings, Queens and Pawns* (New York: George H. Doran, 1915), 137.
40. Rinehart, 154.
41. Rinehart, 160.
42. For a map showing the positions of the lines near the time of Dunn's visit, see Buchan, *Nelson's History of the War*, Volume 4, 110.
43. Robert Dunn, *Five Fronts* (New York: Dodd, Mead, 1915), 177.
44. Dunn, 178.
45. Dunn, 199.
46. Reminiscent of the American politician who admitted to smoking marijuana but not inhaling.
47. Dunn, 200.
48. Dunn, 201.
49. Johnson, 22.
50. Valentine Williams, "Greatest of All Tributes to Christmas," *New York Times*, December 23, 1934, SM 6.
51. Johnson, 23–24.
52. Williams, 12.
53. Halsey, Volume 2, 260.
54. Williams, 12.
55. Halsey, Volume 2, 262.
56. Halsey, Volume 2, 263.
57. Williams, 12.
58. "Fraternizing Between the Lines," *New York Times*, December 31, 1914, 3.
59. The Christmas Truce on the Western Front that occurred in 1914 was unique and never duplicated. Bruce Heydt, "Peace, for a Moment, Breaks Out Along the Western Front," *British Heritage*, January 2005, 14, 16, 60.
60. Williams, 12.
61. Hudson, 93.
62. "American Artist Visits New British Base Camp," *New York Times*, February 21, 1915, SM5.
63. "Allies Win Back Ground; Will Irwin Calls Ypres Hottest Battle of War," *New York Tribune*, April 25, 1915, 1.
64. Hudson, 93.
65. Will Irwin, "Germans Use Blinding Gas to Aid Poison Fumes," *New York Tribune*, April 27, 1915, 1.
66. John Buchan, *Nelson's History of the War*, Volume 7 (London: Thomas Nelson and Sons, 1919), 11–12.
67. Pollard, 69–70.
68. Pollard, 75–76.
69. Buchan, *Nelson's History of the War*, Volume 7, 23–24.
70. Irwin, "Germans Use Blinding Gas to Aid Poison Fumes," 1.
71. Buchan, *Nelson's History of the War*, Volume 7, 17.
72. Pollard, 80–81.
73. Pollard, 83.
74. Pollard, 84.
75. Halsey, Volume 2, 311.
76. Frederick Palmer, *My Year of the Great War* (New York: Dodd, Mead, 1916), 351.
77. Frederick Palmer, 351.
78. Frederick Palmer, 352.
79. Alan Palmer, *The Salient* (London: Constable, 2007), 117.

80. Renamed the American Field Service in 1916. Ed Klekowski and Libby Klekowski, *Eyewitnesses to the Great War: American Writers, Reporters, Volunteers and Soldiers in France, 1914–1918* (Jefferson, NC: McFarland, 2012), 62–63.
81. Folder 29, Archives of the American Field Service and AFS Intercultural Programs.
82. Folder 30, Archives of the American Field Service and AFS Intercultural Programs.
83. *History of the American Field Service in France*, 95.
84. Alan Palmer, 119, 124.
85. Ypres is 20 meters above sea level; the German positions were at 50 meters.
86. Cassar, 248.
87. "French's Chum in U.S.," *Washington Post*, June 27, 1915, 4.
88. "Moore Praises Kitchener," *New York Times*, June 27, 1915, 2.
89. "Detroit Millionaire to sue London Editor," *Boston Globe*, January 30, 1916, 10.
90. "Law Report, March 9," *The Times of London*, March 10, 1916, 3.
91. "Moore Libel Suit Ends in Apology," *New York Times*, March 10, 1916, 12.

Chapter 10

1. Valentin Vermeersch, *Bruges and the Sea* (Antwerp, Belgium: Mercatorfonds, 1982), 235.
2. Karl Baedeker, *Belgium and Holland, Handbook for Travelers* (Leipzig, Germany: Karl Baedeker, 1910), 26.
3. *Murray's Handbook for Travelers in Holland and Belgium* (London: John Murray, 1876,124.
4. *Murray's Handbook for Travelers in Holland and Belgium*, 124.
5. Baedeker, 2.
6. Baedeker, 2.
7. Egbert Hans, "Zeebrugge, the Belgian Coast's U-Boat Nest," *New York Times*, October 21, 1917, 93.
8. Mark D. Karau, *Wielding the Dagger* (Westport, CT: Praeger, 2003), 27–28.
9. Robert M. Grant, *U-Boats Destroyed* (London: Putnam, 1964), 20.
10. Karau, 31.
11. Geoffrey Brooks, *FIPS* (Annapolis, MD: Naval Institute, 1999), translation of Werner Fürbringer.
12. Brooks, 19.
13. Etienne, *The Diary of a U-Boat Commander* (London: Hutchinson, 1920), 41–42; Etienne is a pseudonym for Stephen King-Hall; the diary is that of Karl von Schenk, who served on a UC boat out of Zeebrugge.
14. Karl Neureuther and Claus Bergen, editors, *U-Boat Stories* (New York: Richard R. Smith, 1931), 131— the story of the *UC 70* out of Bruges, April 1918.
15. Paul Kemp, *U-Boats Destroyed* (London: Cassell, 1997), 16.
16. Neureuther and Bergen, 139.
17. Ernst Hashagen, *U-Boats Westward!* (New York: G.P. Putnam's Sons, 1931), 171.
18. Francis Whiting Halsey, *The Literary Digest History of the World War* (New York: Funk and Wagnalls, 1919), 9: 236.
19. Halsey, 9: 236.
20. Karau, 52.
21. Karau, 49.
22. "Submarines Use Canals," *New York Times*, April 8, 1915, 4.
23. De Gerlache de Gomery, *Belgium in War Time* (New York: George H. Doran, 1916), 220.
24. Halsey, 9: 236–237.
25. V.E. Tarrant, *The U-Boat Offensive 1914–1918* (Annapolis, MD: Naval Institute, 1989), 23.
26. Halsey, 9: 247.
27. "Woman New Yorker Lost?" *New York Times*, August 20, 1915, 1.
28. Ibid.
29. "Shocks President Wilson," *New York Times*, August 20, 1915, 1.
30. Karau, 31–32, 54.
31. Etienne, 40.
32. Kenneth Hare, *Guide to Bruges, and Environs*, 3d ed. (Bruges, Belgium: D. Walleyn, 1927), 91.
33. Etienne, 34–35.
34. They resided at 62, rue des Bouchers.
35. Walter Duranty, "American's Banner First in Bruges," *New York Times*, October 30, 1918, 3.
36. Walter Duranty, "U-Boat Officer's Orgies at Bruges," *New York Times*, October 29, 1918, 11.
37. Hashhagen, 233.
38. Duranty, "U-Boat Officers' Orgies at Bruges," 11.
39. Tarrant, 17.
40. Neureuther and Bergen, 131.
41. Edgar von Spiegel, *U. Boat 202* (London: Andrew Melrose, 1919), 81.
42. Hashhagen, 233.
43. Hashhagen, 233.
44. "Sussex Lifebelts Useless," *New York Times*, March 28, 1916, 4.
45. "The German Alibi," *New York Times*, April 13, 1916, 12.
46. Halsey, 9: 330.
47. Halsey, 9: 331.
48. Halsey, 9: 320.
49. Karau, 72.
50. Hashhagen, 233.
51. Neureuther and Bergen, 140–141.
52. Neureuther and Bergen, 141.
53. Etienne, 78.
54. Etienne, 79–80.
55. Tarrant, 145.

56. Francis Whiting Halsey, *The Literary Digest History of the World War* (New York: Funk and Wagnalls, 1919), 4: 7.
57. Tarrant, 47.
58. Halsey, 9: 345.
59. "U-Boat Captain Cynical to Survivors," *New York Times*, February 28, 1917, 2.
60. Virginia Cowles, *The Kaiser* (New York: Harper and Row, 1963), 282–283.
61. Theodore Roosevelt, *America and the World War* (New York: Charles Scribner's Sons, 1915), 200.
62. Roosevelt, 247.
63. Halsey, 4: 14–15.
64. For details of the Zimmermann Telegram and its consequences, the reader is referred to Barbara W. Tuchman, *The Zimmermann Telegram* (New York: Macmillan, 1966).
65. "Zimmermann Defends Act," *New York Times*, March 4, 1917, 1.
66. Halsey, 4: 28.

Chapter 11

1. Romeo Houle, "American Barber's Thrilling War Narrative," *New York Times*, June 11, 1916, SM7.
2. Allan Nevins, *The Letters and Journal of Brand Whitlock: The Letters*, (New York: D Appleton-Century, 1936), 215.
3. Brand Whitlock, *Belgium* (New York: D. Appleton, 1919), 2:734–735.
4. Whitlock, 732–733.
5. Whitlock, 739.
6. Allan Nevins, *The Letters and Journal of Brand Whitlock: The Journal* (New York: D Appleton-Century, 1936), 364–365.
7. Whitlock, 796.
8. Whitlock, 796–797.
9. Arthur Bartlett Maurice, *Bottled Up in Belgium* (New York: Moffat, Yard, 1917), 174–175.
10. Whitlock, 807.
11. Robert Withington, *In Occupied Belgium* (Boston: Cornhill, 1921), 119; Prentiss N. Gray contributed the final chapter describing his experiences in Brussels after the Whitlocks left on April 2, 1917.
12. Withington, 127.
13. "Needs More Ships to Feed Belgians," *Washington Post*, September 7, 1917, 11.
14. Withington, 131.
15. Withington, 134.
16. C.C. Clayton, "Business in Belgium Under German Rule," *World's Work*, 1918, 36: 470.
17. Clayton, 466.
18. Clayton, 468.
19. "Free Two Americans," *New York Times*, September 1, 1917, 2.
20. "Antwerp on Starvation Diet, Says A.D. Whipple," *Boston Globe*, October 23, 1917, 8.
21. "Famous War Poster his Portrait," *Boston Daily Globe*, September 30, 1917, 47.
22. Between 40,000 and 50,000 Americans joined the Canadian, English or French armies. "Americans at Front May Save Citizenship," *New York Times*, April 23, 1917, 8.
23. "First American Legion Off For Flanders," *New York Times*, May 28, 1916, SM2.
24. "Has King's Cigarette Case," *New York Times*, April 11, 1916, 13.
25. Romeo Houle, "American Barber's Grim War Story," *New York Times*, June 4, 1916, SM1.
26. Romeo Houle, "American Barber's Thrilling War Narrative," SM7.
27. On June 29, 1918, President Wilson signed House Joint Resolution 255, which restored citizenship to those Americans who served in the armed forces of the Allies. Congressional Record—House, July 1, 1918, 8570.
28. Alexander McClintock, "Over There," *Washington Post*, June 17, 1917, SM5.
29. McClintock, "Over There," SM5.
30. Arthur Guy Empey, *Over the Top* (New York: G.P. Putnam's Sons, 1917), 85.
31. Empey, 83.
32. Alexander McClintock, "Counting the Age-Long Minutes Before Starting a Bomb Raid," *Boston Daily Globe*, June 24, 1917, 39.
33. "Britain Confers War Medal Here," *New York Times*, August 16, 1917, 3.
34. "To Enlist Americans," *New York Times*, February 14, 1916, 2; The United States government objected to the name, so the "American Legion" became the "so called American Legion." "'American Legion' Barred," *New York Times*, May 9, 1916, 6.
35. "First American Legion Off for Flanders," SM2.
36. "Baltic as a Transport," *New York Times*, March 16, 1916, 4.
37. R. Wherry Anderson, *The Romance of Air-Fighting* (New York: George H. Doran, 1917), 28.
38. Pat O'Brien, *Outwitting the Hun* (New York: Harper and Brothers, 1918), 46.
39. O'Brien, 11–12.
40. O'Brien, 33.
41. O'Brien, 43.
42. O'Brien, 56.
43. O'Brien, 137.
44. O'Brien, 248.
45. Harvey Cushing, *From a Surgeon's Journal 1915–1918* (Boston: Little, Brown, 1936), 111.
46. John Buchan, *Nelson's History of the War* (London: Thomas Nelson and Sons, 1915–1919), Volume 20: 51.
47. Buchan, Volume 20: 65.
48. Philip Gibbs, *Now It Can Be Told* (Garden City, NY: Garden City, 1920), 473.
49. Gary Goldenberg, *Nurses of a Different*

Stripe (New York: Columbia University School of Nursing, 1992), 84.
50. Cushing, 175–176.
51. Goldenberg, 84.
52. W.A.R. Chapin, *The Lost Legion* (Springfield, MA: Loring-Axtell, 1926), 57.
53. Joseph W. Griggs, "American-Manned Hospitals Bombed," *Boston Daily Globe*, August 27, 1917, 12.
54. Goldenberg, 85.
55. "American Nurses Praised by Haig" *Boston Daily Globe*, December 29, 1917, 3.
56. Chapin, 95.
57. Erich von Ludendorff, *Ludendorff's Own Story* (New York: Harper and Brothers, 1919), Volume 2:105.
58. Von Ludendorff, 106.
59. Chapin, 64.
60. Gibbs, 478.

Chapter 12

1. W.A.R. Chapin, *The Lost Legion* (Springfield, MA: Loring-Axtell, 1926), 74.
2. The treaty was signed by the Russian Soviet Federated Socialist Republic and the Central Powers: the German Empire, the Austro-Hungarian Monarchy, the Ottoman Empire and the Kingdom of Bulgaria. The German Empire was the major player.
3. John Toland, *No Man's Land* (New York: Smithmark, 1980), 121.
4. Erich von Ludendorff, *Ludendorff's Own Story* (New York: Harper and Brothers, 1919), Volume 2: 105–106.
5. John Buchan, *Nelson's History of the War* (London: Thomas Nelson and Sons, 1915–1919), Volume 22: 92.
6. Buchan, Volume 22: 94.
7. Holger H. Herwig, *The First World War* (London: Arnold, 1997), 414.
8. Wilhelm II, *The Kaiser's Memoirs* (New York: Harper and Brothers, 1922), 275.
9. Harry A. Bruno, *The Flying Yankee* (Dodd, Mead, 1918), 111.
10. Bruno, 115.
11. Bruno, 118–119.
12. "British Captain Tells Story of Daring Raid on Zeebrugge Mole," *Boston Daily Globe*, April 26, 1918, 11.
13. For a detailed and lucid description of the Zeebrugge and Ostend raids see Mark Karau, "Twisting the Dragon's Tail: The Zeebrugge and Ostend Raids of 1918," *The Journal of Military History*, April 2003, 67: 455–482.
14. Lieut. Col. Repington, "Two Glorious Pages in British History," *Boston Daily Globe*, April 28, 1918, 8.
15. Karau, 472.
16. *Handbook to Belgium and the Battlefields*, 8th ed. (London: Ward, Lock, 1935), 274.
17. Von Ludendorff, Volume II: 226.
18. Walter Duranty, "German Retreat Was Like a Rout," *New York Times*, November 20, 1918, 3.
19. Marshal von Hindenburg, *Out of My Life* (New York: Harper and Brothers, 1921), Volume 2: 222.
20. Elmer A. Murphy and Robert S. Thomas, *The Thirtieth Division in the World War* (Lepanto, AR: Old Hickory, 1936), 81.
21. American Battle Monuments Commission, *27th Division Summary of Operations in the World War* (Washington, D.C.: United States Government Printing Office, 1944), 7.
22. American Battle Monuments Commission, 27th Division Summary of Operations in the World War, 12.
23. American Battle Monuments Commission, *30th Division Summary of Operations in the World War* (Washington, D.C.: United States Government Printing Office, 1944), 10.
24. John Buchan, *Nelson's History of the War* (London: Thomas Nelson and Sons, 1915–1919), Volume 24: 20.
25. "Diary of Retreat from Belgium," *New York Times*, March 23, 1919, 50.
26. Walter Duranty, "American's Banner First in Bruges," *New York Times*, October 30, 1918, 3.
27. Buchan, Volume 24: maps on pages 34 and 71.
28. Probably b. 1842, d. 1919.
29. J.H. Twells, Jr., *In the Prison City* (London: Andrew Melrose, 1919), 263–264.
30. Duranty, "German Retreat was Like a Rout," 3.
31. Twells, 262–263.
32. "Diary of Retreat from Belgium," 50.
33. Twells, 258.
34. Twells, 261.
35. Twells, 265.
36. Wilhelm II, 288–289.
37. Twells, 270.
38. Buchan, Volume 24: 90.
39. Allan Nevins, *The Letters and Journal of Brand Whitlock, The Journal* (New York: D. Appleton-Century 1936), 523.
40. Twells, 285.
41. Twells, 286.
42. Twells, 289.

Chapter 13

1. Pierre Goemaere, *Across America with the King of the Belgians*, trans. by Beatrice Sorchan (New York: E.P. Dutton, 1921), 133–134.
2. William T. Alderson, ed. "The Attempt to Capture the Kaiser, by Luke Lea," *Tennessee Historical Quarterly*, September 1961, 20: 234.
3. Alderson, ed., 20: 226.

4. Nora Bentinck, *The Ex-Kaiser in Exile* (New York: George H. Doran, 1921), 29.

5. T.H. Alexander, "They Tried to Kidnap the Kaiser — and Brought Back an Ash Tray," *The Saturday Evening Post*, October 23, 1937, 210: 86.

6. Robert Welles Ritchie, "Dare-Devil Yanks Try to Kidnap Kaiser," *Boston Daily Globe*, January 17, 1919, 1.

7. Alexander, 210: 86 reproduced the army letter of censure.

8. "Col. Lea is Convicted of Asheville Bank Fraud," *New York Times*, August 26, 1931, 1.

9. Bentinck, 46–47.

10. Frank Pierrepont Graves, "Report on the Dedication of the Library Building at the University of Louvain," July 4, 1928, 23.

11. Chris Coppens, Mark Derez, and Jan Roegiers, eds., *Leuven University Library 1425–2000* (Leuven, Belgium: Leuven University Press, 2005), 220.

12. A lesson seldom learned by architects even today.

13. Coppens, Derez, and Roegiers, eds., 220.

14. Allan Nevins, *The Letters and Journal of Brand Whitlock, The Journal* (New York: D. Appleton-Century, 1936), 697.

15. "Louvain's $1,000,000 Fully Subscribed," *New York Times*, December 14, 1925, 1.

16. Coppens, Derez, and Roegiers, eds., 508–513 for a complete list of inscriptions.

17. Pierre de Soete, *The Louvain Library Controversy* (Concord, NH: Rumford, 1929), 32.

18. Coppens, Derez and Roegiers, eds., 235.

19. "King Albert Roused by Louvain Dispute," *New York Times*, June 27, 1928, 1.

20. De Soete, 7; Pierre de Soete sculpted the inscription.

21. Graves, 26.

22. Coppens, Derez, and Roegiers, eds., 254.

23. "Warren is Checked by Louvain Police," *New York Times*, June 24, 1928, 22.

24. "Mob Tears Down Anti-Hate Pillars in Louvain Dispute," *New York Times* June 28, 1928, 1.

25. Graves, 12.

26. Graves, 13.

27. George Thorne, ed., *War Crimes* (Liège: Belgium War Crimes Commission, 1946).

28. Coppens, Derez, and Roegiers, eds., 319.

29. Robert M. Crunden, *A Hero in Spite of Himself: Brand Whitlock In Art, Politics, and War* (New York: Alfred A. Knopf, 1969), 362.

30. The more complete story is to be found in Brand Whitlock's journal and letters, edited and published after Whitlock's death. Nevins, *The Journal*.

31. Allan Nevins, *The Letters and Journal of Brand Whitlock, The Letters* (New York: D. Appleton-Century, 1936), 250.

32. Crunden, 316.

33. Quoted in Crunden, 365.

34. Crunden, 364.

35. Nevins, *The Journal*, 501–502.

36. Nevins, *The Journal*, 565.

37. William K. Klingaman, *1919* (New York: Harper and Row, 1987), 544–545.

38. "Whitlock Is Ambassador," *New York Times*, October 1, 1919, 20.

39. Frank P. Sibley, "Belgium's Soldier King is Boston's Honored Guest," *Boston Daily Globe*, October 6, 1919, 1.

40. Goemaere, 47.

41. Goemaere, 46.

42. William Lowell Putnam, *The Kaiser's Merchant Ships in World War I* (Jefferson, NC: McFarland, 2001), 165–167.

43. Nevins, *The Journal*, 579.

44. David D. Anderson, *Brand Whitlock* (New York: Twayne, 1968), 149–151 for a bibliography of Whitlock's publications.

45. Mrs. Nell Whitlock returned to the United States in 1937, where she died in 1942. She is buried in Cannes. "Mrs. Brand Whitlock," *New York Times*, July 12, 1942, 36.

46. Crunden, 427.

Bibliography

Books

Album de la Guerre. Paris: L'Illustration, 1922.
American Battle Monuments Commission. *27th Division Summary of Operations in the World War*. Washington, D.C.: United States Government Printing Office, 1944.
American Battle Monuments Commission. *30th Division Summary of Operations in the World War*. Washington, D.C.: United States Government Printing Office, 1944.
Anderson, David D. *Brand Whitlock*. New York: Twayne, 1968.
Anderson, R. Wherry. *The Romance of Air-Fighting*. New York: George H. Doran, 1917.
Austin, Walter. *A War Zone Gadabout*. Boston: R.H. Hinkley, 1917.
Baedeker, Karl. *Belgium and Holland, Handbook for Travelers*. Leipzig, Germany: Karl Baedeker, 1910.
Bentinck, Nora. *The Ex-Kaiser in Exile*. New York: George H. Doran, 1921.
Bernstorff, Count. *My Three Years in America*. New York: Charles Scribner's Sons, 1920.
Bigelow, Glenna Lindsley. *Liége — On the Line of March*. New York and London: John Lane, 1918.
Brooks, Geoffrey. *FIPS*. Annapolis, MD: Naval Institute, 1999.
Brownell, Will, and Richard N. Billings. *So Close to Greatness*. New York: Macmillan, 1987.
Bruno, Harry A. *The Flying Yankee*. Dodd, Mead, 1918.
Buchan, John. *Nelson's History of the War*. Volume 4. London: Thomas Nelson and Sons, 1915–1919.
_____. *Nelson's History of the War*. Volume 7. London: Thomas Nelson and Sons, 1915–1919.
_____. *Nelson's History of the War*. Volume 20. London: Thomas Nelson and Sons, 1915–1919.
_____. *Nelson's History of the War*. Volume 22. London: Thomas Nelson and Sons, 1915–1919.
_____. *Nelson's History of the War*. Volume 24. London: Thomas Nelson and Sons, 1915–1919.
Bullitt, Ernesta Drinker. *An Uncensored Diary from the Central Empires*. Garden City, NY: Doubleday, Page, 1917.
Buxton, Ian. *Big Gun Monitors*. Annapolis, MD: Naval Institute, 1978.
Cammaerts, Emile. *Albert of Belgium*. New York: Macmillan, 1935.
Cassar, George H. *The Tragedy of Sir John French*. Newark: University of Delaware Press, 1985.
Chapin, W.A.R. *The Lost Legion*. Springfield, MA: Loring-Axtell, 1926.
Churchill, Winston S. *The Great War*. London: George Newnes, 1933.
Clark-Kennedy, A.E. *Edith Cavell*. London: Faber and Faber, 1965.
Cobb, Irvin S. *Paths of Glory*. New York: George H. Doran, 1915.
Coppens, Chris, Mark Derez, and Jan Roegiers, Editors. *Leuven University Library 1425–2000*. Leuven, Belgium: Leuven University Press, 2005.
Cowles, Virginia. *The Kaiser*. New York: Harper and Row, 1963.
Cross, Wilbur. *Zeppelins of World War I*. New York: Paragon House, 1991.
Crozier Emmet. *American Reporters on the Western Front, 1914–1918*. Oxford University Press, 1959.
Crunden, Robert M. *A Hero in Spite of Himself: Brand Whitlock In Art, Politics and War*. New York: Alfred A. Knopf, 1969.
Cushing, Harvey. *From a Surgeon's Journal 1915–1918*. Boston: Little, Brown, 1936.
Dane, Edmond. *Hacking Through Belgium*. London: Hodder and Stoughton, 1914.
Davis, Charles Belmont, ed. *Adventures and Letters of Richard Harding Davis*. New York: Charles Scribner's Sons, 1918.
Davis, Richard Harding. *With the Allies*. New York: Charles Scribner's Sons. 1919.
De Gerlache de Gomery, A. *Belgium in War Time*. Trans. by Bernard Miall. New York: George H. Doran, 1916.

The Deportation of Women and Girls from Lille. New York: George H. Doran, 1916.

Derez, Mark. "The Flames of Louvain: The War Experience of an Academic Community," In *Facing Armageddon: The First World War Experienced,* edited by: Hugh Cecil and Peter Liddle. London: Cooper, 1996.

De Soete, Pierre. *The Louvain Library Controversy.* Concord, NH: Rumford, 1929.

Domelier, Henri. *Behind the Scenes at German Headquarters.* London: Hurst and Blackett, 1919.

Dunn, Robert. *Five Fronts.* New York: Dodd, Mead, 1915.

Empey, Arthur Guy. *Over the Top.* New York: G.P. Putnam's Sons, 1917.

Etienne. *The Diary of a U-Boat Commander.* London: Hutchinson, 1920.

Forbes, Edgar Allen. *Leslie's Photographic Review of the Great War.* New York: Leslie Judge, 1920.

Fortescue, Granville. *Front Line and Deadline.* New York: G.P. Putnam's Sons, 1937.

Galet, Emile Joseph. *Albert, King of the Belgians in the Great War.* Boston and New York: Houghton Mifflin, 1931.

Gay, George I. *Public Relations of the Commission for Relief in Belgium: Documents.* Stanford, CA: Stanford University Press, 1929.

Gerard, James W. *My Four Years In Germany.* New York: Grosset and Dunlap, 1917.

Gibbs, Philip. *Now It Can be Told.* Garden City, NY: Garden City, 1920.

_____. *The Soul of the War.* New York: Robert M. McBride, 1915.

Gibson, Hugh. *A Journal from Our Legation in Belgium.* Garden City, NY: Doubleday, Page, 1917.

Gleason, Arthur H., and Helen Hayes Gleason. *Golden Lads.* New York: A.L. Burt, 1916.

Goldenberg, Gary. *Nurses of a Different Stripe.* New York: Columbia University School of Nursing, 1992.

Goemaere, Pierre. *Across America with the King of the Belgians.* Trans. by Beatrice Sorchan. New York: E.P. Dutton, 1921.

Gordon, Lois. *Nancy Cunard.* New York: Columbia University Press, 2007.

Graham, Cooper C., and Ron van Dopperen. "Edwin F. Weigle: Cameraman for the *Chicago Tribune*," in *Film History.* New Barnet, Herts., UK: John Libbey, 2010.

Grant, Robert M. *U-Boats Destroyed.* London: Putnam, 1964.

Green, Horace. *The Log of a Noncombatant.* Boston and New York: Houghton Mifflin, 1915.

Groom, Winston. *A Storm in Flanders.* New York: Atlantic Monthly, 2002.

Halsey, Francis Whiting. *The Literary Digest History of the World War.* Volume 1. New York and London: Funk and Wagnalls, 1919.

_____. *The Literary Digest History of the World War.* Volume 2. New York and London: Funk and Wagnalls, 1919.

_____. *The Literary Digest History of the World War.* Volume 4. New York: Funk and Wagnalls, 1919.

_____. *The Literary Digest History of the World War.* Volume 9. New York: Funk and Wagnalls, 1919.

Handbook for Travellers in Holland and Belgium. London: John Murray, 1876.

Handbook to Belgium and the Battlefields. 8th ed. London: Ward, Lock, 1935.

Hare, Kenneth. *Guide to Bruges, and Environs.* 3rd ed. Bruges, Belgium: D. Walleny, 1927.

Hashagen, Ernst. *U-Boats Westward!* New York: G.P. Putnam's Sons, 1931.

Hedin, Sven. *With the German Armies in the West.* London and New York: John Lane, 1915.

Herwig, Holger H. *The First World War.* London: Arnold, 1997.

_____. *The Marne, 1914.* New York: Random House, 2009.

Hirschfeld, Magnus. *The Sexual History of the World War.* New York: Falstaff, 1937.

History of the American Field Service in France. Volume 1. Boston: Houghton Mifflin, 1920.

Horne, John, and Alan Kramer. *German Atrocities, 1914.* New Haven: Yale University Press, 2001.

Hudson, Robert V. *The Writing Game: A Biography of Will Irwin.* Ames: Iowa State University Press, 1982.

Hunt, Edward Eyre. *War Bread.* New York: Henry Holt, 1916.

Jäger, Herbert. *German Artillery of World War One.* Marlborough, UK: Crowood, 2001.

Johnson, Douglas Wilson. *Battlefields of the World War.* New York: Oxford University Press, 1921.

Judson, Helen. *Edith Cavell.* New York: Macmillan 1941.

Karau, Mark D. *Wielding the Dagger.* Westport, CT: Praeger, 2003.

Keegan, John. *The First World War.* New York: Alfred A. Knopf, 1999.

Kellogg, Charlotte. *Women of Belgium.* New York: Funk and Wagnalls, 1917.

Kellogg, Vernon. *Fighting Starvation in Belgium.* Garden City, NY: Doubleday, Page, 1918.

_____. *Headquarters Nights.* Boston: Atlantic Monthly, 1917.

_____. *Herbert Hoover, the Man and His Work.* New York: D. Appleton, 1920.

Kemp, Paul. *U-Boats Destroyed.* London: Cassell, 1997.

Kittredge, Tracy B. *The History of the Commission for Relief in Belgium, 1914–1917.* London: Crowther and Goodman, 1918.

Klekowski, Ed, and Libby Klekowski. *Eyewitnesses to the Great War: American Writers, Reporters, Volunteers and Soldiers in France, 1914–1918.* Jefferson, NC: McFarland, 2012.

Klingaman, William K. *1919*. New York: Harper and Row, 1987.
Kriegs-Album des Marinekorps Flandern 1914–1917. Berlin, 1918.
Lawson, Anita. *Irvin S. Cobb*. Bowling Green, OH: Bowling Green State University Popular Press, 1984.
Le Bon, Gustave. *The Psychology of the Great War*. London: T. Fisher Unwin, 1916.
Le Goffic, Charles. *Dixmude*. London: William Heinemann, 1916.
Lehmann, Ernst A., and Howard Mingos. *The Zeppelins*. New York: J.H. Sears, 1927.
Liberty's Victorious Conflict. Chicago: Magazine Circulation, 1918.
March, Francis A. *History of the World War*. Chicago: United Publishers of the United States and Canada, 1919.
Maurice, Arthur Bartlett. *Bottled Up in Belgium*. New York: Moffat, Yard, 1917.
McClellan, George B. *The Heel of War*. New York: G.W. Dillingham, 1916.
McCutcheon, John T. *Drawn from Memory*. New York: Bobbs-Merrill, 1950.
Meyer, G.J. *A World Undone*. New York: Delacorte, 2006.
Mokveld, L. *The German Fury in Belgium*. New York: George H. Doran, 1917.
Morgan, J.H. *The German War Book*. London: John Murray, 1915.
Morse, Edwin W. *The Vanguard of American Volunteers*. New York: Charles Scribner's Sons, 1919.
Murphy, Elmer A., and Robert S. Thomas. *The Thirtieth Division in the World War*. Lepanto, AR: Old Hickory, 1936.
Murray's Handbook for Travelers in Holland and Belgium. London: John Murray, 1876.
Nash, George H. *The Life of Herbert Hoover: The Humanitarian*. New York: W.W. Norton, 1988.
Neureuther, Karl, and Claus Bergen. Editors. *U-Boat Stories*. New York: Richard R. Smith, 1931.
Nevins, Allan. *The Letters and Journal of Brand Whitlock, The Journal*. New York: D. Appleton-Century, 1936.
_____. *The Letters and Journal of Brand Whitlock, The Letters*. New York: D. Appleton-Century, 1936.
O'Brien, Pat. *Outwitting the Hun*. New York: Harper and Brothers, 1918.
Palmer, Alan. *The Salient*. London: Constable, 2007.
Palmer, Frederick. *My Year of the Great War*. New York: Dodd, Mead, 1916.
Perris, G.H. *The Campaign of 1914 in France and Belgium*. New York: Henry Holt, 1915.
Pollard, Hugh B.C. *The Story of Ypres*. New York: Robert M. McBride, 1917.
Powell, E. Alexander. *Fighting in Flanders*. New York: Charles Scribner's Sons, 1915.
_____. *Italy at War*. New York: Charles Scribner's Sons, 1917.
_____. *Slanting Lines of Steel*. New York: Macmillan, 1933.
Preston, Diana. *Lusitania*. New York: Walker, 2002.
Putnam, William Lowell. *The Kaiser's Merchant Ships in World War I*. Jefferson, NC: McFarland, 2001.
Rinehart, Mary Roberts. *Kings, Queens and Pawns*. New York: George M. Doran, 1915.
Room, Adrian. *Placenames of the World*. Jefferson, NC: McFarland, 2006.
Roosevelt, Theodore. *America and the World War*. New York: Charles Scribner's Sons, 1915.
Ruhl, Arthur. *Antwerp to Gallipoli*. New York: Charles Scribner's Sons, 1916.
Sinclair, May. *A Journal of Impressions in Belgium*. London: Hutchinson, 1915.
Simmonds, Frank H. *The Great War: The Second Phase*. Kennerly, NY: Mitchell, 1915.
Souttar, H.S. *A Surgeon in Belgium*. New York: Longmans, Green, 1915.
Tarrant, V.E. *The U-Boat Offensive 1914–1918*. Annapolis, MD: Naval Institute Press, 1989.
Thorne, George, ed. *War Crimes*. Liège: Belgium War Crimes Commission, 1946.
Toland, John. *No Man's Land*. New York: Smithmark 1980.
Tuchman, Barbara W. *The Guns of August*. New York: Bantam Books, 1976.
_____. *The Zimmermann Telegram*. New York: Macmillan, 1966.
Twells, J.H., Jr. *In the Prison City*. London: Andrew Melrose, 1919.
Twice in a Lifetime, Belgium 1914–1940. London: Evans Brothers, 1943.
Van Pul, Paul. *In Flanders Flooded Fields*. Barnsley, South Yorkshire, UK: Pen and Sword, 2006.
Vermeersch, Valentin. *Bruges and the Sea*. Antwerp, Belgium: Mercatorfonds, 1982.
Von Bernhardi, Friedrich. *Germany and the Next War*. New York: Chas. A. Eron, 1914.
Von Hindenburg, Marshal. *Out of My Life*. Volume 2. New York: Harper and Brothers, 1921.
Von Ludendorff, Erich. *Ludendorff's Own Story*. Volume 2. New York: Harper and Brothers, 1919.
Von Spiegel, Edgar. *U. Boat 202*. London: Andrew Melrose, 1919.
A War Nurse's Diary. New York: Macmillan, 1918.
Wawro, Geoffrey. *Franco-Prussian War*. Cambridge University Press, 2003.
Waxweiler, Emile. *Belgium Neutral and Loyal*. New York: G.P. Putnam's Sons, 1915.
Weigle, Edwin F. *My Experiences on the Belgian Battlefields*. Chicago: Hamming, 1914.
Whitlock, Brand. *Belgium*. Volume I. New York: D. Appleton, 1919.

_____. *Belgium.* Volume II. New York: D. Appleton, 1919.

_____. *The 13th District: A Story of a Candidate.* Indianapolis, IN: Bowen-Merrill, 1902.

Wilhelm II. *The Kaiser's Memoirs.* New York: Harper and Brothers, 1922.

Williams, Albert Rhys. *In the Claws of the German Eagle.* New York: E.P. Dutton, 1917.

Williams, Wythe. *Dusk of Empire.* London: Charles Scribner's Sons, 1937.

Withington, Robert. *In Occupied Belgium.* Boston: Cornhill, 1921.

Ypres, 1914. London: Constable, 1919.

The Yser and the Belgian Coast. Clermont-Ferrand, France: Michelin, 1920.

Zuckerman, Larry. *The Rape of Belgium.* New York University Press, 2004.

Newspapers and Magazines

Newspapers

Boston Daily Globe
Boston Globe
Boston Herald
Morning Oregonian
New York Times
New York Tribune
Times of London
Washington Post

Magazines

The American Magazine
The Atlantic Monthly
British Heritage
The Catholic Historical Review
Collier's Magazine
The Contemporary Review
Current History
Everybody's Magazine
The Fatherland
Hamburger Fremdenblatt
Harper's Weekly
Illustré 1914
The Journal of Military History
Kansas History
The Literary Digest
Littell's Living Age
Medicine Studies
Le Miroir
National Geographic
The National Review
The New Republic
Nineteenth Century and After
The North American Review
Outlook
Proceedings of the U.S. National Academy of Sciences
The Saturday Evening Post
Technical World Magazine
Tennessee Historical Quarterly
The Unpopular Review
Die Wochenschau
World's Work

Index

Numbers in ***bold italics*** indicate pages with photographs.

Aachen 6, 9, 11, 40, 42, 55, 64, 66, 73
Aerschot 76–78
Aix-la-Chapelle 68; *see also* Aachen
Albert, King of the Belgians 16, 21, 23, 67, 72, 82, 83, 91, 95, 102, 105–107, 170, 237, 248, 253; enters Antwerp 241; enters Bruges 238; enters Brussels ***242***, 243; visits America 257, 258; Wilson visit 256
Allen, J.A. 109, ***110***, 111
Ambulance de l'Océan 107, 108, 126
America enters war 207, 208; C.R.B 209–211
American Ambulance Field Service 187, 188
American Army 229, 236
American Art Students' Club 93
American College of the Immaculate Conception 37
American Consulate (Antwerp) 88
American journalists: Bennett, James O'Donnell 61, 62, 65, 66; Cobb, Irvin S. 26, 30, 33, 45, 60–62, 64–66; Davis, Richard Harding 21–24, 27–29, 38, 40, 41; Dosch, Arno 30, 40, 61, 106, 107; Dunn, Robert 179, 180; Duranty, Walter 200; *Fighting in Flanders* (book) 88, 89; Fortescue, Granville 52, 57; Gerbeault, Maurice 64; Green, Horace 69, 70, 81, 84, 85, 87; Hansen, Harry 61, 62, 65; Irwin, Will 26, 30, 40, 61; Keeley, James 143; Lewis, Roger 61, 62; McCutcheon, John T. 26, 30, 61, 62, 65, 66; Morgan, Gerald 22, 28, 40; O'Reilly, Mary Boyle 42, 43; Palmer, Frederick 22, 153, 154; Porter, George 89; Powell, E. Alexander 25, 71, 72, 74, 76, 78, 82, 87, 88, 92, 93; Wiegand, Karl 194; Williams, Albert Rhys 118, 119; at Ypres 174, 175, 183, 184, 188
American Legation (Brussels) ***17***, 83, 154, 208, 241
American munitions 196, ***197***, 204
Americans in German Army 64, 76, 79;
German-American Reservists 141, 142; Ypres 176, 219
Amerongen Castle 244, 246
Amherst Woman's Club 144
Andenne 56
Antwerp 21, 23, 37, 48, 67–90, 109, 142; Belgian Army leaves 91; forts ***77***, 79, 80, 88; German entry 88, 89; liberation 241; loot 89, 90; refugees to Holland 85, 87, 91; telegraph 87; Zeppelin attack 38, 72–75
Arabic 196, 197
atrocities (justification) 66
Austin, Walter 109, ***110***

Bates, Lindon W. 145
Beaumont 62
Beaux, Cecilia 120
Becelaere 171
Begleitoffizier 157, 162, 167
Belgian economy 131–133
Belgian Field Hospital 80
Belgian neutrality 6, 7
Belgian Red Cross 84, 107, 126
Belgian Relief Fund 134
Belgium plundered 213, 214
Bell Telephone Company 214
Bennett, James O'Donnell *see* American journalists
Bentinck, Godard 244, 246
Berlin 109, 240
Berlin time (vs. Belgian time) 115, 210
Berry, Walter 255
Bigelow, Glenna Lindsley 9–15
Bixschotte 170, 176, 177
Blount, Daniel Lynds 22, 37, 38, 43, 44
Boulogne 188
Brilliant 232
British-American Tobacco Company 76
British Expeditionary Force 175
British Royal Marines 81–83

279

Brooke, Rupert 82
Bruges 95, 151; U-boat base 190, 193, 198, *199*, 229
Bruno, Harry 229; Ostend bombing 230
Brussels 15, 22, 30, 114; German parade *117*; Germans leave 238, 241; *Kneipe* (German bar) *115*; liberation 241; the love station 116, 117
Bullitt, Ernesta Drinker (Ernesta Drinker Beaux) 119, 120
Bullitt, William 119, 120
Bullock, C. Seymour 217
Butler, Nicholas Murray 249

Caesar 55
Calais 96, 97, 107, 109
Callahan, F.F. 223
Canadian Army 186–188; American Legion 217; American volunteers 187, 215, 216; Passchendaele *224*, 225
Canadians in German Army 215
Cantrell, Edgar Allen 93
Carnegie Endowment for International Peace 249
Casualty Clearing Stations (American) 223
Cavell, Edith 126–129; Tir National 129; trial *128*
Channel ports 112, 177, 186, 228
Charleroi 52, 53
Charleville 157–168; Christmas 182; C.R.B. 162; Crown Prince Wilhelm 160, 161; *Grosses Hauptquartier* 157, 159, 160, 195; Kaiser's residence *158*, 161; Lille deportations 167; Place Ducale *162*; prostitution 158, 161, 162
Château Corneau (Charleville) *158*
Château du Neubois (Spa) 235
Château La Farineuse (Spa) 235, 240
Château Nagelmackers (Château d' Angleur) 9, 14
Château Sous-Bois (Spa) 236
Chicago Tribune film 83, 84
Chisholm Gooden-Chisholm, Mairi 93, 102
Christmas 1914 (Brussels) 154, 155
Christmas ship 143, 144, 154
Christmas truce (1914) 182, 183
Churchill, Winston 82, 85, 132
Clayton, C.C. 213, 214
Cobb, Irvin S. *see* American journalists
Cologne 74
Comité Central de Secours et d'Alimentation 132, 138
Comité National de Secours et d'Alimentation 132, 138, 147
Commission for Relief in Belgium (C.R.B.) 134–168, 174, 208; American delegates 138–141; America enters war 209–213; British objections 132, 134, 135; clothing *148*, 150; espionage 153; foodstuff distribution 137, 138, *149*; funding 145, 146, *147*; Infant Ideal Box 145; Little Bees 148; menus 147, 149; Occupied France 151–168; post war 249;

relief ships 144; restaurants 149, 150; Rhodes scholars 135, 141, 154; ships torpedoed 146, 205, 212; state committees 145, 146; summary 168
Courteny, C.E. 144
Crane, Rufus 225
Crouse, Chas. C. 227
Curtis, Edward D. 139, 154
Cushing, Harvey 220

Daffodil 230, 232
Dalton, T.A. 38
Darrow, Clarence 256
Davis, Richard Harding *see* American journalists
de Broqueville, Lieutenant 99
Deerfield, Massachusetts *147*
de Gaulle, Charles 54
Delannoy, Father Paul 35, 36
de Leval, Gaston 129
de Meister, D.H. 83
Depage, Antoine 107
Depage, Marie 126
de Soete, Pierre 252
Dinant 50–55, 62
Dixmude 95, 97–101, *99*, *101*, 104, 106, 170; falls to Germans 108, 109
Dosch, Arno *see* American journalists
Dunkerque 96, 97; *see also* Dunkirk
Dunkirk 95, 103, 107, 109, 188
Dunn, Robert *see* American journalists
Duranty, Walter *see* American journalists
Dutch internment camp 87
Dutch neutrality 89

Edwards, S. Arlent 200, 238
Elizabeth, Queen of the Belgians 21, 42, 83, 91, 95, 106, 108, 241, *242*, 243, 249, 253
Elvertinghe 188
English Channel: minefields 201; tides 192, 193; *see also* Seabed perils
Entente 7
Etappengebiet 113, 151, *152*, 155

Flanders environment 96, 169, 180–182, 223, 225
Flanders U-Boat Flotilla 191–205
Flandria Palace Hotel (Bruges) 94
Fort Broechem 80
Fort Kessel 80
Fort Waelhem 79, 80, 88
Fort Wavre St. Catherine 79, 80
Fortescue, Granville *see* American journalists
Franco-Prussian War 46
Francqui, Emile 133, 134, 138, 153, 212
francs-tireurs 46–49, 66, 78
Franz Ferdinand, Archduke 5, 6
Franz Josef, Emperor 5, *13*
French, Sir John 173; women 174, 175, 189
French Marines 97
French Naval Brigade 95

Fürbringer, Werner 191–193
Furnes 98, 101, 103, 107

Gaity Theater (Brussels) 24; American dancers 24, 25
Garde Civique 23, 31, 93
Gare de Nord (Brussels) 18, 19, 40, 210, 211, 213
General-Gouvernement 113, 151
George V 215, 217, 225
George VI 242
Gerard, James W. 119, 126, 133, 135, 205; *Lusitania* 126; occupied France 156, 166, 167
Gerbeault, Maurice *see* American journalists
German Army disintegrates 237–240
German dugouts in dunes 104
German Legation (Brussels) 20
Gheluvelt 173, 176
Ghent 25, 91, 93, 94, 98, 151, 152; prostitution 116, 117
Gibbs, Philip 99, 100
Gibson, Hugh 9, 16, 21, 23, 25, 26, 37, 38, 43, 44, 61, 153, 154, 253, 255; Cavell trial 129; C.R.B. 133, 141
Gleason, Arthur H. 98–101
Gleason, Helen Hays 93–95, 98, 101, 103; decorated 102
Gray, Prentis, N. (and family) 211, 212, 213
Green, Horace *see* American journalists

Haig, Douglas 173, 221, 224
Hansen, Harry *see* American journalists
Harvard Unit 220, 221, 223
Hector Munro Ambulance Corps 93, 95, 98, 99, 102, 103, 107; Daimler ambulance 102
Hennebert, Victor 64
Highland, Marshall 205
Hill Cottage (Spa) 236
Hoover, Herbert 133–136, 139, 143, 150, 153–155, 157, 168, 174, 175, 252, 253, 255
Hoover, Lou 133, 153
Hotchkiss, Edwin B. 109, 110, 112
Hotel Astoria (Brussels) 120
Hôtel Britannique (Spa) 236
Hôtel de Flandre (Bruges) 199
Hôtel Métropole (Brussels) 118, 119
Hôtel St. Antoine (Antwerp) 70, 71, 74, 81–83, 87, 89, 142
Houle, Romeo 208, 215, 216
House, Colonel Edward 255
House of the Thousand Columns 33, 45
Hoy, Elizabeth 205
Hoy, Mary E. 205
Huis Doorn 247
Humber 96
Hunt, Edward Eyre 83, 85, 141–144
Huy 55, 56, 62

Intrepid 231, 234
Iphigenia 231
Iris 230, 232
Irwin, Will *see* American journalists

Kaiser kidnap attempt 244–247
Kaiser Wilhelm II 6, 10, 45, 54, 65, 83, 113, 157, 173, 205; Charleville 158, 161, 162, 182; discouraged with army 228; Holland refuge 240, 244, 247; Krupp investor 10; *Lusitania* 126; Roosevelt friendship 206; Spa 235, 240; wood chopping 235, 247
Keeley, James *see* American journalists
Kellogg, Vernon 157, 162–165
Kemmel Hill 236
Knocker, Elsie 93, 102
Kriegsbrauch im Landkriege 131, 132
Krupp 42cm mortar (Big Bertha) 11, 58, 60, 75, 77, 79; Ypres 184, 185
Kultur 45

La Panne 106–108, 126, 256
Laconia 205
Ladeuze, Monsignor Paulin 248, 253
Lambert, Léon 133
Langemark 171, 185; *Kindermord bei Ypern* 171
Le Havre 241, 253; Whitlock's description 254, 256
Lea, Luke 244–247
Lehmann, Ernst 73
Lewis, Roger *see* American journalists
Liège 9–15, 22, 55, 58, 67, 73; food shortages 136; forts 10–14
Lille 155, 164, 179; deportations 165–167
Le Lion Rouge 32
Llewellyn, Karl 176
London motor-busses 81, 85, 91, 92
Louvain 26, 30–49, 68, 78; cathedral 34, 48; Hôtel de Ville 39; library 30, 35, 46, 49; railway station 41; refugees 36; tourist destination 44, 45; Wilson visit 257; *see also* Louvain Library reconstruction
Louvain Library reconstruction 247, 250; American underwriters 249, 250; burned again 251, 253, 254; controversy 252, 253; corner stone laying 248, 249; description 250, 252; site 248
Lucey, J.F. 135, 142; C.R.B. grain caper 136, 137, 144
Ludendorff, Erich 235, 236
Lusitania 21, 22, 109, 123, 133, 174; deception 196; sinking 122–126, 216, 229; *U-20* 125
Luther, Willard 69, 70
Lys Battle *see* Operation Georgette
Lytle, Ridgley 140

MacDonald, Beatrice 225
MacDuffie School 80
Mailines 48
Man hat geschossen 47, 50, 56, 60
marks vs. francs 115
Marne River 60
Marquis de Villalobar 19, 23, 129, 132, 135, 154, 211
Maubeuge 60–62, 64, 65, 75
Maverick, Robert V. 138

Max, Adolphe 23
McClellan, George B. 48
McClintock, Alexander 216, 217
McCutcheon, John T. *see* American journalists
Mercier, Cardinal Désiré 249, 252
Mersey 96
Messines 221, 222
Meuse River 50, 51, 56, 158
Mexico 206, 207
Milner, George 109
Mokveld, Lambertus 34, 41, 50, 55, 56
monitors (warships) 96, 97, **98**
Mons 28
Moore, George Gordon 174, 183; friend of Sir John French 175, 189
Morgan, Gerald *see* American journalists

Namur 55, 57–60, 62, 67
Nieuport 95, 97, 103, 104, 106, 151
North Sea 95; minefields 201; tides 201
North Star 232, 234
Northern France *see* Occupied France

O'Brien, Patrick 218, 219; POW escape 219, 220
Occupied France (relief) 150, 155–157; C.R.B. activity 151–168; President of France against relief 156
Okkupationsgebiet 151, **152**, 155
Operation Georgette 227, 228, 236
Operation Michael 227
Operationsgebiet 113, 151, **152**, 155
O'Reilly, Mary Boyle *see* American journalists
Ostend 25, 81, 85, 93, 95, 151; aerial bombardment 198, 229, 230; U-boat canal 191

Page, Walter Hines 133
Palace Hotel (Brussels) **18**, **19**, 22, 24, 25, **27**, 29, 30, 40, 70, 78, 115, 120, 154, 210, 211, 239
Palmer, Frederick *see* American journalists
Passchendaele 221, **224**, 225; *see also* Ypres (Third Battle)
Pervyse 101–103, 105
Place de Meir (Antwerp) 82
Place Rogier (Brussels) **18**, **19**, 19, 40, 211; skirmish 239
Poperinghe 178, 187, 188
Porter, George *see* American journalists
Powell, E. Alexander *see* American journalists
Presbyterian Hospital Unit 223; nurse 224
Prince August Wilhelm 63
Prince Ernst of Saxe-Meiningen 60
Prize Regulations (U-boat) 197, **198**, 201
Prussian Guard 174, 176

Q-ships **198**, 201
Queen's Hotel (Antwerp) 83, 85

Ramscapelle 106
Richards, Lewis 155

Rigle, Jane 223
Rinehart, Mary Roberts 107, 108; Ypres visit 177–179
Rockefeller Foundation 154
Roosevelt, Theodore 118, 189, 206, 248
Rotterdam 134–138, 142, 143, 146, 147, 157
Roulers 111
Royal Army Medical Corps 221; American units 221, 223–225, 227
Royal Flying Corps 217, 218; American volunteers 218, 219, 229
Royal Navy Volunteer Reserve 81–83
Royal tour (America) 257, 258
Rupprecht, Crown Prince 164, 165, 179

St. Giles Prison 127, 128
Sambre River 55
Scheldt River 67, 82, 83, 89; boat (pontoon) bridges 85
Seabed perils 203, **204**
Second Battle of the Marne 229
Second World War 253
Severn 96
Shaler, Millard 132, 133
Sinclair, May 92
Sirus 232
Škoda 30.5cm mortar 11, **12**, **13**, 58, 60, 61, **77**, 79, 88
Social Darwinism 163, 164, 210
Solvay, Ernest 139
Spa GHQ 235, 238, 240; Kaiser escapes 244
Spanish Legation (Brussels) 19
Stevens, Lawrence Stein 64
Sussex 202

Thetis 231, **234**
Thompson, Donald 25, 71, 72, 80, **81**, 85, 88, 92, 98, 142
Thompson's fort 83–85, **86**, 142, 143
Treaty of Brest-Litovsk 227
Turner, William 124, 126; *see also Lusitania*
Twells, Julia Helen **121**, 140, 238, 239, 241; Brussels royal entry 242, 243

U-boats 190–207; losses 200, 204; mine layers 193, 194; radius of action 194; ships sunk 202, 203; travel by canals 195; unrestricted campaigns 195, 201, 202, 205, 229; *see also* Prize Regulations
U.S. 27th Division 236, 237
U.S. 30th Division 236, 237, 244
Uyttebroeck, Marguerette 36

Van Hee, Julius A. 25, 152, 212
Vatican 252
Verpflegungs-Offizer 167
Vindictive 230–232, **233**, 234, **235**
Vlamertinghe 185, 186
von Bellow-Saleski, Karl Konrad 20, 21
von Bernstorff, Johann 189, 205, 206
von Bethmann-Hollweg, Theobald 6

von Bisssing, Moritz 113, 120, 122, 135, 138, 208, 209, 212, 253
von Bülow, Karl 57
von der Goltz, Colmar 25, *57,* 113, 133
von der Lancken, Oscar 118, 129, 208, 209, 212, 213, 253
von Falkenhayn, Erich 162
von Hindenburg, Paul 235
von Jarotzky, Thaddeus 25, 26, 61
von Moltke, Helmuth 10
von Tirpitz, Alfred 194, 195, 205; sleeping U-boats 195
von Zeppelin, Ferdinand 73

war hysteria *7*
war zone gadabouts 109–112; Mercedes (the dreadnaught) 109, *110,* 111, 112
Warren, Whitney 248, 249, *250,* 252
Weel, Alexander 215
Weigle, Edwin F. 83–85
Wellington, Lawrence 166; Lille deportations 166, 167
Western Electric Company 213, 214
Wharton, Edith 255, 258
Whedbee, M. Manly 76, 78
Whipple, A.D. 214
Whitlock, Brand 15–18, *16,* 21, 23, 29, 37, 42, 47, 50, 75, 108, 117–122, 128–130, 132, 133, 135, 141, 142, 153, 154, 208; ambassadorship 257, 258; American royal tour 257, 258; *Belgium* (book) 254, 255; Gibson disappointment 255; last years 258; Le Havre 253, 254; leaves Belgium 210, 211; Louvain Library reconstruction 248, 249; returns to Brussels 241, 243, 245
Whitlock, Nell 17, 20, 129, 210, 241, 248, 254, 258
Wiegand, Karl *see* American journalists

Williams, Albert Rhys *see* American journalists
Wilson, Woodrow 197, 202, 205, 206, 207; Belgian visit 256, 257
Winterbottom, Gladys H. 80, 83, 92; Minerva automobile 80
Winton automobile 245
Wytschaete 221, 222

Ypres 95, 110, 111, 169–189, *178*; cathedral 170, *172*; Cloth Hall 170, *172*
Ypres (First Battle) 112, 169, 171, 175; summary 177
Ypres (Second Battle) 169; American Ambulance Field Service 187, 188; Americans 215–217; Canadians 186, 187; gas 184–188; summary 188–190
Ypres (Third Battle) 169, 221–226; mines 222; Passchendaele *224,* 225; purpose 221, 226
Ypres Canal 95, 106, 185
Ypres Salient 112, 151, 221; English trench *181*
Yser Front (northern most Western Front) 95–98, 151, 170; collapses 237
Yser inundation 104–106, *111*; Cogge, Charles 105; Geeraert, Henry 105
Yser River 95, 101, 103

Zeebrugge 151; aerial bombardment 198; mole 191, 198; U-boat base 190, *193*
Zeebrugge-Ostend Raid 230–235; submarine C-3 *231*
Zeppelins *121*; bomb Antwerp 38, 72–75; cloud car 75; *Sachsen* 73
Zimmermann, Arthur 206, 207
Zimmermann Telegram 206, 207, 209, 210
zur Strassen, Otto 163

www.ingramcontent.com/pod-product-compliance
Lightning Source LLC
Chambersburg PA
CBHW051211300426
44116CB00006B/529